Comprehensive Textbook
of
SURGERY

Comprehensive Textbook
of
SURGERY

Editor-in-Chief
Dinesh Vyas MD MS FICS
Assistant Professor, Department of Surgery
Director, MS Surgery Clerkship
Adjunct Professor, Institute of International Health
Nanotechnology Biomedical Lab
College of Human Medicine, Michigan State University
Lansing, MI, USA

Editors

Nav Yash Gupta MD FACS
Chief, Division of Vascular Surgery
North Shore University Health System
Skokie, IL, USA

Vijay Mittal MD FICS FACS
Clinical Professor
Wayne State University
School of Medicine
Detroit, MI, USA

Associate Editors

Sanjeev V Changgani MBA MD FCCM
Intensivist, Massachusetts General Hospital
Harvard Medical School
Boston, MA, USA

Tarun Kumar MD MCh FICS
Assistant Professor
Department of Pediatrics Surgery
St Louis University, St Louis, MO, USA

Rahul Kalla MBBCh MD MRCP
Small Bowel Disease Unit
Division of Gastroenterology
Sheffield University, Sheffield, UK

Foreword
Craig Coopersmith

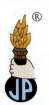

JAYPEE BROTHERS MEDICAL PUBLISHERS (P) LTD

New Delhi • Panama City • London

Jaypee Brothers Medical Publishers (P) Ltd.

Headquarter

Jaypee Brothers Medical Publishers (P) Ltd
4838/24, Ansari Road, Daryaganj
New Delhi 110 002, India
Phone: +91-11-43574357
Fax: +91-11-43574314
Email: jaypee@jaypeebrothers.com

Overseas Offices

J.P. Medical Ltd.,
83 Victoria Street London
SW1H 0HW (UK)
Phone: +44-2031708910
Fax: +02-03-0086180
Email: info@jpmedpub.com

Jaypee-Highlights Medical Publishers Inc.
City of Knowledge, Bld. 237, Clayton
Panama City, Panama
Phone: +507-301-0496
Fax: +507-301-0499
Email: cservice@jphmedical.com

Website: www.jaypeebrothers.com
Website: www.jaypeedigital.com

Comprehensive Textbook of Surgery

First Edition: 2012

ISBN 978-93-5025-052-5

Printed at Gopsons Papers Ltd., Noida

Dedicated to

My brother
Mahesh Vyas, Orthopedics Surgeon and
My father Purshottam Das Vyas
Scientist, Educationist and Social Worker
They both have influenced me to pursue medicine for the most needed

CONTRIBUTORS

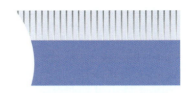

Abhishek Swami MBBS MD
Senior Fellow, Nephrology
Temple University, Philadelphia, PA, USA

Ananya Das MBBS MD
Gastroenterology, Department of Medicine
Mayo Clinic, Scottsdale, AZ, USA

Arpita Vyas MD DCh
Assistant Professor
Pediatric Endocrinology
Michigan State University
Lansing, MI, USA

BB Yeole PhD
Director, Mumbai Cancer Registry
Indian Cancer Society
Parel, Mumbai, Maharashtra, India

Deepa Taggarshe MD
Senior Resident, Department of Surgery
Providence Hospital and Medical Centers
Southfield, MI, USA

Dinesh Vyas MD MS FICS
Assistant Professor, Department of Surgery
Director, MS Surgery Clerkship
Adjunct Professor
Institute of International Health
Nanotechnology Biomedical Lab
College of Human Medicine
Michigan State University, Lansing, MI, USA

Gopala K Yadavalli MD FACP
Chief, Infectious Diseases Clinic, Louis
Stokes Cleveland Department of Veterans
Affairs Medical Center
Associate Program Director
Medicine Residency
Assistant Professor
Division of Infectious Diseases
Case Western Reserve University
Cleveland, OH, USA

Harish Reddy MD
Nephrologist
William Beaumont Hospital
Detroit, MI, USA

Indreesh Ramachandra
MD MBBS FCCP
Assistant Professor
Division of Interventional Cardiology
Department of Medicine
MetroHealth Hospital
Case Western Reserve University
Cleveland, OH, USA

K Kant MBBS MS FACS
Professor, Department of Surgery
Dr SN Medical College
Rajasthan University
Jodhpur, Rajasthan, India

Koji Motsuo MD
Fellow, Gynecology-oncology
Maryland University, MD, USA

Megan Hill MD
Senior Resident, Department of Surgery
Providence Hospital and Medical Centers
Southfield, MI, USA

MP McMonagle MBBCh FRCS
Registrar, Department of Surgery
Selly Oak Hospital, Birmingham University
Birmingham, UK

Nav Yash Gupta MD FACS
Chief, Division of Vascular Surgery
North Shore University Health System
Skokie, IL, USA

Naveen Vyas MD
Specialist, Hematopath
Dubai Hospital, Dubai, UAE

Neelima Rehil MD
Senior Resident
Department of Surgery
Providence Hospital and Medical Centers
Southfield, MI, USA

Norichika Ushioda MD
Department of Obstetrics and Gynecology
Osaka University Graduate School of
Medicine, Osaka, Japan

Pankaj Dangle MD
Department of Surgery
Cardinal Glennon Children Hospital
St Louis University, St Louis, MO, USA

Preet Singh Kang MD
Assistant Professor of Radiology
Case Western Reserve School of Medicine
Cleveland, OH, USA

Puja Van Epps MD
Senior Resident, Department of Medicine
Case Western Reserve University
Cleveland, OH, USA

Rahul Kalla MBBCh MD MRCP
Small Bowel Disease Unit
Division of Gastroenterology
Sheffield University, Sheffield, UK

Rajeev Gupta MBBS MD MRCS
Senior Resident, Department of Surgery
Long Jewish Island Hospital, New York, USA

Richard Englehardt MD
Senior Resident, Department of Surgery
Providence Hospital and Medical Centers
Southfield, MI, USA

RK Vohra MBBS FRCS PhD
Tutor, Royal College of Surgeons
Senior Consultant, Department of
Vascular Surgery, Selly Oak Hospital
Birmingham University, Birmingham, UK

S Rai MBBCh FRCS
Registrar, Department of Surgery
Selly Oak Hospital
Birmingham University, Birmingham, UK

Sanjay Gandhi MD MBBS FCCP
Assistant Professor
Division of Interventional Cardiology
Department of Medicine
MetroHealth Hospital
Case Western Reserve University
Cleveland, OH, USA

Sanjay Porwal MBBS MS
Assistant Professor
Jhalawar Medical College
Rajasthan University
Jhalawar, Rajasthan, India

Sanjeev V Changgani
MBA MD FCCM
Intensivist
Massachusetts General Hospital
Harvard Medical School
Boston, MA, USA

Subhas Gokul MD MRCS
Senior Resident, Department of Surgery
Providence Hospital and Medical Centers
Southfield, MI, USA

Sumeet Virmani MD
Senior Resident, Department of Surgery
Providence Hospital and Medical Centers
Southfield, MI, USA

Tarun Kumar MD MCh FICS
Assistant Professor
Department of Pediatrics Surgery
St Louis University, St Louis, MO, USA

Vijay Mittal MD FICS FACS
Clinical Professor
Wayne State University
School of Medicine, Detroit, MI, USA

Yash Gupta FRCS FCEM
Consultant Surgeon
A and E Departments, King George and
Queen's Hospitals, London
Clinical Lead, Major Incident and
Emergency Preparedness, Joint Chairman
EPBC, Clinical, Governance, London, UK

FOREWORD

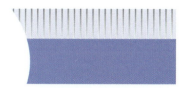

I am honored to have been asked to write the foreword for this exciting new textbook entitled *Comprehensive Textbook of Surgery*, edited by Dr Vyas, Dr Gupta, Dr Mittal, Dr Changgani, Dr Kumar and Dr Kalla. Surgery is an intensely personal endeavor. The bond between surgeon and patient is one of the most intimate known to humanity. A patient trusts a surgeon enough to literally put him into a chemical-induced coma, go inside his body, remove or rearrange vital organs, and stitch them back together, in the hopes of a better future than when he went to sleep. In turn, a surgeon takes expertise obtained from years or decades of training and experience and makes a promise to a patient—"no matter what, I will take care of you."

Increasingly, surgery is also a global endeavor. It is common for surgeons to train and practice in many cities and frequently many countries. In the goal of pursuing what is best for their patients, surgeons will travel far and wide to obtain the requisite skills needed to ensure a positive outcome.

The book sits at the crossroads between the personal and global nature of surgery. The distinguished international editorial board and authors have been carefully assembled to give a view of surgical fundamentals and advanced practice that is not possible in a single city, institution or even country. The lessons taught are universal and are valuable to surgeons everywhere. Each reader of the book is a student of the art of surgery in some way—from a junior medical student on their first rotation to the department, chair in-charge of a major national organization. Each will find something to learn here.

In many ways, the editor-in-chief of this book personifies the lofty goals of the book. Dr Dinesh Vyas' surgical journey began in India, and has found its way through England, France, and the United States, where I was fortunate to work to have him work in my laboratory studying surgical critical care. He brings a perspective that is at once global and at the same time, highly personal. This has led to a book that I believe will be instructive from the most rural communities with a single general surgeon to the most highly specialized academic centers.

I offer my most sincere congratulations to the editors and contributors for putting together this enlightening and comprehensive book.

Craig Coopersmith MD FACS
Professor of Surgery
Director, Surgical ICU
Emory University
Atlanta, USA

PREFACE

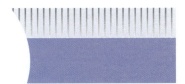

I have brought together contributors, who are experts in their respective fields and are recognized as such. In this process, the editors and contributors remained cognizant of the practical limitations and variances of treating the most general surgical conditions in South-East Asia. This book is a comprehensive review of general surgery that is clinically oriented with a multitude of practical pearls as well as numerous illustrations and charts that summarize information. The main focus of the book is medical and operative management of general surgical conditions. However, there is abundant coverage of medical management and nonoperative treatment of various disease processes.

Comprehensive Textbook of Surgery has been written keeping in mind the disconnect between currently available surgery textbooks and the resources available in the most hospitals in the world. The target audience is medical students, nursing students, surgery residents and surgeons. With simple, easy-to-understand language, it is meant to be an easily accessible resource for surgeons regarding practical advice on the best care available at the present time. A group of six distinguished and accomplished editors with more than thirty contributors have made contributions regarding basic and new surgical diseases, options for diagnosis and treatment of disease processes with the resources avialable to you, the pros and cons of various treatment options, and the management of complications. Emphasis is on common surgical related issues in critical care with chapters on cardiology, renal and infectious diseases. There is an introduction to use of radiology in your practice and a thrust towards lesser invasive interventions with readily available ultrasound machines.

Comprehensive Textbook of Surgery emphasizes trauma management and care. As a surgeon, I have a huge responsibility towards ensuring timely and appropriate care of trauma patients with a systematic approach. The potential for improvement in the care of trauma patients is significant. A textbook such as this is well overdue and will be a refreshing addition to the current cadre of textbooks in this arena.

Dinesh Vyas

ACKNOWLEDGMENTS

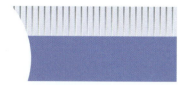

The book has been a brainchild of last 20 years of experience of practicing surgery in various parts of the world and understanding disconnect between the practice, resources and textbooks. There are areas of patient care that have huge need for relevant education and then there are areas of simplification of the textbook.

Surgeons like any physician are overwhelmed with information and at every stage it is important for them to understand and prioritize their reading. In surgery, there are multiple textbooks that have served to some extent all surgeons, but again they leave a lot of areas of question, as the surgeons have lack of global exposure.

I am fortunate to have surgeons from all parts of globe contributing in this text and all are active in their surgical practice at the best institutes of the world.

I wholeheartedly appreciate the efforts of all the editors and contributors of the textbook. There are many others in the publishing that have enabled me to successfully complete this mission. Professor Nav Yash Gupta and Professor Vijay Mittal have been constant support, inspiration and guide in my mission and helped with contributions and editing. I am thankful to the editorial staff and management especially Mr Tarun Duneja (Director-Publishing) and Mr KK Raman (Production Manager), M/s Jaypee Brothers Medical Publishers (P) Ltd, New Delhi, India were extremely helpful with their support and assistance throughout the project.

Lastly, I acknowledge the everlasting strength, support, and vision of my life, Arpita, my mother, Shyama and my daughter, Anoushka for their patience, nurturing personal environment to enable me to complete this vision.

This work is just a start and I have more work in my hand and I think the current team made me more determined to take challenging task and complete them with ease in future.

CONTENTS

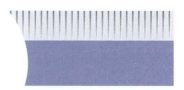

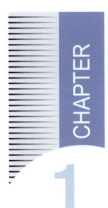

CHAPTER

1

Fluid and Electrolyte

Arpita Vyas, Rahul Kalla

INTRODUCTION

The understanding of body water and electrolyte distribution is paramount in managing surgical patients with electrolyte derangements. These changes can occur preoperative, intra-operative and postoperative and the management is governed by adequate knowledge of the underlying mechanism and appropriate fluid therapy if indicated.

In a normal individual who has not undergone a surgical procedure, there are insensible physiological fluid and electrolyte losses, some of which are outlined in Table 1.1.

A normal individual consumes an estimated 2-3 L of water per day and consumes 3-5 g of salt per day both of which are regulated by the kidneys.

Normal Body Water and Electrolyte Distribution

Total body water (TBW) contributes to 40-60 percent of our total body weight. This may vary with age and sex of the individual. At birth, 80 percent of our body weight comprises of TBW which rapidly decreases with age. It is also known that the percentage of TBW in lean individuals is higher than elderly or obese individuals (10-20% lower). Young adult females also tend to have a lower percentage TBW (50%) compared to aged matched males.

The TBW is compartmentalized in the body with 2/3rd of it being intracellular and 1/3rd being extracellular. An example of TBW distribution in a 60 kg (50% of body weight) female is given in Table 1.2.

The chemical composition of fluid compartments is summarized in the Table 1.3.

The composition of electrolytes within each is governed primarily by the potassium, sodium, chloride and protein content. This is regulated by the ATP driven Na-K pump located within the cell membrane. Therefore, ions and protein movement is restricted, however, water is freely distributed across the compartments. As a result, if excess water is ingested it will be equally distributed amongst the compartments. On the other hand, if sodium containing fluids are given, this will expand the intravascular and interstitial volume.

Although there is free movement of water, the direction of flow into the respective compartments is dependant on the osmotic pressure within the compartment. The ultimate goal of water is to attain osmotic equilibrium.

Osmotic pressure is measured in osmoles (osm) or milliosmoles (mOsm). To calculate osmolality the following equation is used:

$$\text{Serum osmolality} = \frac{2 \text{ sodium} + \text{glucose}}{18 + \text{BUN}/2.8}$$

Table 1.1: Fluid and electrolyte losses in normal individual			
Fluid type	*Volume loss (ml)*	*Potassium loss (mmol)*	*Sodium loss (mmol)*
Feces	300	10	80
Urine	2000	60	–
Other losses	700	–	–
Endogenous	– 300	–	–
Total	2700	70	80

Table 1.2: TBW distribution		
Intracellular fluid volume	*Extracellular fluid volume (ECV) total 10 L*	
2/3rd of total volume 30 L Total = 20 L	Interstitial fluid volume is 3/4th of ECV Total = 7.5 L	Plasma volume is 1/4th of ECV Total = 2.5 L

Table 1.3: Chemical composition of fluid compartments		
Intracellular fluid volume	*Extracellular fluid volume*	
• Na: 10 • K: 150 • Mg: 40 • HCO_3: 10 • Protein: 40	*Interstitial composition* • Na: 144 • K: 4 • Ca: 3 • Mg: 2 • Cl: 114 • Organic acids: 5 • Protein: 1	*Plasma composition* • Na: 142 • K: 4 • Ca: 5 • Mg: 3 • Cl: 103 • HCO_3: 27 • Organic acids: 15 • Protein: 16

The body tries to maintain the osmolality of the ECF and ICF at 290-310 mOsm and any change in the compartments will trigger movement of water across the semipermeable membrane to equalize the osmolalities. The usual travel of water is from a compartment with a low osmolality to a compartment with a relatively higher mOsm. As the calculation above implies that sodium is a major determinant of osmolality, one can say that net movement of water will usually be governed by changes in the concentration of sodium. This theory can be applied clinically when advising patients with hypertension (high intravascular volume) to reduce their salt intake.

ELECTROLYTE DISTURBANCES

Hyponatremia

A low sodium level is usually caused by either depletion of extracellular sodium or excessive dilution.[1] The extracellular volume status is helpful in identifying the cause. In postoperative patients, hyponatremia is commonly a result of over-administration of fluid therapy or a physiological production of ADH as a result of intravascular volume depletion. Figure 1.1 summarizes the causes of a low sodium level.

Symptoms

1. Headache, confusion, seizures
2. Weakness, fatigue, lethargy
3. Vomiting, diarrhea, salivation.

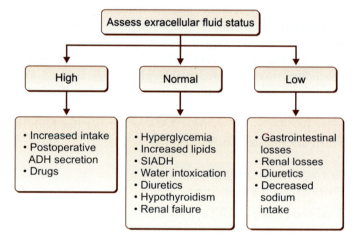

FIGURE 1.1: Syndrome of inappropriate antidiuretic hormone secretion (SIADH)

Signs

1. Signs of raised intracranial pressure, altered deep tendon reflexes
2. Oliguria
3. Hypertension, bradycardia in severe cases.
4. Coma.

Management

• The initial assessment must include fluid status as it will help with the differential diagnoses as mentioned above. The fluid status is assessed by checking blood pressure, peripheral edema, and jugular venous pressure.

- If the patient is hypovolemic due to extrarenal losses, then slow correction Na with isotonic fluids is indicated. It is pertinent that Na levels are corrected slowly as rapid correction may result in permanent demyelination syndrome.[2]
- Over administration of sodium free fluids to post-operative patients is a common cause for hyponatremia, therefore, it is pertinent to review the amount and type of fluid input. Normal saline should be used in these situations. Hypertonic saline is rarely used as it can cause circulatory overload.
- Omit any drugs that may cause a low Na temporarily such as diuretics, proton pump inhibitors, ACE inhibitors.
- If the patient is euvolemic, SIADH should be considered. Note that an increase in ADH secretion postoperatively can be a normal physiological response and is a common cause for hyponatremia in these patients. However, SIADH should be considered. Management includes diagnosis via urinary Na and paired osmolalities of urine and serum and fluid restriction. It is also important to investigate and treat the underlying cause of SIADH.

Hypernatremia (Fig. 1.2)

As in hyponatremia, a high sodium level can be subdivided by the extracellular volume status. Commonly a high sodium level is usually a result of dehydration and low extracellular volume.

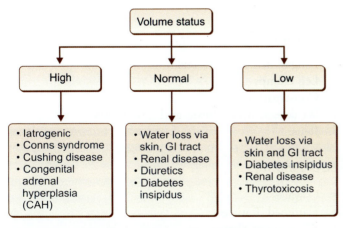

FIGURE 1.2: Causes of hypernatremia

Symptoms

1. Lethargy, thirst, weakness
2. Restlessness
3. Fever
4. In severe cases altered conscious level
5. Note that symptoms rare unless Na more than 160 mEq/l.

Signs

1. Evidence of dry mucous membranes and dehydration
2. Oliguria or increased urine output
3. Fever, tachycardia
4. Signs of Cushing's disease such as buffalo hump, centripetal obesity, moon face
5. Evidence of CAH may include ambiguous genitalia.

Management

- Assess fluid volume status as mentioned previously.
- Monitor fluid input/output chart with daily weights.
- If hypovolemic, the most likely cause is dehydration due to extrarenal losses especially in patients postoperatively. Management involves fluid replacement with isotonic solutions and slow correction of Na to avoid cerebral edema.
- Certain medications can cause hypernatremia such as antacids with sodium bicarbonate, antibiotics such as ticarcillin, salt tablets, intravenous hypertonic saline and should be discontinued.
- If the patient is alert the consider restricting dietary sodium intake temporarily.
- If the above measure fail to correct the Na level one must consider other rare causes such as Cushing's disease, diabetes insipidus and underlying renal disorders.

Hyperkalemia

High potassium level is defined as a value above 5 mEq/L. Severe hyperkalemia is defined as any level above 7 mEq/L. The causes are summarized in Figure 1.3 but usually involves a physiological change of increased absorption, impaired excretion or excessive release from cells.[2] A high potassium level with ECG changes is a medical emergency and should be treated promptly.

Symptoms

1. Mild symptoms include diarrhea, lethargy, nausea and vomiting

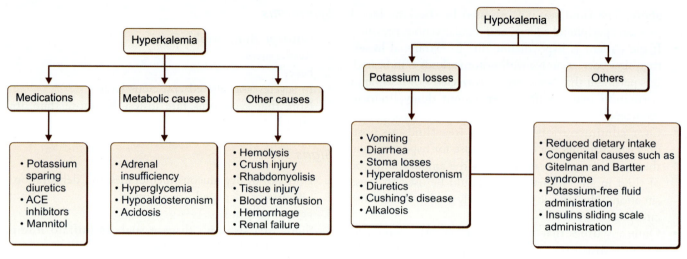

FIGURE 1.3: Causes of hyperkalemia   **FIGURE 1.4:** Causes of hypokalemia

2. Weakness and paralysis may ensue
3. Severe life-threatening symptoms may include chest pain, palpitations, altered conscious level.

ECG Findings

- Flattened P waves
- Prolonged PR interval
- Peaked tented T waves
- Widened QRS complexes
- Sine wave formation
- Arrhythmia such as ventricular fibrillation.

Management

High potassium can be life-threatening but easily correctable and there, at a cellular level, the main goal is to drive the extracellular potassium within the cells to protect cardiac conduction cells from the effects of a raised potassium level.

- If there are ECG changes or in acute severe cases of hyperkalemia, administration of calcium gluconate 10 ml (10%) is required. While administering this drug cardiac monitoring is needed and should be discontinued if bradycardia develops.
- The administration of insulin sliding scale with dextrose will drive the potassium into cells tem porarily (lasts approximately 4 hours).
- In acute situations nebulized salbutamol can also assist in shifting potassium.
- Calcium resins are used to reduce GI absorption of potassium. This is usually given at a 15 g dose orally three times a day but preparations and route vary.

- Treat the underlying cause to prevent recurrent hyperkalemia.
- Bicarbonate can be used in resistant cases with associated metabolic acidosis as high H^+ ions causes a shift of potassium to the extracellular compartment.[3]
- Renal dialysis is usually considered when all medical therapies have been exhausted.
- Once the patient is stabilized assess the medication history and discontinue drugs that may precipitate hyperkalemia. These include potassium sparing diuretics, oral potassium tablets, ACE inhibitors and any other drugs that would precipitate renal failure.
- Ensure that a low potassium diet is encouraged until the potassium is in normal range.

Hypokalemia (Fig. 1.4)

Symptoms/Signs

1. Fatigue, lethargy, anorexia
2. Leg cramps
3. Constipation
4. Weakness, hyporeflexia and paresthesia
5. Ileus.

ECG Findings

- U waves
- Flattened T wave
- ST segment changes
- Arrhythmias and eventually cardiac arrest

Management

- A potassium level below 3 mEq/L potassium replacement should be administered at 20-30 mEq/L with ECG monitoring in severe hypokalemia.
- Potassium levels 3 to 3.5 mEq/L can be replaced orally or intravenous.
- Some patients may be resistant to potassium replacement and in these patients, magnesium levels must be checked as they often co-exist. It will be difficult to correct low potassium if the magnesium level is not corrected first.[4]
- It is also pertinent to omit any drugs that may aid the depletion of potassium temporarily.
- In postsurgical patients, fluid administration must include potassium especially in those who are kept nil by mouth, on insulin sliding scale and stoma patients.

Hypermagnesemia (Fig. 1.5)

- High magnesium levels are rarely seen in surgical patients unless they are known to have renal disease. In these patients, magnesium levels should be monitored closely. Any medications that may increase serum levels such as Mg containing antacids and laxatives should be avoided.
- Symptoms and ECG changes resemble those in hyperkalemia. Symptoms and signs ensue at a level above 6 mEq/L whereas at a level above 10 mEq/L can be fatal.
- Management includes fluid replacement with isotonic saline administration to enhance renal excretion. This management may be ineffective in patients with severe renal failure who would require dialysis.

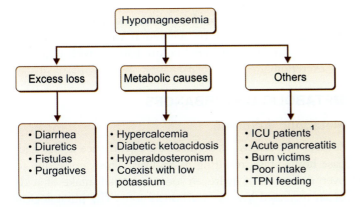

FIGURE 1.5: Causes of hypomagnesemia

Hypomagnesemia

Symptoms/Signs

- Tremors
- Delirium/confusion
- Seizures
- Hyperactive tendon reflexes
- Positive Chvostek's sign.

ECG Findings

- Prolonged QT and PR intervals
- ST segment depression
- Flattening or inversion of P waves
- Torsades de pointes
- Arrhythmias.

Management

- Magnesium depletion is a common problem amongst in-patients and those in the critical care units.[5]
- Magnesium replacements usually come in two preparations. These include sulfates and chlorides.
- Moderately low magnesium levels can be replaced by oral therapy.
- In more severe deficits parenteral replacement is appropriate and should be done cautiously to avoid over-replacement especially in patients with renal failure.
- It is useful to know that hypomagnesemia can occur along with a low potassium and calcium levels and therefore these electrolytes should corrected.

Calcium Homeostasis

- Calcium plays an important role in the neuromuscular function and at a cellular level. The majority of the calcium is stored in the skeletal system with only 1 percent in the extracellular fluid.
- Calcium is distributed as three forms: Ionized (40%), albumin-bound (50%) and anion-bound (10%).
  The serum calcium concentration (4.2–5.2 mEq/L) is regulated by three hormones chiefly vitamin D, parathyroid hormone and calcitonin. These hormones have direct and indirect effects on three major organ systems as shown in Figure 1.6.
- The acid-base balance also alters the calcium concentration. Acidosis increases the serum calcium concentration as it reduces the protein binding whereas low serum calcium is seen in alkalosis.
- The ionized calcium concentration is important in the postoperative surgical patient especially post-

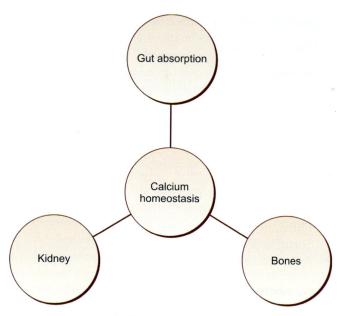

FIGURE 1.6: Effects on organ systems by hormones

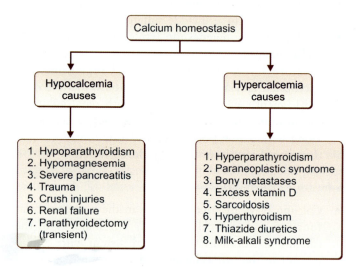

FIGURE 1.7: Causes of calcium abnormalities

parathyroidectomy patients. The disturbance, although transient can cause clinical signs and symptoms that would require correction.

- Figure 1.7 lists some of the important causes of calcium abnormalities.

Hypocalcemia

- Clinical manifestations include lethargy, abdominal and muscle cramps, carpopedal spasm and in severe cases convulsions are also seen.

- Important clinical signs to elicit are exaggerated tendon reflexes, Chvostek's sign (spasm on tapping the facial nerve) and Trousseau's sign (spasm resulting from a blood pressure cuff applied to the upper limb).
- QT interval prolongation and T wave inversion are seen on the ECG. In severe cases conduction blocks and arrhythmias are seen.
- Management initially involves investigating and correcting pH abnormalities. In patients with an acute transient low calcium level, intravenous calcium gluconate or chloride can be given while monitoring the ECG. In patients with chronic low calcium, oral vitamin D and calcium supplements can be given.
- Malignancies associated with increase osteoclastic activity can result in hypocalcemia as a direct result of increased bone formation.[7]

Hypercalcemia

- Clinical symptoms include fatigue, muscle weakness, depression, abdominal pains, constipation and nausea, and symptoms of renal calculi.
- Severe hypocalcemia (level above 12 mg/dL) is a medical emergency as it can cause coma and death.
- ECG abnormalities include shortened QT interval, prolonged PR and QRS, flattened T waves and in severe cases conduction blocks and cardiac arrest.
- Malignancy and parathyroid abnormalities account for the majority of symptomatic hypocalcemia.[6]
- Treatment initially involves aggressive fluid replacement to enhance the excretion. If this is ineffective then furosemide, IV pamidronate and IV sodium sulfate are methods of reducing serum calcium. Management depends on the protocols within the local trust/hospitals.
- Corticosteroids can be used in patients where the cause is sarcoidosis, vitamin D intoxication or Addison's disease.
- Plicamycin can be used in metastatic disease.
- Hemodialysis may be needed if there is refractory hypocalcemia or in renal failure patients with impaired excretion.

METABOLIC DISTURBANCES

Metabolic Acidosis

A metabolic acidosis is defined as a disturbance in the acid-base homeostasis resulting in acidosis. This can be due to overproduction of hydrogen ions, increased intake of acids or an increased loss of bicarbonate ions. The physiological response is to counteract this and restore homeostasis. This is done by the following methods:

- Hyperventilation in order to remove more CO_2 (Kussmaul respirations)
- Increased production/reabsorption of bicarbonate ions via kidneys
- Increase the secretion of hydrogen ions.

A lot can be determined by working out the anion gap in these patients. In normal individuals there is an anion gap of less than 12 mmol/l and is usually due albumin and the gap must be adjusted accordingly.[8] Any value above this represents unmeasured ions which would be due to ingestion or generation within the body. The formula involves subtracting cations from anions:

$$\text{Anion gap} = (Na + K) - (Cl + HCO_3)$$

Causes of a High Anion Gap Acidosis

- Lactic acidosis
- Diabetic ketoacidosis
- Ingestion of acids, e.g. methanol, ethylene glycol
- Salicylate poisoning
- Organic acid production in renal failure.

Causes of Normal Anion Gap Acidosis

- Loss of bicarbonate ions via kidneys, GI tract or fistulae
- Medications such as acetazolamide
- Renal tubular acidosis.

Of these causes lactic acidosis and GI tract losses post-surgery are the commonest causes. Lactic acidosis develops as result of reduce tissue perfusion resulting in the production of lactic acid which can be corrected once perfusion is restored. GI tract losses are above the normal insensible losses that occur in the body and bicarbonate ions are lost. The body maintains the anion gap by restoring chloride ions.

Metabolic Alkalosis (Fig. 1.8)

Metabolic alkalosis is a common problem amongst surgical patients as many of them are volume deplete postoperatively. In order to correct the metabolic alkalosis it is pertinent to fluid resuscitate these patients with normal saline and adequately replace potassium via KCL solutions as these patients are also chloride deplete. This will negate the need for the kidneys to reabsorb bicarbonate and will allow acid-base homeostasis.

Respiratory Alkalosis

Hyperventilation and loss of CO_2 from the alveoli is the physiological phenomenon that results in respiratory

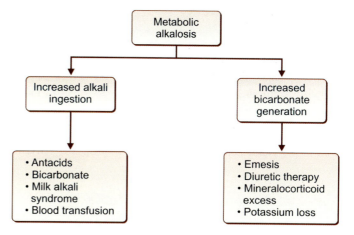

FIGURE 1.8: An algorithm for metabolic alkalosis

alkalosis. It results in a high pO_2, low pCO_2 with or without metabolic compensation. This pattern of breathing can be seen in the following clinical scenarios:

- Pain, anxiety
- Early stages of septicemia
- Neurological disorders like head trauma, meningitis
- Medications such as salicylates
- Hypoxia
- Thyrotoxicosis.

Hyperventilation causes electrolyte shift into cells primarily potassium and enhances binding of calcium to albumin resulting in symptomatic hypocalcemia and hypokalemia. Treatment generally involves correcting the underlying cause.[9]

Respiratory Acidosis

Any illness that will cause the patient to hypoventilate will result in respiratory acidosis. This can be diagnosed by a high pCO_2, low pO_2 with or without metabolic compensation. The list below summarizes some of the causes:

- *Lung related*: Effusion, atelectasis, pneumonia, mucus plug, COPD exacerbation
- *Postoperative pain*: Intra-abdominal or thoracic preventing optimal lung expansion
- CNS pathology
- Abdominal distension/compartment syndrome.

Treatment involves correcting the underlying problem and optimizing lung expansion if possible. If medical therapy fails to recover the acidosis then invasive ventilation should be considered in the context of the clinical case.

Table 1.4: Types of parenteral solutions

Type of infusion	Contents in mEQ/L				
	Na	K	Cl	HCO₃	Osm
0.9% saline	154	0	154	0	308
Ringer lactate	130	4	109	28	278
0.45% saline	77	0	77	0	407
3% saline	513	0	513	0	1026
5% dextrose	0	0	0	0	253
Normal body extracellular fluid	142	4	103	27	280

Types of Parenteral Solutions (Table 1.4)

There are a number of different parenteral solutions used in practice. Ringer lactate and normal saline are isotonic solutions and are usually used to replace insensible losses. It is, however, important to bear a few points in mind when considering the type of fluid replacement:

- The volume deficit
- The electrolyte abnormality present postoperatively
- Any potassium deficit
- Replacement of any ongoing insensible loss.

Hypertonic solutions are reserved only in situations where there is severe hyponatremia. Care must be taken to correct Na level slowly in order to prevent cerebral pontine myelinolysis.

Hypertonic saline solutions have been used in closed head injuries as it has shown to increase the cerebral perfusion, reduce cerebral edema and improve the overall outcome.[9-11] This is not the case for trauma patients as hypertonic saline solutions have not shown to be more beneficial than isotonic solutions.[12]

The other subset of parenteral therapy is colloids and this includes albumin, gelatins and dextrans. These are primarily used to expand intravascular volume in postoperative shock. Albumin is derived from blood hence it can cause allergic reactions and it has been shown in studies that it may cause renal and pulmonary failure when used during hemorrhagic shock.[13,14] Gelatins are derived from bovine collagen whereas dextrans are produced by bacteria grown on sucrose media. Both are volume expanders but dextrans are now only used to reduce plasma viscosity.

SPECIAL CONSIDERATIONS

Burns

Burns involve damage to the epidermis, dermis or the subcutaneous tissue causing permanent disfigurement, pain and electrolyte imbalance. The severity depends on the cause, degree, body parts affected and the presence/absence of inhalation injury.[15] Patient's age and co-morbidities can also influence the severity. There are four essential features in managing patients with thermal injury. These are prevention of burn shock by adequate fluid resuscitation, adequate ventilation, removal of necrotic tissue with wound closure and metabolic support. In this section we will concentrate on the fluid resuscitation needs.

Fluid resuscitation is a crucial step in managing a patient with thermal injury and an adequate fluid administration without causing overload can be difficult at times as these patients have burn associated edema which can be mistaken for overload to the inexperienced clinician. The physiological mechanism of adequate intravascular volume allowing optimal tissue perfusion can be disturbed in these patients.[16,17] Many texts describe urine output as the sole sensitive indicator in determining tissue perfusion. Lab studies have shown that kidneys are the first organs to experience hypoperfusion.[18] Therefore, renal function and urine output are useful indicators in assessing organ perfusion. The extent of burns is determined by the rule of nines where body parts injured are expressed as a percentage (Fig. 1.9), with 9% for each limb, 9% for the head and neck and the remaining divided equally between the front and back of the body.

There are a number of resuscitation fluid formulae but the commonly used regime is the modified Brooke formula.[19]

Figure 1.10 summarizes the management.

The electrolyte abnormalities in burn injury patients occur in phases which are categorized as below:[21-23]

1. *Fluid accumulation phase:* This occurs within 36 hours of the injury and causes fluid shift from the vascular compartment to the interstitial space causing high potassium, hyponatremia, hypovolemia, hypocalcemia and metabolic acidosis.

2. *Fluid remobilization phase:* This usually occurs 2 days after the injury and causes fluid shift back to the vascular compartment causing low potassium, hypervolemia, hyponatremia, metabolic acidosis.

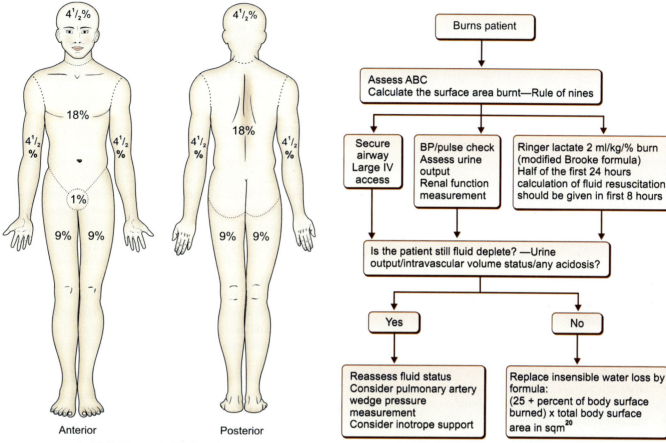

FIGURE 1.9: Rule of nines
(*Courtesy*: Diagram taken from UW health website)

FIGURE 1.10: Management of burns patient

3. *Recovery phase*: May cause further electrolyte disturbance due to inadequate dietary intake or enteral feeding.

Burns patients are prone to infected wounds, pulmonary edema, airway compromise and gastrointestinal complications such as Cushing's ulcer and paralytic ileus. Therefore, apart from correcting electrolyte abnormalities, one must undertake a thorough clinical assessment and manage any associated complications.

GASTRIC OUTLET OBSTRUCTION (GOO)

Gastric outlet obstruction is a pathological obstruction of the free flow of gastric contents into the duodenum. The causes include peptic ulcer disease, tumor, polyps, pyloric stenosis, or any extrinsic compression such as pseudocysts, gallstones.

Nausea and projectile vomiting are cardinal features of this surgical presentation. There may be associated abdominal pain. The characteristic electrolyte abnormalities include:

- Increased urea and creatinine levels
- Low potassium which may be severe
- Hypochloremic metabolic alkalosis due to acid (HCl) loss from the stomach.

Definitive treatment involves correcting the underlying cause for GOO; however, in the interim the electrolyte abnormalities must be corrected.

Biliary Fistula

Biliary fistulae are any abnormal communication with the bile duct system. They are usually internal as communication with the abdominal wall is rare. The fistulae are the result of chronic inflammation, adhesions and erosions of the visceral surfaces. This communication is usually with the gastrointestinal tract and is usually caused by gallstones,[24] but can be due to bile duct malignancy, chronic cholecystitis and inflammatory bowel disease.[25,26]

Patients with this fistula present with abdominal pain, nausea, dyspepsia, steatorrhea and rarely gallstone ileus. Frequently they can cause electrolyte abnormalities. These include:

- Hyponatremia which can be profound in external biliary fistulae
- Hypokalemia
- Hypomagnesemia
- Malabsorption of fat soluble vitamins.

Colonic Diarrhea

Diarrhea is a change in bowel habit to become more loose and/or an increased frequency. It is also defined as stool weight in excess of 200 g/day and having more than 3 bowels movements a day. It is a common problem and its causes are vast. Diarrhea can be of acute or chronic in nature and is divided into the following types (with a few examples):

- Infective   - Bacterial, viral and protozoal
- Inflammatory - Autoimmune, radiation and micro-scopic colitis
- Neoplastic   - Colorectal, pancreatic and VIPoma
- Metabolic   - Thyrotoxicosis, carcinoid syndrome
- Drug related - Antibiotics, laxatives. Many other drugs have diarrhea as a side effect
- Malabsorption - Coeliac disease, Whipple's disease and tropical sprue.

Diarrhea results in a number of electrolyte disturbances along with dehydration if the total output exceeds the total fluid intake. This results in the following electrolye disturbances:

1. Hypokalemia
2. Hyponatremia[27]
3. Metabolic acidosis due to bicarbonate loss.

These are the major electrolyte abnormalities and replacement of the electrolytes should be prioritized by the severity of the disturbance and its effect on the body. Associated electrolytes such as magnesium levels can also be affected and therefore, it is pertinent to check and correct these.

Liver Cirrhosis

Cirrhosis is a histological change of normal liver tissue into fibrosed nodular liver as a result of chronic irreparable liver injury. There are a number of causes to chronic liver disease, however, alcohol and viral hepatitis are the leading causes worldwide.

Symptoms can develop and are usually a result of impaired hepatic synthetic function. This includes coagulopathy, hepatic encephalopathy and variceal bleeding. Cirrhosis is a major problem worldwide and with scarcity of transplants, many of them have recurrent admissions with complications of their illness. One of the factors that warrant medical review is electrolyte disturbance. The electrolyte disturbances are summarized during cirrhosis phase and post-liver transplant phase.

- *Cirrhosis phase:* Cirrhosis impairs the normal synthetic function of the liver resulting in a scarcity of albumin in turn resulting in a reduced oncotic intravascular pressure. This causes fluid shift into the extravascular space resulting in ascites, peripheral edema. These patients have a number of electrolyte abnormalities resulting from the disease as well as the diuretic therapy:
  1. Diuretic related hyponatremia, hyper/hypokalemia, renal impairment, hypomagnesemia and hypocalcemia.
  2. Hepatorenal syndrome causing renal impairment and refractory hyponatremia. Definitive treatment usually involved transplantation. Transjugular intrahepatic portosystemic shunting can be used (TIPS).
  3. Raised ammonia levels resulting in hepatic encephalopathy. This is precipitated by infection, constipation, medications, variceal bleeding, renal failure and a high protein diet.
  4. Other abnormalities include uremia and hypoglycemia.
- *Liver transplantation phase:* One must fulfill strict criteria in order to be eligible for a liver transplantation. Once eligible the workup for transplantation involves minimizing any perioperative and postoperative complications. A number of electrolyte disturbances can occur some of which are summarized below:
  1. *Calcium:* Hypocalcemia is evident preoperative however, severe hypocalcemia is evident postoperatively as the new liver metabolizes citrate, massive blood transfusion during transplant releases citrate. This is transient (36 - 48 hours) and should be treated with intravenous fluid replacement.
  2. *Potassium:* Hypokalemia is common preoperatively but immediately post-op the potassium level rises due to reperfusion, this however is transient (10 minutes). Later on hypokalemia may be a feature due to bile, ascitic and nasogastric drainage loss.
  3. *Magnesium:* Low magnesium is a feature throughout pre- and post-liver transplantation phases. Cyclosporin given postoperatively further increases renal magnesium loss.

4. *Sodium:* Hypernatremia is a feature intra- and post-operatively as blood products are frequently administered. Overzealous correction of this can cause neurological signs also known as central pontine myelinolysis.

5. *Phosphate:* Low phosphate levels are a feature post-operatively due to fluid administration, cyclosporine administration, carbohydrate administration.

REFERENCES

1. Miller M. Syndromes of excessive antidiuretic hormone release. Crit Care Clin 2001;17:11.
2. Laureno R, Karp BI. Myelinolysis after correction of hyponatremia. Ann Med 1997;126:67.
3. Kapoor M, Chang G. Fluid and electrolyte abnormalities. Crit Care Clin 2001;17:571.
4. Adrogue HJ, Lederer ED, Suki WN, et al. Determinants of plasma potassium in diabetic ketoacidosis. Medicine 1986;65:163.
5. Kobrin SM, Goldfarb S. Magnesium deficiency. Semin Nephrol 1990;10:525.
6. Aguilera IM, et al. Calcium and the anaesthetist. Anaesthesia 2000; 55:779.
7. Wong ET, Rude RK, Singer FR, et al. A high prevalence of hypomagnesaemia and hypomagnesaemia in hospitalized patients. Am J Clin Pathol 1983;79:348.
8. Fisken FA, Heath DA, Somers S, et al. Hypercalcemia in hospital patients: clinical and diagnostic aspects. Lancet 1981;1:202.
9. Krapf R, et al. Chronic respiratory alkalosis. The effect of sustained hyperventilation on renal regulation of acid-base equilibrium. N Engl J Med 1991;324:1394.
10. Bushinsky DA, Monk RD. Calcium. Lancet 1998;352:306.
11. Gluck SL. Acid-base. Lancet 1998;353:474.
12. Moore FA, Mckinley BA, Moore EE. The next generation in shock resuscitation. Lancet 2004;363(9425):1988-96.
13. Shackford SR. Effects of small-volume resuscitation on intracranial pressure and related cerebral variables. J Trauma 1997;42:S48.
14. Moore EE. Hypertonic saline dextran for post-injury resuscitation: Experimental background and clinical experience. Aust NZ J Surg 1991;61: L732.
15. Wade CE, Kramer GC, Grady JJ, et al. Efficacy of 7.5% saline and 6% dextran-70 in treating trauma. A meta-analysis of controlled clinical studies. Surgery 1997;122:609.
16. Lucas CE. The water of life. a century of confusion. J Am Coll Surg 2001;192:86.
17. Lucas CE, Ledgerwood AM, Higgins RF, et al. Impaired pulmonary function after albumin resuscitation from shock. J Trauma 1980;20:446.
18. Shirani KZ, Pruitt BA Jr, Mason AD Jr. The influence of inhalation injury and pneumonia on burn mortality. Ann Surg 1987; 205:82.
19. Horton JW, Baxter CR, White DJ. Differences in cardiac responses to resuscitation from burn shock, Surg Gynaecol Obstet 1989; 168:201.
20. Cioffi WG, De Meules JE, Gamelli RL. The effects of burn injury and fluid resuscitation on cardiac function in vitro. J Trauma 1986;26:638.
21. Asch MJ, Mersol PM, Mason AD Jr, et al. Regional blood flow in the burned anaesthetised dog. Surg Form 1971;22:55.
22. Pruitt BA Jr. The burn patient: initial care. Curr Probl Surg 1979;16:23.
23. Harrison HN, Moncrief JA, Duckett JW, et al. The relationship between energy metabolism and water loss from vaporization in severely burned patients. Surgery 1964;56:263.
24. Noskin EA, Strauss AA, Strauss SF. Spontaneous internal biliary fistula: a review of literature and report of two cases. Ann Surg 1949;130:270.
25. Chandar VP, Hookman P. Choledocolonic fistula through a cystic duct remnant: a case report. Am J Gastroenterol 1980;74:179-81.
26. LeBlanc KA, Barr LH, Rush BM. Spontaneous biliary enteric fistulas. South Med J 1983;76:1249-52.
27. Pizzoti NJ, Madi JC, Iamanaca AI, et al. Hyponatremia: Study of its epidemiology and mortality. Rev Hosp Clin Fac Med 1989;4: 307-311.

BIBLIOGRAPHY

1. Adrogue HJ, et al. Hypernatremia. N Engl J Med 2000;342:1493.
2. Adrogue HJ, et al. Hyponatremia. N Engl J Med 2000;342:1581.
3. Adrogue HJ, et al. Management of life-threatening acid-base disorders. N Engl J Med 1998;338:26,107.
4. Greenberg A. Hyperkalemia: treatment options. Seminal Nephrol 1998;18:46.
5. Reber PM, Heath H. Hypocalcemic emergencies. Med Clin North Am 1995;19:93.
6. Shepard MM, Smith JW 3rd. Hypercalcemia. Am J Med Sci 2007; 334:381.
7. Shires GT, Williams J, Brown F. Acute changes in extracellular fluids associated with major surgical procedures. Ann Surg 1961; 154:803.

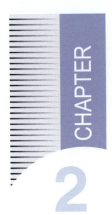

2

History of Surgery: Origin and Propagation of Plastic Surgery

Yash Gupta

INTRODUCTION

The problem of caring for injured and diseased is as old as human race. What was practiced in the prehistoric period is not clearly understood because of lack of written records. However, historical records available from India support the evidence that in ancient times India had a civilization in which medical and other sciences were well developed.

A brief history of Indian civilization would illustrate the knowledge and skills used in general surgery, trauma and plastic surgery.

The main knowledge base for Aryan culture was four sacred books, the 'Vedas'. These were written in Sanskrit. The text had prayers, incantations, chants and mantras. Although scholars have not been able to clearly go back to the origin of the Vedas, it is well accepted that they were compiled around 3500 BC. The most ancient of the 4 Vedas is the *Rig Veda*. There are descriptions of lacerated limbs being sutured in a manner that the patients could walk after the surgery. The Ashwini Kumara's, the Divine Physicians of Vedic Period cured cases of paralysis and successfully repaired severed limbs. Ayurveda [The science of life has been recognized as subdivision of *Atharva Veda* (Chapter 1 verse 6 of *Sushruta Samhita* (Fig. 2.1)]. This has revolutionized our knowledge of the art and science of Medicine (inclusive of all branches of medicine and surgery as we know today). Although the original script of the Ayurveda are not available, most of its contents are well described in the classic treatise by eminent ancient Indian physician Charak (1000 BC) and Sushruta (600 BC), the original plastic surgeon. The treatise of Ayurveda is fully described in the historic Indian text of *Sushruta Samhita*.

Ayurveda literally means science of life and the aim was to '*treat the disease and to preserve the health of the healthy*'. It has been divided in 8 subgroups:

1. Surgery
2. Medicine
3. Ophthalmology
4. ENT
5. Obstetrics
6. Psychiatry
7. Pediatrics
8. Toxicology.

Sushruta (600 BC) described the earliest known work on plastic surgery in the *Sushruta Samhita*. The book has 186 chapters written in Sanskrit language and chapter 16 deals with some fundamental techniques of plastic surgery. The book has been translated in Arabic (Kitab-e-Susrud, around 800 AD), in Latin (by Hessler, 1844-55), in German (by Vellurs), in English (by Bhishgratna, 1907; by Singhal et al. 1984). Present day Varanasi, India, was known as Kashi in 600 BC. A highly evolved civilization was already flourishing. King Bimbisara ruled Magadha and later his son Ajatshatru fought many battles and established himself as Emperor of India. Sanskrit was universal language and scholars came from far and wide to study at the University of Kashi. Sushruta worked at Kashi mainly as a Surgeon and wrote his Samhita based on the Ayurveda.

सुश्रुतसंहिता

SUSRUTA¹ SAMHITA²,³

सूत्रस्थानम् ।

SUTRA—STHANA⁴

प्रथमोऽध्यायः ।

Chapter One

1.   ORIGIN OF AYURVEDA

अथातो वेदोत्पत्तिमध्याय व्याख्यास्यामः ॥१॥

FIGURE 2.1: Opening verse of *Sushruta Samhita* (Sanskrit text with English translation)

14. ROTATION OF PEDICLED SKIN FLAP

गण्डादुत्पाट्य मांसेन सानुबन्धेन जीवता ॥
कर्णवालीमपालेस्तु कुर्यान्निर्लिख्य शास्त्रवित् ॥ १४ ॥

In the absence of the ear lobule, the expert (plastic surgeon) should elevate a living flap from the cheek², connected at its base and should reconstruct the ear lobule after scraping³.

FIGURE 2.2A: Rhinoplasty technique by Sushruta

27.20/1—32. RHINOPLASTY
27.20/1. Introduction

विश्लेषितायास्त्वथ नासिकाया बध्यामि सन्धानविधिं यथावत् ।

Now I would describe the proper method of rhinoplasty when the nose has been cut off.
27.20/2,28. THE PEDICLE FLAP FROM THE CHEEK

नासाप्रमाणं पृथिवीरुहाणां पत्रं गृहीत्वा त्ववलम्बि तस्य ॥ २७ ॥
तेन प्रमाणेन हि गण्डपार्श्वादुत्कृत्य बद्धं त्वथ नासिकाग्रम् ।
विलिख्य चाशु प्रतिसंदधीत तत् साधुबद्धं भिषगप्रमत्तः ॥ २८ ॥

FIGURE 2.3A: Rhinoplasty technique by Sushruta

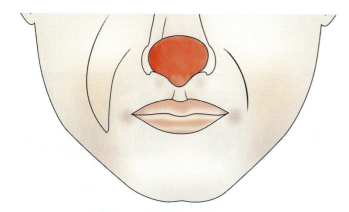

FIGURE 2.2B: Author's graphic interpretation

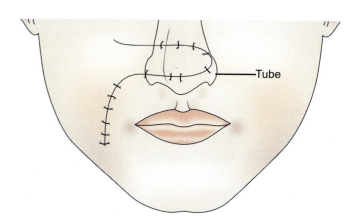

Tube

FIGURE 2.3B: Author's graphic interpretation

Chapter 16 of *Sutra-sthana* Sushruta Samhita specifically describes the reconstruction of lost ear lobe using a piece of skin which is attached to cheek and is alive by continuation! This is the first ever description of a flap in the world literature. He also describes the cheek (naso-labial) flap to reconstruct defects of nose and cleft lip. Figures 2.2A and B to 2.9 are a translation of relevant verses.

He was dealing with small mutilations, predominantly punitive, and was able to use the nasolabial flap effectively. It was quick and simple to raise and left minimal donor scar. He also used this flap to repair cleft lips.

Figure 2.10 shows a conceptual painting of Shushruta performing surgery

Sushruta Instruments and Techniques (Figs 2.11 and 2.12)

Supremacy of surgery is described in verses 18-19 of chapter 1 of the *Sushruta Samhita*. This part (*shalya*) is regarded as the best of all parts of *Ayurveda*, because it gives quick results, uses blunt and sharp instruments, caustics and cauteries and its help is sought for all other sections of the medical sciences. This part is eternal, sacred and a means of obtaining heavenly life, reputation, long life and also livelihood.

Taking a tree leaf of the size of the nose and placing it (on the cheek), a flap should be raised of the same size from the side of the cheek maintaining its continuity; it should then be approximated to the front part of the nose after (making the nose raw) and then the vigilant surgeon should quickly suture the same by the correct technique.

FIGURE 2.4

29,30. POST-OPERATIVE CARE

सुमहित सम्यगतो यथावत्रातिद्वयेनासिकमीद्य बद्ध्वा ।
प्रोद्रम्य चैनामवचूर्णयत् पत्तुद्भयटीमूकाश्वनेश्च ॥ २९ ॥
संछाद्य सम्यक् पिचुना सितेन तैलेन विश्वेदनकृतिलानाम् ।
पूत च पाय्यः स नरः सुसीरो स्निग्धो विरेक्यः न यवौदनेन ॥ ३० ॥

Having examined the nose which has been properly sutured and correctly shaped, the same should be fixed by two tubes and elevated. Then, the powder of red sandal wood, *madhūka* and *rasāñjana* should be sprinkled on the nose after elevating it.

It should be dressed properly with white cotton and should be soaked repeatedly with sesamum oil; *ghrta* should be administered to the patient after the previous meal has been properly digested and a purgative should be prescribed as instructed.

FIGURE 2.5

FIGURES 2.4 and 2.5: Rhinoplasty technique by Sushruta

31. FINAL APPEARANCE

रूढं च सन्बानमुपागतं स्यात्तदर्बशेषं तु पुनर्निकृन्तेत् ।
हीनां पुनर्बंर्धयितुं यतेत समां च कुर्यादतिवृद्धमांसाम् ॥ ३१ ॥

When the graft has properly taken up, base of the same should be snapped. The short graft should be elongated and the long graft should be made uniform.

FIGURE 2.6: Rhinoplasty technique by Sushruta

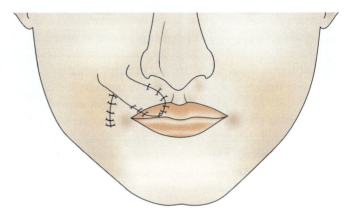

FIGURE 2.9: Author's graphic interpretation

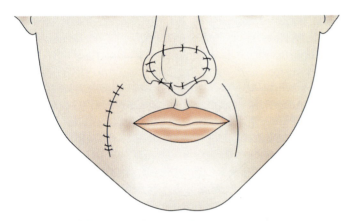

FIGURE 2.7: Author's graphic interpretation

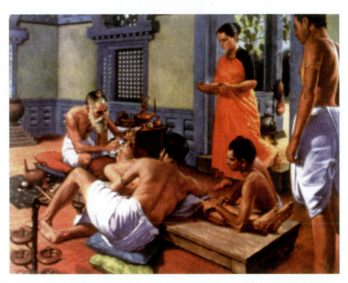

FIGURE 2.10: A conceptual painting of Sushruta performing surgery

32. CLEFT-LIP SURGERY

नाडीयोगं विनौष्ठस्य नासासन्धानबद्विधिम् ।
य एवमेव जानीयात् स राज्ञः कर्तुमर्हति ॥ ३२ ॥

Plastic surgery of the harelip should be done similar to that of rhinoplasty but without the use of two tubes. Only he who knows these (techniques) is entitled to be the royal physician.

इति सुश्रुतसंहितायां सूत्रस्थाने कर्ण्यव्यधबन्धविधिर्नाम पोडशोऽध्यायः ॥ १६ ॥

Thus ends the sixteenth chapter entitled 'The Techniques of Ear Puncture and Plastic Surgery' of *Sūtra-sthāna* of *Suśruta Samhitā.*

FIGURE 2.8: Cleft lip repair technique by Sushruta

Sushruta recommended that a surgeon keep his nail short, be clean, wear a white dress, have good manners and be accompanied by a dependable assistant. Operations were done on auspicious days and preceded by religious ceremonies and prayers by the surgeon. The operating rooms were cleaned and fumigated with vapors of white mustard and Neem (an Indian tree with antiseptic properties) leaves. In the diagnosis of a case inspection, palpation, percussion, smell and taste played important part. The affected area was shaved usually before an operation because presence of hair was associated with wound. He describes several types of surgical instruments both blunt and sharp.

Sushruta describes the instruments in Chapters 7-9 of the Sushruta Samhita. He makes detailed observation on the metal used for instruments, their shape according to usage. In verse 14 of Chapter 8, he says:

'When the blade of the knife has been made so sharp that it can slice the hair into two, the different parts of the instrument

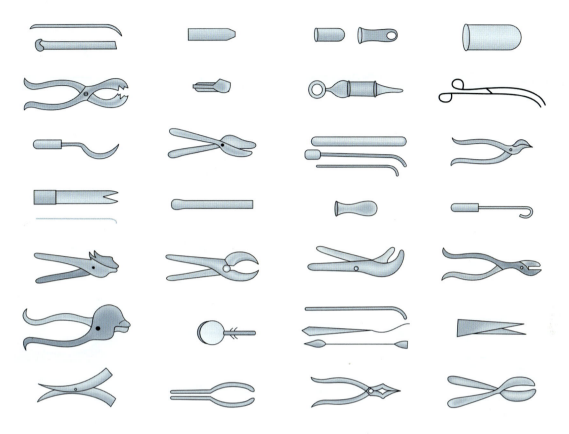

FIGURE 2.11: Selection of blunt instruments

have been fixed properly, the adjustments regarding the measurements have been done correctly and the instrument has been held in the proper way only then it should be used in surgical operations'.

He also describes the importance of hand as the most important instrument. Verse 3 Chapter 7 of *Sutra-sthana* is quoted here:

'Yantras (instruments) are one hundred and one; here, it should be noted that the hand is the most important amongst Yantras. Why So? Because in the absence of the hand, the instrument cannot be even used; and because the application of instruments is dependent upon it'.

The qualities of surgeon are described in verse 10 of Chapter 5 of *Sutra-sthana*:

'Boldness, swiftness in action, sharpness of his instruments, no sweating or trembling of hands and confidence are praiseworthy qualities of a surgeon at the time of operation.'

Silk, cotton and horse hair were used as suturing materials and opium was used as analgesic and sedative. He also describes various ointments for wound care. The enormity and the scientific excellence of his work can only be fully appreciated after reading the Sushruta Samhita in detail.

Propagation of Plastic Surgery from Ancient India to Europe

Gupta (1988), carried out extensive research at Oxford, whilst working in the Department of Plastic Surgery at the Radcliff Infirmary. The work was presented at the Royal College of Surgeons in London in 1988. The cheek flap Rhinoplasty was traced to be the originally described by Sushruta around 600 BC (Fig. 2.13). Then the technique was traced to Vagbhata in 400 AD.

Vagbhata (400 AD) described the cheek flap rhinoplasty in even greater detail in his book *Astang Hridyans*. Verses 59-65 of Chapter 18 of *Uttarsthana* describe this elegantly:

'Do as follows for a clean youth whose nose has been cut. Having cut a pattern of leaf to the size of nose, cut similarly on cheek. Protect the skin and flesh (attachment of that flap) near the nose so that it remains his part. Then suture the cheek with a sharp needle and cotton thread and then having incised the edge of the

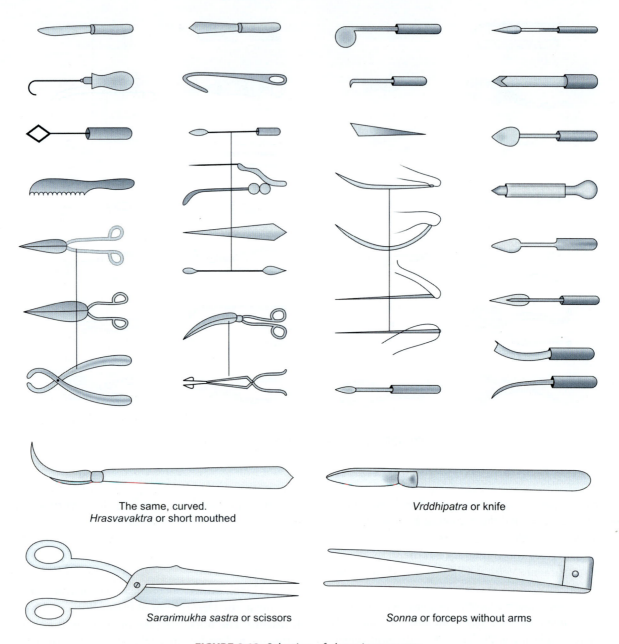

The same, curved.
Hrasvavaktra or short mouthed

Vrddhipatra or knife

Sararimukha sastra or scissors

Sonna or forceps without arms

FIGURE 2.12: Selection of sharp instruments

nasal opening, turn the outer skin. Then unite the strap of skin from the cheek, suturing it to the nose with care. Lift it with two tubes so that he may breathe nicely. Then having wetted the wound with oil, cover it with fine paste of.patanga and madhuka. Then having tied it with ghee and honey, keep an attendant (to watch the patient). Subsequently treat the wound as required after knowing the developments. Excise the excess of flesh and skin near the nostril and suture it nicely. If short then develop it again'.

By 400 AD, trade routes were well established for export of gems and spices from India to Persia, Greece and Italy (Fig. 2.14). After the fall of Gupta empire, the Ayurvedic Medicine and Surgery lost much of its strength and its practice became more of a family tradition. Nonetheless Sushruta's teachings disseminated along the trade routes. The art of Sushruta's cheek flap rhinoplasty reached Sicily via Persia.

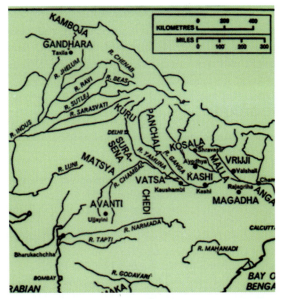

FIGURE 2.13: Sixteen major states of northern India (600 BC)

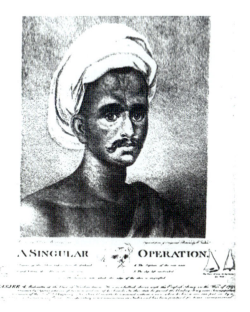

FIGURE 2.15: Cowasjee operation in Gentlemen's Magazine (1794)

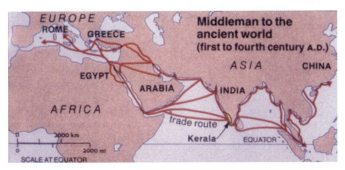

FIGURE 2.14: Trade and silk routes from India to the West

Zeis (1863) documented the accounts of Branca, the father, using cheek flap rhinoplasty around 1450 AD:

'Moreover the flesh was cut by his father from cheek of the mutilated man, he (Branca) himself cut from man's arm ...'

Upper arm flap rhinoplasty was later observed on mainland Italy in the region of Calabria where Vineo family used it with good results. This was further popularized by Professor Gasper Taglicozzi (1597). He specifically rejected the use of forehead and cheek skin for rhinoplasty. Thus suggesting that he was well aware of the previous work in this field. For various reasons of misuse and misinterpretations, rhinoplasty as an art became almost forgotten after the death of Taglicozzi.

Gentlemen's Magazine (1794) Carried a Sensational Article

Cowasjee a bullock cart driver with British army was taken prisoner by Tippoo Sultan and punished him by cutting his nose off. He later returned to Poona in this disgraced state. British resident Sir Charles Mallet had previously met an oil cloth merchant who had his nose reconstructed by Artist of Poona. Sir Charles then sent for this Kumhar who was famous as a nose restorer. Two surgeons from Bombay army, Thomas Cruso and James Findlay with Colonel Ward witnessed the operation.

'A pattern of wax was shaped like a nose and flattened and outlined marked on forehead. Skin flap was quickly raised leaving it attached at 5. The nasal defect was scrapped and flap approximated to it. No sutures were used. On 25th day a final tidy up was carried out ...' It was later reported that nose was so strong that he could blow or sneeze without fear of dropping off (Fig. 2.15)!

This article appeared in 1793 in Bombay and Madras gazette and later in the Gentlemen's Magazine with initials 'B.L.'. Some believed that it was a typographical error for C.L. pertaining to CL Lucas who was a surgeon at Madras around that time. This misconception was further enhanced by assuming that he performed the first reported case of forehead flap Rhinoplasty. Patterson (1971) has tried to clarify some of the confusion. It is now quite clear that though

CL Lucas performed some rhinoplasties, he did not reconstruct Cowasjee's nose. The initials B.L. stood for B. Longmate who did the engraving and sent the article for publication to the Gentlemen's Magazine.

Carpue (1816) described two operations of rhinoplasty using Indian forehead flap. Rhinoplasty operations were freely performed and described by Diefenbach and Tribhuvandas Shah. Keegan (1900) made full reference to Shah in his book. He emphasized the importance of using local turned in flaps to provide lining thereby preventing contractures. Indian forehead rhinoplasty was developed into a fine art by Sir Harold Gilles.

From Sushruta to Vagbhata, the nasal defects were mostly small punitive mutilations and cheek flap was well used. Later, with more wars and bigger weapons, bigger defects were encountered and treated with forehead flap and passed down as family tradition over many centuries. A written original description of forehead flap still evades us. Perhaps when another 1500 ancient Sanskrit medical text have been translated, we may have some answers.

Tribute to Sushruta by McDowell (1975)

'.. Through all of Sushruta's flowery language, incantations and irrelevancies, there shines the unmistakable picture of a great surgeon. Undaunted by his failures, unimpressed by his success, he sought the truth unceasingly and passed on to those who followed. He attacked disease and deformity definitively, with reasoned and logical method. Where path did not exist, he made one....'

BIBLIOGRAPHY

1. Carpue JC. An account of two successful operations for lost nose, Longamn, London, 1816.
2. Gentlemen's Magazine. London, 1794.
3. Gupta Y. Origin and propagation of rhinoplasty, presented at the Royal College of Surgeons, London, 1988.
4. Keegan DF. Rhinoplasty operations, Ballier Tindall and Cox, London, 1900.
5. McDowell F. The source book of plastic surgery. The William & Wilkins Company Baltimore, 1975.
6. Pandya SK. British Medical Journal 1987;295:1662.
7. Patterson TJS. Plastic and Reconstructive Surgery 1971;48:71.
8. Singhal GD, Tripathi SN, Chaturvedi GN. Fundamental and plastic surgery considerations in ancient Indian surgery, Singhal Publications, Varanasi, India, 1984.
9. Sushruta, 600 BC, Sushruta Samhita, Sutra-sthana, Chapters 1-27.
10. Taglicozzi G. 1597, De curtom chirurgie per isitioneum, Bologna, Italy, Chapter 13.
11. Vagbhata, 400 AD, Astang Hridyans, Uttarsthana, Chapter 18.
12. Zeis E. Die Literature und Geschichte der Plastischen chirurgie, Englemann, Leipzig; 1863. p.213.

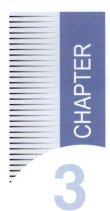

CHAPTER

3

Preoperative Cardiac Risk Stratification

Sanjay Gandhi, Indreesh Ramachandra

INTRODUCTION

One of the guiding principles of surgery is "do no harm". Every surgeon wants to ensure that every patient has a successful outcome after the surgical procedure without any complication. In reality, there is always an inherent risk for potential complications with every procedure. The prudent surgeon tries to anticipate and if possible minimize the inherent risks to the greatest possible extent in the available time frame.

Nearly 100 million surgical procedures are performed worldwide annually. Approximately 1 million of these patients have cardiovascular complications. Cardiovascular complications impact mortality and morbidity in the short term as well as up to 2 years in some studies. The incidence of major cardiovascular complications in patients undergoing elective major surgical procedures is 1.9–4 percent and accounts for 10–40 percent of all postoperative fatalities.

AIM OF PREOPERATIVE RISK STRATIFICATION

The purpose of preoperative evaluation is not to give medical clearance but rather to perform an evaluation of the patient's current medical status; make recommendations concerning the evaluation, management, and risk of cardiac problems over the entire perioperative period; and provide a clinical risk profile that the patient, primary physician, and non-physician caregivers, anesthesiologist, and surgeon can use in making treatment decisions that may influence short- and long-term cardiac outcomes.

EVALUATION

Patient Characteristics—Identifying the High-Risk Patient

A great deal of clinical research has been focused on identifying this high-risk group and on strategies to minimize cardiovascular risk. Even in a group of high-risk patients, the majority of patients undergo surgical procedures successfully. The challenge is to identify the small group of patients at high-risk of cardiovascular complications in the perioperative period. This group has received great attention and consequently consumes significant resources. Given that the background complication rate is low for the vast majority of patients, any strategy to identify a high-risk group has to be both highly sensitive and highly specific. In this regard, so far the clinical history of the patient yields the greatest number of clues to help evaluate the magnitude of risk.

History

A good history is a crucial component of preoperative evaluation and provides a basis for assessment of perioperative risk, further testing, if required and management perioperatively. Focused history should be obtained to identify high-risk cardiac conditions specifically unstable coronary syndromes, decompensated heart failure, significant arrhythmia or significant valvular heart disease (Table 3.1). The second important component of history is assessment of functional capacity of the patient. The ability to perform a spectrum of daily tasks has been shown to correlate well

Table 3.1: Active conditions for which patient should undergo evaluation and treatment of cardiac conditions before noncardiac surgery	
Condition	*Examples*
Unstable coronary syndromes	Canadian Cardiovascular Society class III or IV angina, acute or recent myocardial infarction (> 7 days but </= 30 days)
Decompensated heart failure	New York Heart Association class IV heart failure or new onset or worsening heart failure
Significant arrhythmias	High grade atrioventricular blocks—Mobitz II, third degree AV block
	Symptomatic bradycardia
	Supraventricular arrhythmias including atrial fibrillation with poorly controlled ventricular rate (HR >100 bpm at rest)
	Symptomatic ventricular arrhythmias
	New ventricular arrhythmia
Severe valvular heart disease	Severe aortic stenosis (aortic valve area <1.0 cm^2 or mean pressure gradient >40 mm Hg or symptomatic)
	Symptomatic mitral stenosis

Adapted from: ACC/AHA 2007 guidelines on perioperative cardiovascular evaluation and care for noncardiac surgery

with assessment by more sophisticated treadmill testing and is an important prognostic marker for cardiovascular outcomes. A functional capacity of >/= 4 metabolic equivalents (METs) is used in the preoperative algorithm. In a more simpler terms, if a patient is able to do light work around the house like dusting or cleaning clothes, or able to walk up a hill or on level ground at 4 mph he can exercise for =/>4 METs on a treadmill. Next the history should include an assessment of modifiable risk factors and evidence for associated diseases including peripheral arterial disease or cerebral vascular disease. The cardiovascular evaluation must be undertaken within the framework of patient's overall health including consideration for pulmonary disease, diabetes mellitus, renal insufficiency (serum creatinine level greater than 2 mg per dL) and hematological disorders as these co-morbid conditions have been shown to affect cardiovascular outcomes. In addition to perioperative management this evaluation may provide an opportunity to affect the long-term management of patients with or at risk of cardiac disease.

Physical Examination

A focused cardiovascular examination including general appearance, vitals, peripheral pulse and cardiac examination complements a good history. The examination provides clues to clinical evidence of heart failure (rales, elevated jugular venous pressure, peripheral edema, third heart sound), associated vascular disease (carotid bruit, decreased distal pulses) which heightens the suspicion for cardiac disease and murmurs suggestive of valvular heart disease.

Diagnostic Studies

The history and physical examination should guide the physician's decision to order further testing. These may include blood chemistries for metabolic or electrolyte disturbance, hematological tests for anemia, X-ray and ECG.

Preoperative ECG: The current guidelines recommend a resting 12 lead ECG in patients with at least one clinical risk factor who are undergoing vascular surgical procedures or patients with known coronary heart disease, peripheral arterial disease or cerebrovascular disease undergoing intermediate risk surgical procedures (Class I). However, a resting ECG is not recommended in asymptomatic persons undergoing low-risk surgical procedures.

Stress test: Stress test should only be considered in a limited subgroup of patients (Fig. 3.1). These are patients with poor or uncertain functional capacity and 3 or more clinical risk factors for CAD, undergoing intermediate or high-risk surgery. Majority of patients undergoing noncardiac surgery do not need stress testing prior to surgery.

Exercise: An exercise stress test can provide an objective measure of functional capacity, identify the presence of myocardial ischemia or arrhythmia and estimate risk for perioperative cardiovascular complications and long-term prognosis. The onset of myocardial ischemia at low workload is associated with significantly increased risk for perioperative and long-term cardiac events (Table 3.2). In ambulatory patients this is the test of choice.

Pharmacological: Stress testing for patients who cannot exercise can be accomplished by dobutamine stress echo (DSE) or

Risk level	Ischemic response gradient
Table 3.2: Prognostic gradient of ischemic responses during an ECG monitored exercise test in patients with suspected or known coronary artery disease	
High	Ischemia induced by low-level exercise (less than 4 METs or heart rate less than 100 bpm or less than 70% of age-predicted heart rate) manifested by 1 or more of the following: – Horizontal or downsloping ST depression greater than 0.1 mV – ST-segment elevation greater than 0.1 mV in noninfarct lead – Five or more abnormal leads – Persistent ischemic response greater than 3 minutes after exertion – Typical angina – Exercise-induced decrease in systolic blood pressure by 10 mm Hg
Intermediate	Ischemia induced by moderate-level exercise (4 to 6 METs or heart rate 100 to 130 bpm [70 % to 85% of age-predicted heart rate]) manifested by 1 or more of the following: – Horizontal or downsloping ST depression greater than 0.1 mV – Persistent ischemic response greater than 1 to 3 minutes after exertion – Three to 4 abnormal leads
Low	No ischemia or ischemia induced at high-level exercise (greater than 7 METs or heart rate greater than 130 bpm [greater than 85% of age-predicted heart rate]) manifested by: – Horizontal or downsloping ST depression greater than 0.1 mV – One or 2 abnormal leads
Inadequate test	Inability to reach adequate target workload or heart rate response for age without an ischemic response. For patients undergoing noncardiac surgery, the inability to exercise to at least the intermediate risk level without ischemia should be considered an inadequate test.

bpm: beats per min; CAD: coronary artery disease; MET: metabolic equivalent

dipyridamole/adenosine myocardial imaging with thallium-201 or technetium -99m. The DSE involves increased myocardial demand by pharmacological stimulation with dobutamine while intravenous dipyridamole or adenosine induce hyperemic response by vasodilatation. Overall sensitivity of DSE for prediction of perioperative death or MI is 85 percent with a specificity of 70 percent. Beattie and colleagues examined the predictive value of stress testing with echocardiography versus nuclear perfusion imaging including 25 studies with stress echo and 50 studies of stress nuclear imaging. The likelihood ratio for the primary endpoint of perioperative death or MI with a positive stress echo was twice that of a positive stress nuclear imaging. However, the finding of moderate to large ischemia by either pharmacological modality was highly predictive of perioperative death or MI but such abnormality was only present in 15 percent of all the patients tested.

Coronary angiography: Coronary angiography should only be considered if there is a clinical indication independent of the need for surgery. This would include patients with unstable angina or recent myocardial infarction or patients in whom noninvasive evaluation reveals a large area of myocardial ischemia.

Surgery Characteristics

The risk of perioperative complications are due to an interaction between factors unique to the patient (age, CAD, valvular heart disease, renal disease, etc.); factors specific to the surgical procedure (endoscopic versus open, revascularization versus amputation, etc.); and the factors specific to the situation under which the surgery is being performed (emergently, academic center, rural hospital, etc.).

If adequate time is available to assess the patient prior to the surgery, the assessment may reveal factors that predict the short- and long-term outcomes for the patient. The ability to predict such outcomes may alter the decision for surgery.

For example, identifying the presence of significant left ventricular dysfunction may make the surgeon choose a laparoscopic approach to an open approach in a patient with chronic gallstone disease. The decision to operate on a patient with asymptomatic uterine fibroids discovered on an Ultra sonogram may change to one of monitoring. The ability to predict long-term outcomes is important when the specific surgery is being performed based on the expectation that the patient will live long enough to experience the benefit from the surgery, such as a hemicolectomy for multiple polyps in a patient with severe CAD.

Urgency of Surgery

Patients undergoing emergent surgery have a 2 to 4 fold higher mortality than patients undergoing elective surgery. This has been shown to be true for vascular surgery such as for AAA surgery. A patent with a ruptured has > 40 percent risk of mortality than elective AAA repair. Patients with an emergent medical condition need surgery immediately for saving their lives. In this situation, there is usually little or no time for a cardiac evaluation. In some situations, surgery may be needed to be done quickly but not necessarily emergently such as in the case of a malignancy or limb gangrene or acute cholecystitis due to gallstone. In these situations, cardiac evaluation should be done rapidly and optimization of medical therapy can be done. However, the delay due to additional cardiac testing should not delay the surgical procedure so much that it results in an overall worse prognosis for the patient.

Stepwise Approach for Perioperative Cardiac Assessment (Fig. 3.1)

Step 1: Urgency for noncardiac surgery—if the surgery is deemed emergent, it may not allow for further cardiac assessment and in this case the role of consultant would be to optimize perioperative medical management and postoperative follow-up. However, if the surgery is non-urgent further evaluation can be done preoperatively.

Step 2: Evaluation for active cardiac conditions—including unstable coronary syndrome, arrhythmia, uncompensated heart failure or severe valvular disease. If any of the above is

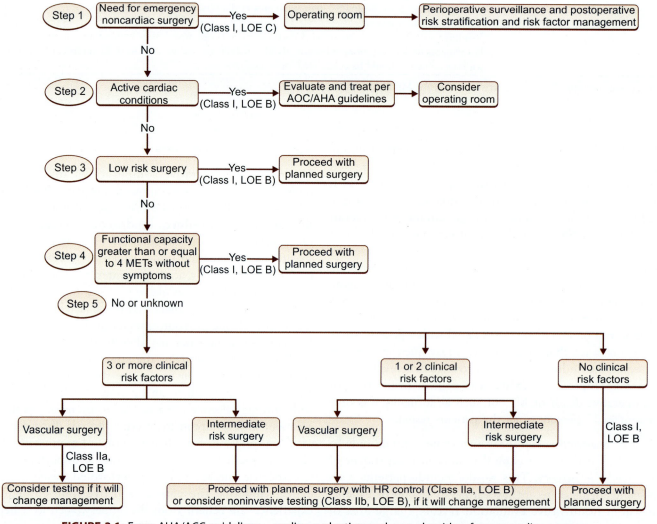

FIGURE 3.1: From AHA/ACC guidelines—cardiac evaluation and care algorithm for noncardiac surgery

present, it would require management by a cardiology consultant as per standard guidelines.

Step 3: Low risk surgery—if the cardiac risk from proposed surgery is low, further testing usually does not add any incremental benefit and is not recommended.

Step 4: Patients functional capacity—if the patient has a functional capacity of greater than or equal to 4 METs without symptoms, management will rarely be changed by further testing and it is therefore appropriate to proceed with planned surgery.

Step 5: If the patient has poor functional capacity, is symptomatic or functional capacity cannot be determined, further management is guided by presence or absence of clinical risk factors. If patient has no risk factors, it is appropriate to proceed with planned surgery. If that patient has one or two risk factors, it might be appropriate in most patients to proceed with surgery. If the patient has 3 or more risk factors further testing may be considered if this will change management.

In essence, majority of patients undergoing non-cardiac surgery do not require stress testing. However, careful clinical evaluation of the patient, in context of proposed surgery, can guide further testing in moderate to high-risk patients when it is likely to change management.

Anesthesia Consideration

All inhaled volatile anesthetic agents have adverse cardiovascular effects including myocardial depression and after load reduction. However in several clinical trials, the use of volatile anesthetics was associated with decreased troponin release or preserved LV systolic function or decreased late cardiac events, compared with use of balanced anesthesia techniques with opiates. Regional or local anesthesia may be considered in high-risk patients. However, both epidural and spinal approaches cause sympathetic blockade with reduction in preload and after load. For lower extremity or lower abdominal surgery these may be considered. However, higher dermatomal level of neuraxial anesthesia may result in hemodynamic consequences. MASTERS trial (Multicenter Australian Study of Regional Epidural Anesthesia) randomized 915 patients undergoing abdominal surgery to epidural or general anesthesia. There was no difference in outcomes of death or MI in the two groups. However, there were fewer pulmonary complications in patients randomized to neuraxial anesthesia.

Medical Therapy to Reduce Perioperative Cardiac Events

A variety of pathophysiologic mechanisms are triggered during the postoperative state including inflammatory cytokines, elevated circulating catecholamine, altered hemodynamic stress, hypercoaguability and altered energy substrate metabolism. A single therapeutic intervention cannot alter all the different potential triggers for myocardial ischemia and infarction. Combination of measures may reduce perioperative ischemia.

Perioperative Beta Blockade

It is widely believed that heightened sympathetic tone plays a significant role in perioperative cardiovascular complications and attenuation of this response will lead to improved outcomes. Based on several small and moderate sized studies, beta blockers gained wide acceptance for reduction of perioperative cardiovascular complications in patients undergoing noncardiac surgery despite limitations of these studies. The ACC/AHA/ESC guidelines regarding use of beta blockers is given in Table 3.3. The recent publication of the POISE trial and a meta-analysis by Bangalore et al has raised concerns about "automatic" or "universal" beta blockade use in the perioperative setting.

The POISE trial is the largest trial of perioperative beta blockade that used a fixed dose of long acting metoprolol in patients 2–4 hours before undergoing noncardiac surgery. It showed a significant reduction in nonfatal MI but an overall increased risk of mortality and nonfatal strokes in the treatment group. A meta-analysis by Bangalore et al[10] of 33 trials involving over 12000 patients, showed that perioperative beta blockers was not associated with any significant reductions in all cause mortality, cardiovascular mortality or heart failure. Treatment of 1000 patients with beta blockers results in 16 fewer nonfatal MI in survivors but at the expense of 3 nonfatal disabling strokes and 104 hemodynamic events needing treatment.

Thus trials have shown heterogeneity in the effects of perioperative beta blockade on outcomes when beta blockade is administered to all patients. When effects of beta blockade were studied as stratified by surgical risk, those in the highest risk category had a 63 to 73 percent relative risk reduction compared to the intermediate risk category.

Hence, all patients cannot be treated as a homogeneous group. In addition, the beta blockers studied included atenolol, bisoprolol, esmolol and metoprolol. We

Table 3.3: AHA/ACC guidelines for beta blocker use

Class I

1. Beta blockers should be continued in patients undergoing surgery who are receiving beta blockers to treat angina, symptomatic arrhythmias, hypertension, or other ACC/AHA class I guideline indications (Level of Evidence: C)
2. Beta blockers should be given to patients undergoing vascular surgery who are at high cardiac risk owing to the finding of ischemia on preoperative testing (Level of Evidence: B)

Class IIa

1. Beta blockers are probably recommended for patients undergoing vascular surgery in whom preoperative assessment identifies CHD. (Level of Evidence: B)
2. Beta blockers are probably recommended for patients in whom preoperative assessment for vascular surgery identifies high cardiac risk, as defined by the presence of more than 1 clinical risk factor (Level of Evidence: B)
3. Beta blockers are probably recommended for patients in whom preoperative assessment identifies CHD or high cardiac risk, as defined by the presence of more than 1 clinical risk factor, who are undergoing intermediate-risk or vascular surgery (Level of Evidence: B)

Class IIb

1. The usefulness of beta blockers is uncertain for patients who are undergoing either intermediate-risk procedures or vascular surgery, in whom preoperative assessment identifies a single clinical risk factor (Level of Evidence: C)
2. The usefulness of beta blockers is uncertain in patients undergoing vascular surgery with no clinical risk factors who are not currently taking beta blockers (Level of Evidence: B)

Class III

Beta blockers should not be given to patients undergoing surgery who have absolute contraindications to beta blockade (Level of Evidence: C)

Adapted from: ACC/AHA 2007 guidelines on perioperative cardiovascular evaluation and care for noncardiac surgery

recommend that beta blockers should not be used in low risk and intermediate patients undergoing low risk procedures if they do not have any other indication for beta blockers. Further, beta blockers, if indicated, should be commenced at least 1 week and preferably even earlier in order to titrate the dose for the individual patient to achieve resting heart rates less than 70 beats per minute based on the fact that up regulation of beta receptors takes time and that lower heart rates were associated with greater protection. This period also allows for detection of side-effects including bradycardia or hypotension in a given patient. Ultra short acting esmolol would allow for rapid response to changes in the hemodynamic status of the patient in the intraoperative and immediate postoperative period. Once adequate stability has been established and recovery is proceeding as expected, switch from IV to oral beta blockade should be made. Long acting oral beta blockers should be preferred at this time. In the long-term, beta blockers should be continued if there is any indication for using a beta blocker. If not, then the beta blocker should be gradually withdrawn over a period of weeks.

Perioperative Calcium Channel Blockers

The few studies of calcium channel antagonists showed no significant reduction in mortality or cardiovascular events

in patients undergoing noncardiac surgery. However, there were too few events in these studies to draw any meaningful conclusion.

Perioperative Alpha Agonists

A meta-analysis of 12 trials of alpha-2 adrenergic agonists showed a significant reduction in total mortality and myocardial infarction in patients undergoing vascular surgery. The results of this meta-analysis were primarily driven by the results of one trial of mivazerol. A trial of clonidine did not show any reduction in perioperative MI in patients undergoing noncardiac surgery but showed a trend towards reduction in mortality at 2 years. The trial, however, had very few events in the perioperative period. Alpha-2 agonists may be added for hypertension control or in a patient with hypertension and one clinical risk factor.

Perioperative Statins

Lipid lowering therapy using statins have shown to be beneficial in secondary prevention of cardiovascular events. In addition, statins have been shown to stabilize atherosclerotic plaque, improve endothelial function and alter inflammation. Observational and retrospective studies have suggested a statistically significant reduction in perioperative cardiac mortality in patients undergoing vascular surgery. One randomized study of statins in 200 patients undergoing noncardiac surgery showed a statistically significant reduction in cardiac events and the composite endpoint of cardiac death, unstable angina, MI and stroke (Table 3.4). At this time, available data suggests a beneficial effect of statins for reducing perioperative cardiac events in patients undergoing high and intermediate risk surgery.

If the patient meets guidelines for statin therapy but is not on a statin, the preoperative assessment should consider this an opportunity to add statin therapy to reduce lifetime risk of cardiovascular events. However, the dose and targets for statin therapy are unclear.

Perioperative Nitroglycerin

Nitroglycerin causes systemic venodilation and reduces preload. It also reduces myocardial ischemia in patients with angina. In the perioperative setting, Nitroglycerin can potentiate hypotension in conjunction with other anesthetic agents.

Nitroglycerin has not been shown to reduce cardiac events in patients undergoing noncardiac or cardiac surgery. It is reasonable to continue nitroglycerin in the postoperative period in patients who are on it preoperatively after taking into account potential hemodynamic effects of nitroglycerin. If nitroglycerin is needed perioperatively for controlling hypertension, it is reasonable to use a continuous infusion for more predictable action than other routes.

Coronary Revascularization to Reduce Perioperative Cardiac Events

Routine coronary revascularization in patients with stable cardiac symptoms before noncardiac surgery does not significantly alter the short-term risk of death or MI or the long-term outcome. In a large, randomized trial of coronary artery revascularization before elective major vascular surgery (CARP trial) 510 patients with significant coronary artery disease (defined as one or major artery with at least 70% stenosis) among 5859 patients undergoing vascular surgery were randomly assigned to coronary revascularization or no coronary revascularization prior to surgery. Of the 225 patients in revascularization group, 59 percent had PCI (PTCA and bare metal stent) and 41 percent had CABG. There was no difference in 30 day death (3.1% versus 3.4%) or postoperative MI (12% versus 14%) or long-term mortality at 2.7 years (22% versus 23%) in the revascularization group compared with non-revascularization group.

Preoperative CABG

The purpose of CABG prior to a surgery is not only to lower perioperative risk but also to provide long-term benefit. In a series of 1001 patients undergoing coronary angiography prior to elective vascular surgical procedures, 251 patients met the criteria for surgical revascularization. Of these 216 patients underwent CABG. The mortality rate for CABG was 5.3 percent and the mortality rate after vascular procedures was 1.5 percent. The overall mortality rate for the entire cohort was 1.4 percent for patients with normal coronary arteries, 1.8 percent for patients with moderate CAD, and 3.6 percent for patients with advanced CAD and 14 percent for patients with severe, uncorrected or inoperable CAD. However, patients undergoing low risk procedures like skin, breast or urological surgery have a very low mortality rate of less than 1 percent and may not benefit from preoperative revascularization. In subset of patients undergoing higher risk surgical procedures, CABG reduces the rate of death (1.7% vs. 3.3%) and nonfatal MI (0.8% vs. 2.7%). These data suggest that patients undergoing low risk procedures are unlikely to derive benefit from CABG before low risk surgery but patients with multi-vessel disease or severe angina undergoing high risk surgery may benefit from revascularization prior to noncardiac surgery. Further, CABG may provide long-term benefit of survival in patients with three vessels CAD especially those with low ejection fraction and diabetes as compared to medical therapy.

Preoperative PCI

The role of preoperative PCI to reduce perioperative events is very limited. Only patients with ST elevation MI, unstable angina and non-ST elevation MI benefit from early invasive management. The balance of evidence to date suggests that routine preoperative revascularization in patients with stable coronary artery disease is of no value in preventing perioperative death or MI.

Coronary revascularization is recommended in patients with acute ST elevation myocardial infarction or patients with high risk unstable angina or non-ST elevation myocardial infarction. Coronary revascularization with coronary artery bypass graft surgery (CABG) or percutaneous intervention (PCI) before noncardiac surgery is recommended for patients with stable angina who have significant left main disease, three vessel coronary artery diseases or two vessel coronary artery disease with proximal left anterior descending artery involvement especially if the ejection fraction is less than 50 percent.

Table 3.4: AHA/ACC guidelines for statin use
ACC/AHA guidelines for statin therapy

Class I
For patients currently on statins (e.g. due to CAD, DM or hyperlipidemia), and scheduled for noncardiac surgery, the statin should be continued in the postoperative period.

Class IIa
For patients undergoing elective vascular surgery with and without clinical risk factors, it is reasonable to start a statin therapy.

Management of Patients with CAD

1. *Patient with prior angioplasty (PTCA) without stent:* It is recommended that in patient with recent PTCA without stent, the surgery be carried out at 2-8 weeks post-PTCA. Early surgery (2-4 weeks) should be avoided to allow for endothelialization at site of angioplasty and delayed surgery (>8 weeks) increases the risk of re-stenosis and is therefore not recommended.

2. *Patients with PCI with bare metal stents:* Bare metal stent thrombosis risk is highest in the first two weeks following stent implantation and is exceedingly rare after 4 to 6 weeks and requires dual anti-platelet therapy (aspirin and thienopyridine) for at least 4 weeks. Therefore, it is reasonable to delay elective cardiac surgery for 4 to 6 weeks following implantation of a bare metal stent. Daily aspirin therapy should be continued perioperatively, if possible.

3. *Patient with drug eluting stents:* Drug eluting stents are effective in reducing the risk of re-stenosis. However, due to effects of drugs the endothelialization is delayed and in addition to risk of subacute stent thrombosis there is a small but significant risk of late (up to 1 year) and very late (>1 year) stent thrombosis. The current guidelines recommend to continue dual anti-platelet therapy with aspirin and thienopyridine for at least 12 months. Therefore any elective surgery should be delayed for at least one year. It is strongly recommended to continue with aspirin perioperatively. There is no evidence that use of heparin or anti-thrombin or intravenous anti-platelet agents or coumadin will reduce the risk of stent thrombosis after discontinuation of oral anti-platelet agents.

Table 3.5: Criteria for detecting perioperative MI

At least one of the following:

Criterion 1 Typical rise and fall of biomarkers (especially Troponin) with the peak occurring after surgery in a patient without an alternative explanation. CK-MB should be used if Troponin assay is unavailable along with one of the following:
- New Q waves or ST T wave changes of ischemia
- Symptoms compatible with ischemia
- Coronary artery intervention
- New wall motion abnormality on ECHO cardiographic imaging or new fixed defect on radionuclide imaging.

Criterion 2 New pathologic Q waves if biomarkers were not obtained or were obtained at times that an MI could be missed.

Criterion 3 Pathologic evidence of a new or healing MI.

MONITORING AND SURVEILLANCE

Detecting Perioperative MI

The diagnosis of perioperative MI is associated with 30 to 50 percent short-term mortality and reduced long-term survival. During the perioperative period, a myocardial infarction may go unrecognized. Most perioperative MIs occur during the first 72 to 96 hours after the noncardiac surgery. During this period, patients may have altered perception due to the post-surgical state, being in unfamiliar ICU settings or due to use of upload analgesics. Up to half the patients with a perioperative myocardial infarctions do not have typical symptoms. A low index of suspicion is necessary to detect the infrequent perioperative MIs. There are no criteria established yet for diagnosis of MIs following noncardiac surgery. Table 3.5 lists the criteria proposed by Devereaux et al. Routine intra- and postoperative ST-segment monitoring can be useful in patients with known CAD or those undergoing vascular surgery or patients with single or multiple risk factors for CAD. Postoperative troponin measurement is recommended in patients with ECG changes of chest pain typical of acute coronary syndrome and is not well established in clinically stable patients. In patients with high or intermediate clinical risk factors with known or suspected CAD, undergoing high or intermediate risk procedures, ECG should be done at baseline, immediately after surgery and for the first 2 days after surgery. Cardiac specific troponin should be used to supplement the diagnosis in these symptomatic patients.

Role of Echocardiography

In patients with persistent hemodynamic instability, a bedside transthoracic echocardiogram can provide useful information about LV and RV function, wall motion, valvular function and the status of the pericardium. If needed transthoracic windows are suboptimal, a trans-esophageal echocardiogram can provide the necessary information which can guide therapy. There is minimal data regarding the utility or cost effectiveness of TTE or TEE in the perioperative setting for noncardiac surgery.

Role of Pulmonary Artery Catheter

The decision to place a pulmonary artery catheter must be weighed carefully in terms of the benefit versus the potential risks, which include pulmonary embolism, infection, pneumothorax and potential for misinterpretation leading to wrong therapy. Studies have shown no role for routine use of pulmonary artery catheters for hemodynamic monitoring in noncardiac surgery.

In specific patients with unstable hemodynamics or those with systolic LV dysfunction and coexisting renal dysfunction, pulmonary artery catheters may aid management if expertise in interpreting the hemodynamic data is available at the institution.

MANAGEMENT OF SPECIFIC SITUATIONS

Hypertension

Hypertension is common in patients undergoing non-cardiac surgery. While long-term treatment of hypertension reduces morbidity and mortality, stage 1 or 2 hypertension (BP < 180/110) is not an independent predictor of perioperative cardiovascular complications. For patients on antihypertensive therapy, the medications should be continued perioperatively especially beta blockers and clonidine to avoid withdrawal hypertension. If the BP is <180/110 a delay in surgery is not recommended. However, for patients with BP >/= 180/110 consideration should be given to better blood pressure control prior to elective surgery. Beta blockers appear to be an effective drug for blood pressure management in this setting. Oral antihypertensive medications should be restarted cautiously postoperatively with care to avoid perioperative hypotension especially in patients who have decreased vascular volumes.

Valvular Heart Disease

Cardiac murmurs are commonly recognized in patients undergoing noncardiac surgery. A good history and physical examination to quantify the severity of the valvular disease and echocardiographic evaluation may be warranted for significant murmurs as per AHA/ACC guidelines.

1. *Severe aortic stenosis* increases the risk of perioperative myocardial infarction. For patients with symptomatic severe aortic stenosis, aortic valve replacement should be considered prior to elective noncardiac surgery. For patients who are not candidates for aortic valve replacement, balloon angioplasty may be considered.

2. *Mitral stenosis*: Significant mitral stenosis increases the risk of heart failure perioperatively. Mitral balloon valvuloplasty or open surgical repair should be considered in patients who would need these procedures independent of need for noncardiac surgery or in patients with severe mitral stenosis who are undergoing high risk surgery. Further, patients with mitral stenosis benefit from aggressive control of tachycardia to avoid pulmonary congestion.

3. *Aortic regurgitation*: In patients with severe aortic regurgitation, attention to after load reduction and volume control is recommended to minimize the risk for pulmonary congestion.

4. *Mitral regurgitation*: Patients with severe mitral regurgitation also benefit from after load reduction and judicious use of diuretics.

5. *Mechanical prosthetic valve*: For patients who require minimally invasive surgery (e.g. dental procedure, superficial biopsies), the recommendation is to briefly decrease the INR to low therapeutic range and resume normal dose of anticoagulation post-procedure. However, unfractionated heparin is recommended for patients with high risk of thromboembolism or those undergoing surgery with high risk of bleeding.

6. *Antibiotic prophylaxis* is no longer recommended for most procedures in patients with aortic and mitral stenosis or regurgitation unless the patient has prior history of infective endocarditis or prosthetic cardiac valve.

VENOUS THROMBOEMBOLISM PROPHYLAXIS

The risk for venous thromboembolism (VTE) is increased in patients with the following risk factors: increased age, prolonged immobility, prior VTE, malignancy, major surgery especially procedures on abdomen, pelvis or lower extremity, obesity, heart failure, myocardial infarction, fractures and hypercoaguable state. The choice of prophylactic therapy—graded compression stockings, low dose subcutaneous heparin, low molecular weight heparin or intermittent

Table 3.6: Levels of thromboembolism risk in surgical patients and management

Level of risk	Calf DVT %	Proximal DVT%	Clinical PE %	Prophylaxis
Low				
Minor surgery in <40-year-old	2	0.4	0.2	Early mobilization
Moderate	10-20	2-4	1-2	LDUH (every 12 hours), LMWH (<3400 units daily), GCS or IPC
Minor surgery with risk factors				
Surgery in 40-60-year-old with no risk factors				
High	20-40	4-8	0.4-1	LDUH (every 8 hours), LMWH (>3400 units daily) or IPC
Surgery in >60-year-old or 40-60-year-old with additional risk factors				
Highest	40-80	10-20	0.2-0.5	LMWH (>3400 units daily), fondaparinux, oral vitamin K antagonist or IPC/GCS plus LMWH/LUDH
Surgery in patients with multiple risk factors				
Hip or knee arthroplasty				
Major trauma or spinal cord injury				

Additional risk factors: Prior venous thromboembolism (VTE), cancer, hypercoaguability. GCS: graduated compression stockings; IPC: intermittent pneumatic compression; LDUH: low dose unfractionated heparin; LMWH: low molecular weight heparin

pneumatic compression should be considered depending on the risk of thromboembolism and type of surgery (Table 3.6).

MANAGEMENT OF ANTICOAGULATION

Many patients are on long-term anticoagulation. The common reasons for long-term oral anticoagulation with vitamin K antagonists (warfarin and its derivatives) include prosthetic heart valves, atrial fibrillation, pulmonary embolism and recurrent DVT.

Management of the anticoagulation regimen is important not only for reducing the risk of bleeding perioperatively but also to minimize the risk of thromboembolism peri-operatively. There are limited data available regarding specific management strategies. Most of the data is derived from retrospective examination of patients who are on anticoagulation and underwent noncardiac procedures. The detailed recommendations derived from a consensus of expert opinion and the limited data available have been published. Specifically, the risk of thrombosis on holding anticoagulation for 7 to 10 days has been extrapolated from randomized

controlled trials of anticoagulation for atrial fibrillation, pulmonary embolism and DVT. This has been balanced against the risk of bleeding during surgical procedures.

The specific recommendations include:

1. Indication for anticoagulation for each patient and their risk for thromboembolism should be carefully reviewed and therapy tailored to particular patient.
2. The oral anticoagulant (warfarin and its derivatives) should be withheld for a period of at least 3 to 5 days prior to the surgical procedure.
3. An INR should be measured day 3 to day 5. If the INR < 2.0, then the surgical procedure can be performed safely.
4. In patients who are at the highest risk of thrombo-embolic events; such as those with prosthetic mechanical valves, prior stroke or homozygous for genetic predisposition to thrombosis; oral anticoagulation should be substituted with either unfractionated heparin intravenously or low molecular weight heparin subcutaneously, especially once their warfarin has been held and their INR is sub-therapeutic.

5. If unfractionated heparin is used, appropriate dosing guidelines should be followed with adjustment as per PTT values measured at 6 hour intervals. The intravenous unfractionated heparin should be discontinued 4 to 6 hours prior to the surgical procedure.

6. If low molecular weight heparin (LMWH) is used, appropriate weight based dosing regimen should be used and corrected for estimated GFR (eGFR) values to minimize bleeding risk. The last dose of LMWH should be given 12 hours before the procedure. The last dose should be half the usual dose for the patient.

7. High-risk patients, who are candidates for preoperative bridging with either unfractionated intravenous heparin or subcutaneous LMWH, are also likely to be appropriate candidates for postoperative bridging.

8. In the western world, the costs of hospitalization far outweigh the costs of subcutaneous low molecular weight heparin, either self-administered or administered by a visiting nurse specialist. In the majority of cases in the developing world, postoperatively most patients remain in the hospital until both the physician and patient feel reassured of the safety of being discharged home. In these circumstances, often patients stay long enough in the hospital such that a therapeutic level of anticoagulation can be achieved with oral vitamin K antagonists. Bridging can be achieved with intravenous unfractionated heparin using a weight-based regimen in most patients. The intravenous heparin should be commenced 12 to 24 hours after adequate hemostasis has been achieved. A loading dose is not recommended. Further adjustment of doses should be made using frequently monitored PTT levels.

Subcutaneously administered LMWH heparin offers some advantages over continuous intravenous unfractionated heparin. It is easy for nurses to administer. It does not require frequent PTT monitoring and so avoids the discomfort of frequent blood draws. Many hospitals may not be able to obtain PTT levels every 6 hours. If started in the hospital and if the patient is sub-therapeutic at the time of discharge, the patient is likely to find it easier to accept the need for subcutaneous twice daily injections and therefore continue it at home until therapeutic INR is achieved.

ARRHYTHMIAS

Patients undergoing surgical procedures not infrequently have arrhythmias. Both atrial and ventricular arrhythmias can occur.

Acute supraventricular or atrial tachyarrhythmia that are hemodynamically unstable need to be immediately treated with electrical or pharmacological cardioversion. A consultation with a cardiologist may be needed for further arrhythmia specific management.

Premature atrial complexes (PACs), atrial bigeminy or short runs of atrial tachycardia respond favorably to beta blockers.

Patients with hemodynamically stable atrial flutter or atrial fibrillation need to have adequate control of the ventricular rate, usually achieved by beta blockers. Other agents include calcium channel blockers and digitalis. Beta blockers are the most effective, especially given at every 2 to 4 hours intervals. If beta blockers are unable to control the ventricular rates, cardiology consultation is needed to evaluate patient for antiarrhythmic agents such as short-term amiodarone infusions.

Reentrant supraventricular tachyarrhythmia (SVT) can be treated either pharmacologically or with ablative therapy. The timing of therapy for the SVT should be based on the patient's symptoms and the reasons for the elective surgery. SVTs can be safely dealt with either before or after the elective surgical procedure.

Ventricular ectopics, bigeminy, complex ventricular ectopy and runs of nonsustained ventricular tachycardia, especially if asymptomatic usually do not need additional therapy unless they are occurring in the setting of an underlying MI or decompensation of heart failure. Treatment directed to the underlying cause is usually all that is needed.

However, sustained VT warrants consultation with a cardiologist and urgent electrical cardioversion is needed for hemodynamically unstable rhythms. The cause for sustained or symptomatic ventricular tachycardia must be searched for prior to the elective surgical procedure. These patients may need amiodarone in the perioperative period. Other useful agents for this include lidocaine or procainamide.

Bradyarrhythmias in the preoperative period may contraindicate or limit the dose of beta blockers that can be used in the perioperative setting. Asymptomatic sinus bradycardia, 1st degree AV block, right bundle branch block, bi-fascicular block and left bundle branch block usually do not need any specific therapy in an asymptomatic patient.

In a patient with more advanced conduction system disease such as second degree or third degree heart block or in patients with syncope, the bradycardia would need to be addressed prior to the elective procedure. Patients may need a temporary pacemaker to help them get through the surgery. Rarely do patients need a permanent pacemaker prior to their elective procedure. Once again the timing is dependent upon the patient's symptoms and the reason for the surgical procedure.

PACEMAKERS AND DEFIBRILLATORS

Perioperative Management of Implantable Cardiac Devices

More patients are undergoing device implantation - pacemakers for symptomatic bradyarrhythmias, ICDs for primary or secondary prevention of sudden cardiac death and biventricular devices for heart failure. These same patients have significant co-morbidities putting them at risk for a variety of illnesses, some of which need noncardiac surgery (Table 3.7).

Intraoperatively, the main issue confronting the surgeon is the potential interaction between diathermy and the device. Electromagnetic interference (EMI) of cardiac devices is an uncommon but well-described phenomenon. Any external source capable of producing strong electromagnetic fields can potentially interfere with the implanted cardiac device. The interaction is unpredictable. It can alter device programming temporarily or permanently. The result may be an inhibition of device output or a triggering of the device output. Sometimes it can result in overdrive pacing or even trigger the delivery of a shock.

For these reasons, the following recommendations have been made:

1. The output of the diathermy must be kept to the lowest effective. Diathermy should be used in short, intermittent bursts. These techniques minimize the amount of far-field signals generated, lessening the likelihood of EMI.
2. The grounding patch of the diathermy device is usually placed far from the device. In abdominal surgeries, it is usually placed on the thigh. For head and neck surgeries, placing the patch on the scapular region opposite the side of the cardiac device directs the current vector away from the cardiac device. If that cannot be done, the grounding patch should be placed at a distance of at

least 10 cm or greater from the cardiac device. The strength of the electromagnetic field varies inversely with the square of the distance from the site of flow of current. At distances > 10 cm and with the usual power settings of the diathermy device, the amount of EMI generated is likely to be small.

3. A magnet can be used to temporarily alter device programming. Placing a magnet over the device activates a reed switch that changes the pacing mode to asynchronous ventricular pacing in single chamber devices or asynchronous dual chamber pacing in dual chamber devices. Asynchronous pacing refers to the device pacing the cardiac chambers ignoring the underlying intrinsic rhythm. In the case of pacemakers, the effect of placing a magnet over the device during surgery may be all that is needed, but however the effects of an external magnet on pacemakers vary from manufacturer and even between models from the same manufacturer. It is best to contact the particular manufacturer to obtain accurate information.

With regard to ICDs, almost all ICDs are reprogrammed to a monitor only mode when an external magnet is placed. Thus, the device would not shock or pace the patient even in the case of a true clinically significant VT or VF. The surgeon and anesthesiologist should be aware of this. These patients should be connected to an external defibrillator so that emergent defibrillation can be rapidly accomplished should the need arise.

In biventricular devices, placing a magnet causes the device to pace asynchronously. If the device has defibrillation capacity as well, the magnet converts the device to a monitor mode only and these patients would need to be connected to an external defibrillator as well.

4. In addition, in some instances reprogramming of the device should be considered prior to the surgery, especially if the anesthetist or surgeon is unfamiliar with perioperative device management.

One important thing to recognize is that many monitoring devices count a pacer spike in calculating the heart rate. In this situation, if a patient is asystolic, the monitor will not detect asystole as it counts the pacing spikes as intrinsic cardiac electrical activity.

HEART FAILURE

Heart failure is increasing in prevalence throughout the developing and developed world. This is related to several

Table 3.7: Surgical checklist for implantable cardiac devices		
Is patient pacemaker dependent	Yes	No
Has patient experienced shock for VT/VF	Yes	No
Has the device been evaluated in last 6 months	Yes	No
Any interval change in cardiac status since last interrogation	Yes	No

factors—an aging population, increasing prevalence of diabetes and hypertension in most parts of the developed and developing countries. Several studies have shown that these same patients are at the highest risk for perioperative complications during noncardiac surgery. Lee Goldman in his study in 1977 of factors that influence perioperative mortality assigned the highest score to the physical finding of S3 on auscultation which is a marker for decompensated heart failure. In the Revised Cardiac Index, a history of heart failure is a risk factor. The ACC guidelines consistently have suggested deferring elective noncardiac surgery in the presence of decompensated heart failure.

Recently retrospective analysis of a large Medicare database showed that patients who had a diagnosis of heart failure had a greater risk of complications in the perioperative period following noncardiac surgery including mortality and readmission for heart failure. The magnitude of risk was higher than the magnitude of risk associated with known CAD in that same cohort. This fact that even with current pharmacologic therapies, heart failure continues to be a significant risk factor is sobering. Unfortunately there are no studies attempting to identify specific therapies or treatment strategies to manage heart failure in the perioperative setting.

In general, these patients should be actively managed by a cardiologist with experience in the management of heart failure (Table 3.8). Fluid management with and without diuretics, doses of after load reducing agents, dose adjustments for any change in renal function as well as the hypotensive effects of narcotic agents are all challenges that require experience as well as a great deal of anticipation.

Generally, perioperatively it is better to cut down on the dose of diuretics and allow the patient to be mildly hypervolemic prior to the surgery in anticipation of fluid loss and shifts. The dose of ACEI may have to be cut in half on the night prior to the surgery and may have to be held on the morning of the surgery to minimize accentuation of the hypotensive response to anesthetic agents. Postoperatively, if patients are not able to take oral medications,

then Intravenous enalapril every 6 to 8 hours can be used based on the BP response. These patients benefit by continuation of beta blockers. It may be prudent to hold spironolactone to minimize hyperkalemia which is frequently seen in this perioperative setting due to tissue injury. Discontinuing digoxin until the patient is able to take medications orally later on is prudent and unlikely to cause any deterioration in the patient's cardiac condition.

A pulmonary artery catheter may be useful in managing patients with severely compromised systolic function who are likely to experience significant fluid shifts. The risks and benefits have to be individualized for each patient. Even more useful is accurate record of daily weight changes and frequent input/output monitoring. In general trends in these changes are likely to give a clue to the shift in the patient's overall condition than any one time value.

As soon as the patients are capable of taking medications orally, their preoperative regimen should be reinstated. Usually the doses of the medications are likely to be different from their immediate perioperative doses but that is usually titrated over a period of weeks on an outpatient basis.

An important issue is the use of blood products in these patients. There is debate regarding the threshold for transfusion of blood products. There is no absolute number of hemoglobin for which transfusion is mandatory. Usually many physicians will transfuse for a hemoglobin < 8.0 g/dl, especially if the change is rapid or if the patient has symptoms that are likely to be ameliorated with transfusion. Small randomized trials of transfusion in the perioperative setting have shown that patients who are transfused for symptoms are more likely to benefit compared to automatic transfusions triggered by a specific hemoglobin value.

Patients who have a history of heart failure with preserved systolic function are physiologically different from those with depressed systolic function. In these patients, the key to management is the adequate control of hypertension, heart rate and appropriate fluid balance. Patients who have advanced pericardial disease or infiltrative diseases need active involvement of a cardiologist in the

Table 3.8: Surgical checklist for heart failure		
1. Any change in symptoms in recent 2 weeks?	Yes	No
2. Any weight gain of > 3 lbs over baseline in last week?	Yes	No
3. Any change in medications in last 2 weeks?	Yes	No
4. SBP < 90/55 mm Hg	Yes	No
5. BP > 130/90 mm Hg	Yes	No
6. Rales > ¼ of both lung bases	Yes	No

If the answer to any of these is yes, a consultation with a cardiologist should be obtained for managing any potential acute decompensation.

perioperative management for non-cardiac surgery. These patients need adequate preload and hence diuretics have to be used very cautiously.

SYSTEMS ISSUES

Perioperative risk assessment should be addressed both at the systems level, team level and the patient level by the entire medical team.

1. All patients scheduled for elective procedures should have had a preoperative assessment of cardiac, pulmonary and renal risk.
2. The patient's data should be appropriately color coded so that providers are immediately alerted when certain high-risk features are present. If electronic charts are used, appropriate alerts should be triggered.
3. Specific alerts should trigger an automatic referral to a physician with experience in perioperative cardiac management.
4. This risk assessment should be communicated during handoffs at every stage of care transition, i.e. from the clinic to the OR, OR to the ICU and to the step-down units. In some institutions, standardized sign out sheets have been used to reduce the risk of omission of data.
5. Internists or cardiologists should be involved early on in the postoperative period in the care of patients undergoing high-risk surgery or those with complex cardiovascular conditions.
6. Chain of Responsibility for care should be clearly established for the perioperative period.
7. Protocols for drug concentrations and dosages should be standardized for the hospital and should ideally be identical between the OR, ICU and step down areas to minimize drug administration errors.
8. Protocols for use of perioperative medications such as beta blockade, heparin and analgesia should be established for nursing including cutoffs and indications for escalating therapy or alerting other team members.
9. Protocols for measuring biomarkers and performing ECGs should be well established.
10. Nonphysician members should be allowed to escalate care if physicians are immediately unavailable.
11. Hospitals need to track the outcomes of surgery to detect patterns of care that may be improved through systems design.
12. Protocols for perioperative anticoagulation including indications for bridging and postoperative resumption for anticoagulation should be established. The importance of following instructions regarding anticoagulants preoperatively as well as postoperatively should be emphasized to the patient as well as their immediate family involved in the care of the patient. It is important to discuss the risks and benefits related to bleeding and anticoagulation. The need for any blood products should be discussed as well so that the patient and their family can make necessary arrangements for blood products.

At the team level the greatest emphasis should be on complete communication during handoffs between providers and between stages of care.

Nurses and junior physicians should be familiar with the protocols at the institution so as to be able to give appropriate orders for timely provision of care.

BIBLIOGRAPHY

1. ACC/AHA Guideline.
2. Bonow. Braunwald's heart disease—a textbook of cardiovascular medicine, 9th edn. Saunders, An Imprint of Elsevier, 2011.
3. Goldberger. Clinical electrocardiography: a simplified Approach, 7th edn. Mosby, An Imprint of Elsevier, 2006.

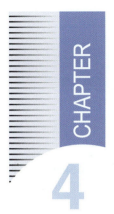

Surgical Critical Care

Sanjeev V Changgani

INTRODUCTION

Critical care medicine or Intensive care medicine is a discipline of medicine concerned with provision of specialized care to the critically ill patients. The origin of critical care began with close monitoring of the wounded soldiers in the Crimean war by Florence Nightingale and evolved through polio epidemic in 1952 into its current multidisciplinary and multiprofessional model. Current multiprofessional model of critical care utilizes team approach (intensivist, nurse, respiratory therapy, pharmacy, physical therapy, nutrition, etc.) to deliver timely, safe, and efficient patient-centered care.

Critical care involves immediate stabilization of abnormal physiology and organ support, followed by definitive therapy and continued care. End-of-life care is part of critical care. Critical illness or injury acutely impairs one or more vital organ systems such that there is a high probability of imminent or life-threatening deterioration in the patient's condition. Although critically ill is typically cared for in an intensive care unit (ICU) where high degree of monitoring, attention and therapy is provided, critical care can be initiated at any place where the patient is determined to be critically ill. Some of the common conditions and concepts in the surgical critical care are presented in this chapter. The reader is referred to many treatises in this area for an extensive review.

ACUTE RESPIRATORY FAILURE AND MECHANICAL VENTILATION

Acute respiratory failure is one of the common reasons for admission to ICU and is associated with increased postoperative mortality. Acute respiratory failure, defined as inability of the lungs to oxygenate the blood and/or

eliminate carbon dioxide (CO_2) due to inefficiency of oxygenation and imbalance of respiratory load and capacity, is a nonspecific condition and often associated with an underlying process (local: injury/trauma, pneumonia, worsening chronic lung disease; systemic: inflammation, injury/trauma, sepsis). The nature of the underlying process often determines prognosis.[1,2] Two common types of acute respiratory failure and their common causes are shown in Figure 4.1.

Clinical Signs and Symptoms

Tachypnea is an important sign of critical illness and should not be ignored. Dyspnea as a result of compensatory increased work of breathing and cyanosis are commonly present. Crackles and other adventitious breath sounds may be heard on auscultation of the chest. These signs and symptoms are a result of decrease in functional residual capacity (FRC) and lung compliance and increase in intrapulmonary shunting due to interstitial and alveolar edema and gravity and weight-based dependent atelectasis. Other signs and symptoms of associated systemic disease may be present. Risk factors for postoperative respiratory failure are listed in Table 4.1. Phosphorus level should be evaluated as hypophosphatemia can play a significant role in postoperative respiratory failure in a patient with poor respiratory reserve.

Diagnosis

Initial diagnosis is made clinically, based on good history and physical examination. This is complemented by laboratory and radiological testing. An important goal in diagnosis of acute respiratory failure is to determine degree of its severity and compensation. Pulse oximeter is a useful

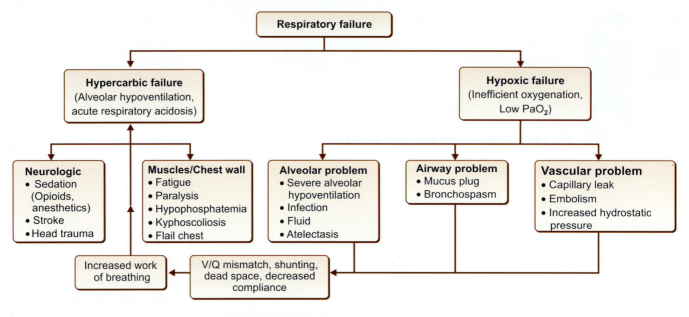

FIGURE 4.1: Common types of respiratory failure

Table 4.1: Risk factors for postoperative respiratory failure
• Advanced age
• High BMI
• Smoking history
• Pre-existing lung disease
• Poor functional status
• Malnutrition
• History of cancer and/or chemo-radiation
• Obstructive sleep apnea
• Transfusion
• Neurologic disease
• Alcohol abuse
• Hypophosphatemia

BMI= Body mass index (kg/m^2)

Table 4.2: Acute lung injury/acute respiratory distress syndrome	
ALI	Acute onset of respiratory failure New onset bilateral infiltrates on CXR or CT scan Noncardiogenic (absence of left ventricular failure; clinical, echocardiographic, or PAOP < 18 mm Hg) PaO_2/FiO_2 < 300 mm Hg independent of PEEP
ARDS	All of the above, except PaO_2/FiO_2 < 200 mm Hg

CXR: chest radiograph; CT: computed tomography; PAOP: pulmonary artery occlusion pressure; PEEP: positive end expiratory pressure

monitor to assess adequacy of peripheral arterial hemoglobin saturation. Pulse oximetry however does not assess adequacy of ventilation. An arterial blood gas (ABG) is useful in this regard.

Alveolar-arterial (A-a) oxygen gradient can be calculated using the equation:

$$\text{(A-a) oxygen gradient} = FiO_2 (P_B - PH_2O) - \frac{PaCO_2}{R} - PaO_2$$

FiO_2 = fraction of inspired oxygen; P_B = barometric pressure; PH_2O = partial pressure of water; R= respiratory quotient; $PaCO_2$= partial pressure of carbon dioxide in arterial blood; PaO_2 = partial pressure of oxygen in arterial blood.

A normal alveolar-arterial (A-a) oxygen gradient (less than 10 mm Hg on room air) supports pure hypercapnic respiratory failure due to hypoventilation. An increased (A-a) oxygen gradient is present in presence of hypoxemia due to ventilation/perfusion (V/Q) mismatch, diffusion defect or intrapulmonary shunt. Criteria for diagnosis of acute lung injury (ALI) and acute respiratory distress syndrome (ARDS) are summarized in Table 4.2. ALI/ARDS is acute inflammatory condition of the lungs caused by direct (pneumonia, aspiration, contusion, inhalation of toxic gases, drowning) or indirect (sepsis, massive trauma, ischemia, cardiopulmonary bypass, systemic inflammation due to major surgery) injury. The ABG in ALI/ARDS will typically show hypoxemia with acute respiratory alkalosis (low $PaCO_2$) due to hyperventilation. The presence of acute respiratory acidosis in ALI/ARDS is a late sign and indicates respiratory decompensation and impending respiratory arrest. In contrast, respiratory acidosis is common in acute-on-chronic respiratory failure and hypoxemia is a late sign.

Chest radiograph and computed tomography (CT) are commonly performed in the diagnosis of acute respiratory failure. Chest radiograph, in ALI/ARDS, commonly shows bilateral interstitial infiltrates, often diffuse and fluffy and basal atelectasis. CT scan can accurately define lung pathology (distribution of infiltrates, consolidation, effusions, atelectasis, and pneumothorax).[3] The radiological findings are subject to change due to evolving nature of the disease process and effects of PEEP and lung recruitment.

Management

The primary goal in the management of acute respiratory failure is to restore adequate oxygenation and ventilation. Supplemental oxygen should be immediately provided to improve oxygenation. Treatment of underlying cause of respiratory failure is initiated simultaneously. The need for low-flow/low FiO_2 (nasal cannula or face mask) Vs high-flow/high FiO_2 (nonrebreathing mask with reservoir) delivery system is dependent on the degree of hypoxemia and the patient's flow demand. A patient with severe hypoxemia and high minute ventilation, for example, should receive high-flow/high FiO_2 nonrebreathing mask with reservoir. Ventilatory assistance in acute respiratory failure can be provided noninvasively (noninvasive positive pressure ventilation, NIPPV) or invasively (mechanical ventilation).

Noninvasive Positive Pressure Ventilation (NIPPV)

NIPPV is administered using an interface to the upper airway and does not require endotracheal intubation. NIPPV has a significant role in the management of acute respiratory failure, especially in certain settings. There is strong evidence to support use of NIPPV in acute respiratory failure due to COPD exacerbation,[4-6] acute cardiogenic respiratory failure,[7-9] in immunocompromised patients, and to facilitate ventilator weaning in intubated COPD patients. Several studies and meta-analyses have shown significant reductions in intubation and mortality rates and reduced hospital length of stay in patients treated with NIPPV through respiratory muscle unloading and improvement in gas exchange.[5,6] NIPPV may be considered in postoperative respiratory failure, patients with do-not-intubate (DNI) status, and as a bridge to extubation and prevent extubation failure.[10,11] Although NIPPV has been shown to be effective in the above settings, its use in acute hypoxic respiratory failure remains controversial.[12,13] Contraindications to NIPPV are

Table 4.3: Contraindications to NIPPV

- Uncooperative/Agitated patient
- Apnea
- Hemodynamic instability
- Obtundation
- Copious secretions
- Postsurgical, e.g. esophagectomy, spit fistula, facial surgery/trauma
- Undrained pneumothorax

listed in Table 4.3. The patient on NIPPV should be monitored for improvement or deterioration in respiratory status based on close clinical examination and blood gases.

Interface and Settings

Success of NIPPV depends on a multitude of factors; interface (or mask), ventilator setting, and skills of providers (physician, nursing, respiratory therapy). Nasal and full face (oronasal) masks are commercially available. Both masks perform equally well, although nasal mask may be associated with excessive leak from the mouth. When using these interfaces, the bony facial prominences and ear cartilage should be well padded and closely monitored for erythema and pressure necrosis. Most critical care ventilators are designed to deliver invasive or noninvasive ventilation. Pressure-limited (pressure support) mode is most commonly used and is well accepted by patients. This can be delivered in a continuous (continuous positive airway pressure, CPAP) or bi-level (Bi-level positive airway pressure, BiPAP) mode. Whatever the chosen mode, initial settings should be low (8-10 cm H_2O) for better patient tolerance and can be titrated in 2 cm H_2O increments. Typical starting BiPAP setting consists of inspiratory pressure (inspiratory positive airway pressure, IPAP) of 8-10 cm H_2O and EPAP (expiratory positive airway pressure, EPAP) of 4-5 cm H_2O. IPAP may be increased to improve ventilation and EPAP may be increased to improve oxygenation or prevent upper airway collapse or apnea. Other advanced modes such as mandatory backup minute ventilation (set tidal volume and rate) and proportional assist ventilation (PAV) are available on some critical care ventilators. Although gastric decompression using a nasogastric tube is not routinely advised in a patient receiving NIPPV, it should be strongly considered to prevent possibility of abdominal compartment syndrome when high settings (e.g. $\geq$ 20 cm H_2O) are used during NIPPV.[14]

Mechanical Ventilation

The goals of mechanical ventilation include provision of adequate gas exchange (arterial oxygenation and carbon

Table 4.4: Indications for intubation and mechanical ventilation

- Cardiorespiratory arrest
- Impending respiratory arrest, e.g. progressive respiratory acidosis, fatigue, or decline in mentation
- Airway protection, e.g. impaired or loss of consciousness
- Refractory hypoxemia
- Failure of conservative or noninvasive support, e.g. supplemental oxygen, adjuvant therapy or NIPPV
- Intracranial hypertension, e.g. hyperventilation

dioxide clearance), reduce work of breathing, and prevent iatrogenic harm to the patient. Often, the goals are conflicting and depend upon the clinical setting. Specific therapy for the underlying cause of respiratory failure is instituted simultaneously. The decision to intubate and institute mechanical ventilation is most often clinically based. Indications for mechanical ventilation are listed in Table 4.4.

Ventilation Strategy Vs Modes

It is important to consider that mechanical ventilation strategy, and not the mode(s), determines the outcome in a mechanically ventilated patient. Protective mechanical ventilation strategy should include considerations for the following:

Tidal volume: Tidal volume (V_T) used in mechanical ventilation is based on predicted body weight (PBW), and not actual body weight, especially in the obese patient. In patients with ALI/ARDS, V_T of 6 ml/kg PBW when compared with V_T of 12 ml/kg PBW has been shown to reduce mortality, release of inflammatory makers, and dependence on mechanical ventilator.[15-17] In at risk patients, one should not, however, wait for ALI/ARDS to occur before considering low V_T strategy. In most circumstances low V_T allows to keep plateau pressure (P_{plat}) lower than 30 cm H_2O. Application of high V_T and P_{plat} has been associated with high mortality in critically ill patients requiring mechanical ventilation in a variety of non-ALI/ARDS setting, e.g. pulmonary edema, COPD, CHF, trauma, aspiration, and following surgery. Low V_T strategy may also result in many positive circulatory effects (improved venous return and cardiac output) by reducing intrathoracic pressure and right ventricular afterload, and resultant hypercapnia. Consequences of low V_T and P_{plat} include hypercapnia, atelectasis, and hypoxia if respiratory rate and PEEP are not sufficiently increased.

Positive end expiratory pressure (PEEP): PEEP, when applied appropriately, should prevent atelectasis and improve oxygenation in a mechanically ventilated patient. Therefore, PEEP may have protective effect by preventing lung derecruitment and promoting alveolar recruitment. Unfortunately, the effects of PEEP on arterial oxygenation and pulmonary mechanics are not as simple as it may seem. High PEEP/low FiO_2 compared with low PEEP/high FiO_2 in ARDS net trial failed to improve mortality in patients with ALI/ARDS.[18] Alternatively, in ALI/ARDS PEEP may be titrated using static pressure-volume (P-V) compliance curve or by measuring lung compliance (or elastance). It is difficult to identify lower inflection point on P-V compliance curve in every patient with ALI/ARDS. Similarly, effect of PEEP on lung compliance (or elastance) depends upon the underlying etiology of ALI/ARDS (pulmonary or extra-pulmonary). Therefore, strategy to select adequate level of PEEP is quite complex in an individual patient.

Patient-ventilator synchrony: Ideally, patient's inspiratory time (neural input) and ventilator inspiratory time should be matched to establish patient-ventilator synchrony. During spontaneous ventilation patient-ventilator interaction is complex and dependent upon respiratory drive, muscle strength, timing, and respiratory mechanics. In order to optimally reduce work of breathing and provide sufficient alveolar ventilation, mechanical breaths must proportionally support patient's spontaneous inspiratory effort and respiratory rate/minute ventilation. These features are available as assist-controlled ventilation (ACV), automatic tube compensation (ATC), pressure support ventilation (PSV), and proportional assist ventilation (PAV) in most contemporary mechanical ventilators. Providing optimal sedation, sleep, and anxiolysis are also important in ensuring patient-ventilator synchrony.

Spontaneous breathing and weaning: Using partial support and less sedation encourages spontaneous breathing in a patient on mechanical ventilator. Spontaneous ventilation improves V/Q matching, reduces atelectasis and results in better gas exchange and oxygenation. Cardiovascular effects of spontaneous ventilation include better venous return, cardiac output and oxygen delivery. Therefore, encouraging spontaneous breathing during mechanical ventilation is associated with better perfusion and organ function, less need for sedation and quicker weaning and discontinuation from mechanical ventilator support. Patients with left ventricular dysfunction should be watched closely during spontaneous breathing trial as depressed left ventricle may not tolerate increase in ventricular filling and afterload associated with spontaneous breathing.

Modes: Positive-pressure mechanical ventilatory support, partial or total, provides pressure and flow to the airway. The basic ventilator modes are classified based on three features of a mechanical breath: *trigger* (ventilator or patient), *target* (volume or pressure), and *cycle* (transition from inspiration to exhalation). Commonly utilized modes of mechanical ventilation in clinical practice are listed in Table 4.5. Commercially available ventilators offer combination of these modes. Desired goals and mechanical ventilator settings in common clinical conditions are summarized in Table 4.6.

Table 4.5: Common modes of mechanical ventilation				
Mode	*Trigger*	*Target*	*Cycle*	*Parameters set*
Volume-control Assist-control	Ventilator Ventilator	V_T	Time and V_T	RR, V_T, I:E, Flow rate, FiO_2, PEEP
	Patient	V_T	Time and V_T	RR, V_T, I:E, Flow rate, FiO_2, PEEP
SIMV	Ventilator Patient	V_T	Time and V_T	RR, V_T, I:E, Flow rate, FiO_2, PEEP
Pressure-control	Ventilator Patient	Inspiratory pressure	Time	RR, IP, I:E, FiO_2, PEEP
Pressure-support	Patient	Inspiratory pressure	Flow	RR, IP, FiO_2, PEEP

V_T: tidal volume; SIMV: synchronized intermittent mandatory ventilation; PEEP: Positive end expiratory pressure; I:E: inspiratory expiratory ratio; IP: inspiratory pressure

Table 4.6: Mechanical ventilation: Clinical conditions	
Clinical condition	*Goals and settings*
ALI/ARDS	Protect healthy portions of lungs Mode: PC or VC V_T: 6 ml/kg (PBW), RR: to maintain pH >7.25 (permissive hypercapnia) PEEP: to keep FiO_2 <0.6, I:E 1:2 or 2:1 P_{Plat} <30 cm H_2O
Chronic obstructive pulmonary disease (asthma)	Prevent auto-PEEP and barotrauma Mode: Assist-control I:E 1:3- 1:4 (low RR and inspiratory time, high inspiratory flow rate, low V_T) P_{Plat} <35 cm H_2O, Low PEEP
Neuromuscular disease (stroke, cervical spine injury, myasthenia gravis)	Mode: VC or PS or PC V_T 8-10 ml/kg, RR: to maintain pH >7.30, I:E 1:2 PEEP: to keep FiO_2 <0.6
Restrictive lung disease (pulmonary fibrosis, kyphoscoliosis)	Prevent barotraumas Mode: VC or PC Low V_T (5-8 ml/kg PBW), I:E 1:2, low PEEP
Unilateral pulmonary disease (lobar pneumonia, aspiration, bronchopleural fistula)	Protect healthy lung, permissive hypercapnia, and prevent hyperinflation Mode: VC or PC Low V_T and PEEP High RR and inspiratory flow rates
Intracranial hypertension	Prevent hypercapnia, hypoxia Mode: VC or PC V_T: 5-8 ml/kg, RR: to keep $PaCO_2$ 35-40 mm Hg PEEP <10 cm H_2O

Weaning and extubation: All patients supported on mechanical ventilator should be evaluated on a daily basis for ability to breathe spontaneously, weaning, and eventually for extubation. Weaning process involves decreasing support from ventilator and allowing the patient to increase work of breathing. Common criteria for weaning include reversal or resolution of acute respiratory failure, ability to make inspiratory effort, cardiovascular stability, and adequate gas exchange indicated by pH (>7.25), PaO_2 (> 60 mm Hg, FiO_2 < 0.6), PEEP < 10 cm H_2O.[19] Patients considered weanable should undergo a short period (30-120 minutes) of spontaneous breathing trial (SBT). SBT may include breathing with a T-tube, CPAP, or PS. Close clinical observation is important during SBT. Rapid shallow breathing index [RR ÷ V_T (L)] between 60 and 105 has been shown to be highly predictive of weaning success. Weaning does not necessarily mean that the patient can be extubated. Adequate mental state and amount of secretions should be evaluated before extubation. Tight fluid balance or forced diuresis, bronchodilators and physiotherapy may improve weaning success during SBT.

HEMODYNAMIC SUPPORT AND RESUSCITATION

Shock is a state of inadequate supply or inappropriate utilization of oxygen and nutrients by the cells. Unless reversed by resuscitation, this can lead to multiple organ failure, irreversible tissue damage and death. The goal of hemodynamic support and resuscitation is to restore the balance between oxygen supply and utilization and prevent tissue death. Multiple studies have shown that perioperative hemodynamic optimization and early goal-directed resuscitation improves outcome in high-risk surgery patients.

Clinical Presentation and Characterization

The classical clinical picture of shock such as hypotension and altered tissue perfusion (oliguria, altered mental state, decreased skin perfusion) may not be present in all patients, especially the young and during compensatory phase. "Cryptic shock" is present with normotension despite decreased tissue perfusion. Elevated blood lactate level is one of the important biochemical markers of shock. Weil and Shubin classification of shock is based on underlying pathophysiological mechanism. *Hypovolemic shock* is the most common form of shock seen in surgical and trauma patients. Common causes of hypovolemic shock include hemorrhage and dehydration. Capillary leak with loss of intravascular volume can result in hypovolemic shock in the early postoperative period. *Cardiogenic shock* is the result of cardiac pump failure. This may be due to postoperative myocardial infarction, cardiomyopathy, cardiac valvular disease, or arrhythmia. *Obstructive shock* is the result of obstruction to the flow of blood into or out of the heart. The common causes include massive pulmonary embolism and cardiac tamponade. *Distributive shock* may be due to capillary leak due to mediator-induced systemic inflammation, vasodilation and loss of sympathetic tone. Sepsis, anaphylaxis, neurogenic, and acute adrenal insufficiency are causes of distributive shock. Shock due to sepsis is complex in nature and includes features of all four types of shock.

Management

Management of shock includes treatment of the underlying cause, resuscitation and hemodynamic monitoring to evaluate guide and response to therapy. Supplemental oxygen should be provided to treat hypoxemia. Intubation and mechanical ventilation when considered should be performed early. Importance of initial fluid loading is common to all types of shock irrespective of its underlying cause. In patients with hemorrhagic shock, bleeding must be stopped. Often the source of bleeding is obvious from drains in the postoperative period. Correction of coagulopathy and hypothermia must be actively pursued in a patient with postoperative bleeding. In patients with postoperative myocardial infarction, anticoagulation and thrombolytic therapy must weigh the risk of bleeding. Percutaneous coronary intervention and intraaortic balloon counterpulsation may be used as appropriate. In patients with obstructive shock, percutaneous pericardiocentesis for cardiac tamponade may be performed at beside under echocardiography, and thrombolytic therapy or surgical thromboendarterectomy may be considered for massive pulmonary embolism. In patients with septic shock, timely administration of antibiotics and removal of source are crucial.

Hemodynamic Monitoring and Resuscitation

Basic noninvasive monitoring with electrocardiogram (ECG), arterial blood pressure (BP), and pulse oximetry (SpO_2) is initiated in all patients with shock. Invasive hemodynamic monitoring, in addition to repeated clinical assessment, may be required for assessment of global and regional tissue perfusion. Early goal-directed therapy using hemodynamic monitoring has been shown to improve outcome in septic shock.[20] Direct beat-to-beat BP monitoring using an intrarterial catheter is indicated in presence of persistent severe hypotension despite fluid loading and when frequent sampling of arterial blood gases and titration of vasoactive drugs is required. Exact target value for arterial pressure (systolic or mean arterial pressure) is not known and should be determined for an individual patient based on age, comorbidites, and adequacy of global oxygen delivery. Measurement of oxygen delivery and consumption, cardiac output (flow) or their surrogate or determinants may be considered in a patient with persistent signs of organ hypoperfusion with or without hypotension. Key determinants of oxygen delivery include hemoglobin [total (gm/dl) and percent saturation (SaO_2)] and cardiac output. The role of pulmonary artery catheter, a gold standard cardiac output monitor, for hemodynamic management in critical care practice has been extensively scrutinized in the literature and even considered as harmful. Central venous pressure (CVP) alone may be used as a trend monitor for assessment of right heart preload and volume responsiveness. Both, CVP and pulmonary artery occlusion pressure (PAOP), however, is reliable only half the time as a guide for fluid therapy. Therefore, approximately 50 percent of the patients may receive excessive amounts of fluids based on CVP or PAOP as preload monitor. Often, simple straight leg raising test may demonstrate fluid responsiveness in a spontaneously breathing patient with hemodynamic instability. Dynamic physiological parameters [pulse pressure variation (PPV), systolic pressure variation (SPV), and stroke volume variation (SVV)], derived from arterial pressure waveform analysis has been shown to be more sensitive indicators of preload/fluid responsiveness in mechanically ventilated patients. There has been recent insurgence of plethora of minimally invasive cardiac output monitors. Although based on good physiological principles, their clinical application is fraught with lack of accuracy, precision, and outcome data. Measurement of mixed venous oxygen saturation (S_VO_2) can provide information on adequacy of resuscitation and systemic oxygenation, i.e. balance between oxygen consumption and oxygen delivery. More recently, based on a landmark study by Rivers et al.,[20] central venous oxygen saturation $(S_{CV}O_2)$ monitoring, as compared with true S_VO_2 from pulmonary artery, is used as an endpoint $(S_VO_2 > 65\%)$ to guide goal-directed resuscitation in the critically ill patient.

Since no single hemodynamic parameter can provide all the information necessary to determine adequacy of resuscitation in a critically ill patient with shock, integrated multiple hemodynamic parameters along with repeated clinical examination should be used to assess response to

therapy. The Surviving Sepsis Campaign Guidelines recommend that the goals of initial resuscitation in septic shock should include a CVP of 8-12 mm Hg, an MAP > 65 mm Hg, a urine output of > 0.5 ml/kg/hr, and a $S_{CV}O_2$ > 70 percent.[21] These endpoints of resuscitation can also be applied in high-risk patients undergoing major surgery.

More recently attention is drawn to the state of microcirculation in patients with shock, independent of systemic hemodynamics. Microcirculatory alterations, such as decreased capillary density, stagnation, sludging and shunting of blood, can result in tissue hypoperfusion and hypoxia. Impairment of microcirculation is more severe in non-survivors and its persistence is associated with development of organ failure and death. Technology to visualize and assess microcirculation has improved over the years. Nevertheless, it is not readily available in most ICUs. Lactate measurement has been used to assess tissue hypoperfusion and is considered a biochemical marker of the state of microcirculation. Although hyperlactatemia could be due to aerobic and anaerobic pathology, mitochondrial dysfunction and oxygen supply dependency in severe sepsis and septic shock is commonly associated with hyperlactatemia. Increased blood lactate level, and a lack of decrease during therapy, carries poor prognosis in critically ill patients.[22,23] Therefore, blood lactate level should be used in goal-directed therapy and may be used as a resuscitation endpoint.

Fluids Vs Pressors

Fluid administration is the first line of treatment in most types of shocks. The goal of fluid administration is to improve cardiac output by increasing preload (plasma volume). Fluids should be given as a "bolus". Crystalloid solutions are commonly used for fluid resuscitation. The common considerations in fluid administration include, crystalloid solution (250-1000 ml) infused rapidly over 30 minutes with physiological endpoints (BP, HR, urine output, CVP, etc.) and keeping safe limits in mind. The total amount of fluids required for adequate resuscitation is variable in each patient. One must carefully watch for potential complications of excessive fluid administration, such as pulmonary edema, hypoxemia, and abdominal compartment. Biological properties of crystalloids and colloids may be considered when choosing fluids for resuscitation. Normal saline and synthetic colloids have been shown to induce inflammation by neutrophil activation. Starch solutions may cause coagulopathy by inhibiting platelet function and impairing fibrin polymerization and should be avoided in perioperative period in patients with coagulopathy, severe sepsis or at risk for bleeding.[24]

Vasopressor therapy may be required in patients with shock to treat hypotension refractory to or in addition to fluid therapy and to maintain adequate perfusion pressure. Central venous access should be established as early as possible when vasopressor use is considered in the treatment of shock. The choice of vasopressor agent may vary with the underlying etiology of shock. Current Surviving Sepsis Guidelines recommend dopamine or norepinephrine in the initial management of septic shock.[21] Phenylephrine, epinephrine or vasopressin is not considered as the initial vasopressor in septic shock. Physiological doses of vasopressin (max. dose 0.04 units/min) may be used in addition to norepinephrine infusion to treat persistent hypotension due to septic shock. A prospective, randomized controlled trial performed by Levy et al. compared the effects of norepinephrine and dobutamine to those of epinephrine in dopamine-resistant septic shock.[25] Despite equal hemodynamic response, deleterious effects on splanchnic perfusion and rise in lactate were more likely observed with epinephrine infusion. Epinephrine is, however, the drug of choice in anaphylactic shock. Inotropic agents are used to treat conditions associated with reduced myocardial contractility. Dobutamine is considered the inotrope of choice to improve cardiac output in patients with impaired ventricular function due to septic shock.

Adjuvant Therapy in Shock

Drotrecogin alfa (activated) and low dose steroids have been used with improved outcomes in most severe forms of septic shock. Intraaortic balloon counter pulsation may be used to improve coronary perfusion in patients with cardiogenic shock. Renal replacement therapy (RRT) is considered to manage fluid overload and electrolyte abnormalities associated with acute kidney injury in patients with shock and multiple organ dysfunction. However, correct timing, mode, and dose of RRT remain controversial. Physiological doses of steroids may be considered in the patient with vasopressor dependent septic shock.

ABDOMINAL COMPARTMENT SYNDROME

The abdomen is a closed space lined by compliant (abdominal wall and diaphragm) and noncompliant (ribs, spine and pelvis) structures. Normally, intra-abdominal contents include solid organs, hollow viscera, and little fluid (ascites). Abdomen behaves as a hydraulic system whereby the pressure measured at one point may be assumed to represent the intra-abdominal pressure (IAP) throughout the abdomen. IAP, measured in mm Hg, is the intrinsic pressure within the abdomen at steady-state. Normal IAP ranges from subatmospheric to 0 mm Hg. Morbid obesity and pregnancy may be associated with chronic elevations in IAP (10-15 mm Hg). IAP is slightly elevated (5-7 mm Hg) in critically ill adults on mechanical ventilator. Normally, IAP varies with respiration (increases during inspiration and decreases during exhalation) and body position (increases with elevation of head of the bed or reverse Trendelenburg). Clinical understanding and research into effects of elevated IAP (intra-abdominal hypertension, IAH) on physiology and organ function as well as morbidity and mortality in the critically ill has increased significantly over the past decade. Development of intra-abdominal hypertension and abdominal compartment syndrome during ICU period is an independent risk factor for death. Although initially considered a disease of traumatically injured, IAH/ACS is now recognized as a cause of significant organ failure, morbidity and mortality in all critically ill populations. This section presents a brief review of diagnosis and management of abdominal compartment syndrome (ACS). In 2007 The World Society of Abdominal Compartment Syndrome (WSACS, www.wsacs.org) published definitions and recommendations from the international conference of experts on ACS.[26,27]

Definitions related to IAP and its critical care implications are summarized in Table 4.7. Due to its simplicity and minimal cost, bladder pressure measured after instillation of 25 ml volume of sterile saline via Foley catheter is considered the reference standard for intermittent IAP measurement. IAP is expressed in mm Hg and measured at end-expiration in supine position and with the transducer zeroed at the level of midaxillary line. Bladder pressure should be measured intermittently every 4 hours in patients at risk of developing IAH/ACS. Sensitivity of physical examination in detecting IAH has been demonstrated to be too low.

Diagnosis

Incidence and prevalence of IAH and ACS is reported to be high and can occur in a wide variety of critically ill populations. Numerous risk factors for the development of IAH/ACS have been identified in large-scale prospective trials. Common risk factors for IAH/ACS are listed in Table 4.8. High index of suspicion and low threshold for serial IAP measurement should be considered in high-risk postsurgical patients with acute onset organ dysfunction.

Table 4.7: Intra-abdominal pressure: Definitions and critical care implication	
Definitions	*Critical care implication*
IAP: Intrinsic pressure within abdominal cavity Normal: subatmospheric to 0 mm Hg	5-7 mm Hg in critically ill on mechanical ventilator
IAH: Intra-abdominal hypertension Sustained elevation in IAP ≥ 12 mm Hg	Potential for organ dysfunction (decrease in venous return and cardiac output).
Grading of IAH: Grade I: IAP 12-15 mm Hg Grade II: IAP 16-20 mm Hg Grade III: IAP 21-25 mm Hg Grade IV: IAP > 25 mm Hg	Urgent medical disease Increasing risk for ACS and organ failure
ACS: Abdominal compartment syndrome Sustained IAP > 20 mm Hg + New organ dysfunction/failure	Documented new organ dysfunction/failure Emergent surgical condition
Primary ACS: Condition associated with injury, surgery or disease in the abdominopelvic region (peritonitis, inflammatory or oncologic bowel disease, abdominal trauma)	Frequently requires early surgical or interventional radiological intervention
Secondary ACS: Condition originating outside abdominopelvic region (medical or burn patient, polytrauma, septic shock)	Surgical decompression should be considered Mortality higher than primary ACS
Recurrent ACS: ACS following resolution of I[ry] or II[ry] ACS	Can occur despite "open abdomen" or following closure of abdomen. Significant morbidity and mortality
APP= MAP- IAP	Predictor of visceral and intrabdominal organ perfusion Target ≥ 60 mm Hg
FG= MAP- 2 × IAP	Predictor of renal perfusion and AKI

IAP: intra-abdominal pressure; IAH: intra-abdominal hypertension; ACS: abdominal compartment syndrome; APP: abdominal perfusion pressure; MAP: mean arterial pressure; FG: filtration gradient; AKI: acute kidney injury

Unrecognized and untreated ACS has been shown to be associated with progressive multiorgan failure and high risk of death. End-organ squelae of ACS are summarized in Table 4.9.

Management

The best treatment for ACS is prevention. Screening patients at risk for ACS, monitoring IAP, goal-directed fluid resuscitation guided by defined end-points and early recognition of ACS, and possibly keeping the abdomen open in some situations are useful preventative strategies. The reader is referred to an algorithm for the management of IAH/ACS proposed by the World Society of Abdominal Compartment Syndrome. Key principles in the management of IAH/ACS include resuscitation for optimization of systemic and splanchnic perfusion, serial monitoring of IAP (bladder pressure), medical management to reduce IAP, and early surgical decompression of IAH/ACS refractory to medical therapy.

Resuscitation: Fluid resuscitation to maintain adequate intravascular volume and preload is important in IAH/ACS, and should be initiated early. Combination of hypovolemia (relative or absolute) and elevated intrathoracic pressure due to positive pressure ventilation tends to aggravate hypotension in IAH/ACS. Total amount of crystalloid administered must be closely monitored. Interactions between heart and lung become more complex in IAH/ACS due to changes in lung mechanics. It is important to keep in mind that CVP and PAOP may be falsely elevated in IAH/ACS and are not reliable monitors to guide fluid therapy. Dynamic measures of volume responsiveness (SVV, PPV, or SPV) may be considered to guide fluid therapy in IAH/ACS. There is some evidence that the use of hypertonic saline may be associated with significantly decreased fluid

Table 4.8: Risk factors for IAH/ACS	
Category	Examples
Metabolic	Acidosis (pH < 7.2)
	Hypothermia (core temperature < 33°C)
	Hypotension
Hematologic (coagulopathy)	Platelets < 55, 000/mm^3, INR> 1.5
	Disseminated intravascular coagulation (DIC)
	APTT > 2 x normal
Shock/massive resuscitation	Capillary leak
	Sepsis
	Crystalloids > 5 L/24 hours
	Massive transfusion (> 10 units of blood/24 hour)
Surgical	Major trauma/Burns
	Abdominal surgery with primary fascial closure
	Damage control laparotomy
Abdominopelvic etiology	Fluid (hemoperitoneum, ascites)
	Air (pneumoperitoneum, acute massive visceral distension)
	Increased intraluminal contents (gastroparesis, ileus, colonic pseudo-obstruction, toxic mega colon, massive bowel edema)
Medical	Acute respiratory failure with elevated intrathoracic pressure
	Prone positioning

APTT: activated partial thromboplastin time; INR: international normalized ratio

Table 4.9: End-organ consequences of IAH and ACS		
Organ system	Physiologic sequelae	Consequences
Cardiovascular	↓preload, CO, SvO$_2$, BP	↓tissue perfusion (hypovolemic shock)
	↑ afterload	↑ lactate
	↑ CVP, PAOP (falsely elevated)	Cardiac arrest
	Venous stasis	↑ risk for DVT
Respiratory	Diaphragm elevation	↓FRC, ↑ atelectasis
	↑ ITP, pleural pressure swing	↑ intrapulmonary shunt
	↓compliance (↑ PIP on VCV,	Hypoxia, hypercarbia
	↓V$_T$ on PCV	↓PaO$_2$/FiO$_2$ ratio
Hepatosplanchnic	↓hepatic and intestinal perfusion	Ischemia, necrosis
	↑ hepatic and intestinal congestion and edema	Bacterial translocation
Renal	Renal ischemia	Oliguria/anuria
	↓GFR and FG	AKI
Brain	↑ Intracranial pressure	Cerebral edema and hypoxia
	↓CPP	

requirement, lower inspiratory pressure, and higher abdominal perfusion pressure (APP). Inotropes may be considered to improve cardiac output and myocardial contractility in patients with LV dysfunction. The concept of APP, defined as MAP minus IAP, is an important consideration for resuscitation in IAH/ACS. The goal is to maintain adequate splanchnic perfusion. APP has been studied as a resuscitation end-point in several trials. APP value of ≥ 50-60 mm Hg is suggested as an appropriate resuscitation goal. This can be achieved through a balance of judicious fluids and vasoactive drugs. Maintaining adequate APP appears to predict improved survival from IAH/ACS.

Mechanical ventilation: IAH/ACS is associated with increased intrathoracic pressure, pleural pressure and chest wall stiffness with resultant alveolar collapse, atelectasis and hypoxemia. Peak inspiratory pressures rise with volume-control and tidal volume drops during pressure-control mode of ventilation due to decreased lung compliance in IAH/ACS. Plateau pressure and ΔP (P_{Plat} – PEEP) should be closely monitored. High airway pressures are usually needed to maintain adequate ventilation due to stiff chest wall. Titrating PEEP to overcome atelectasis and improve oxygenation can be challenging in IAH/ACS. Probably the best strategy includes incrementally increasing the PEEP to the level equal to IAP (which closely reflects pleural pressure). As opposed to ALI/ARDS, high airway pressure (P_{Plat}) is less concerning in ACS because the transpulmonary swing in pressure (ΔP-PEEP) is less when PEEP is equal to IAP. Frequent blood gas monitoring and close attention to intravascular volume status is required with this strategy. PEEP and P_{Pla} should be immediately reduced once abdomen is decompressed and ACS has resolved.

Surgical decompression: Surgical decompression of the peritoneal cavity (decompressive laparotomy) coupled with open abdomen management technique remains the gold standard for management of ACS. A variety of temporary abdominal closure techniques have been described. Whatever the technique used, commercial or customized, it is important to avoid tension on fascia, provide sufficient sterile cover over abdominal contents, and prevent recurrent ACS by allowing visceral expansion during on-going resuscitation. Timing and method of abdominal closure following resolution of the ACS and improvement in organ failure is variable for each case.

Medical management: Several nonsurgical (medical) treatments may be used in the treatment of IAH/ACS. These are usually temporarizing measures, especially for lower grades of IAH and to facilitate transport of the patient. Stomach and rectum may be decompressed using a nasogastric and rectal tube. Prokinetic motility agents (erythromycin, neostigmine, or metoclopramide) may be considered to improve ileus and evacuate intraluminal contents. Pseudomembranous colitis or surgical etiology of ileus, however, should be excluded before using prokinetic agents. Fluid management using diuretics or venovenous hemofiltration or ultrafiltration may be considered once fluid and vasopressor requirement has ceased. Controlled paracentesis may be used in patients with chronic ascites. Sedation and neuromuscular blockade may be helpful by decreasing airway and IAP, especially during transport.

PREVENTING ERRORS AND IATROGENIC COMPLICATIONS

"Primum non nocere", first do no harm, is one of the fundamental aspects of medical practice. Reports, such as "To Err is Human" and "Crossing the Quality Chasm", have shown that medical errors are common and adversely affect patient outcomes.[28,29] *Napoleon Bonaparte (1820)* once said "I do not want two diseases—One nature made, one doctor made". Safety and performance has become a main focus of attention in recent years in healthcare, including ICU. An ICU, where multiple, often complex, interventions by multiple providers occur, is a stressful and error prone environment. It is not uncommon to have a situation in the ICU similar to the holes in a stack of "Swiss Cheese" to line up resulting in an error.[30] The holes represent failures. Most errors result from a combination of active failures and latent conditions (system). Fortunately, not all errors result in a complication or patient harm. This is often called "near miss" or "sentinel event". Patient safety is the result of a series of checks and balances that ensures safe practices within the framework of an ICU. Establishing a culture of safety is among the major challenges faced by current ICUs.

Several approaches have been advocated by many Quality and Safety organizations and evidence-based research to improve safety and quality of care in ICU. First and foremost, the ICU must create a safety culture, as proposed by Pronovost, whereby collective attitudes and beliefs of the caregivers take into account the effect of local culture on safety outcomes.[31] All caregivers must be empowered to speak up without hesitation, increase awareness and create protective barrier whenever they notice safety practices being breached by another provider. Secondly, structure (how care is organized) and process (how it is delivered) of care is important in quality of care. Intensivist led multidisciplinary and mutli-professional ICU team recognizes each team member's contribution towards patient care. Recently, there is increased emphasis on organizing the goals and process of care in the form of goal-sheet, checklist and bundles. This ensures that the team has shared and common goals of care for the patient and important elements of treatment plan and procedure are followed consistently. This has been

Table 4.10: Common strategies to reduce errors and complications in ICU	
Category	*Strategies*
ICU Organization	Multiprofessional model Daily goals Anonymous error reporting
Infectious disease	Handwashing and infection control practices Local antibiogram and antibiotic selection Timely administration Proper specimen sampling and labeling Invasive catheter care, sepsis and VAP bundle Procedure checklist
Respiratory	Lung protective ventilation Sedation interruption Daily spontaneous breathing trial
Cardiovascular and resuscitation	Early goal-directed therapy Crystalloids over colloids for fluids Guidelines for ACS and CHF CPR: effective least interrupted chest compressions Therapeutic hypothermia
Metabolic	Conservative glycemic management (BG 150-180 mg/dl)
Pharmacy/Medications	Clinical pharmacist Pharmacokinetic dosing Avoiding deliriogenic drugs

shown to reduce errors and complications and improve patient outcomes. Examples include daily goal-sheet, procedure checklist, and various disease bundles (e.g. sepsis, central line care, and ventilator associated pneumonia bundle). Although this may at first seem very labor intensive, however, once incorporated in the daily practice it becomes part of the ICU safety culture and daily routine. Finally, one must recognize that errors are bound to occur and each ICU should have a system of measuring, reporting and analyzing errors in a non-threatening manner. Table 4.10 lists common strategies to reduce errors and complications in the ICU.

FUTURE DIRECTION

Critical care has made significant advancements over last 50 years and is still evolving. In addition to providing excellent clinical care, the current focus is on ICU organization and management, communication, accountability, and error prevention. In future, the practice of critical care medicine will be collaborative, recognizing regional and cultural differences; see no geographic boundaries or barriers to communication. Future critical care will utilize technology in the diagnosis and delivery of critical care, e.g. telemedicine. In future, accountability will be important in every aspect of care for the critically ill in the ICU. Finally, it is important to create a balance between professional and spiritual aspect of critical care.

REFERENCES

1. Brun-Buisson C, Minneli C, Bertolini G, et al. ALIVE Study Group. Epidemiology and outcome of acute lung injury in European intensive care units. Results from the ALIVE study. Intensive Care Med 2004;31(1):51-61.
2. Rubenfeld GD, Caldwell E, Peabody E, Weaver J. Incidence and outcomes of acute lung injury. N Engl J Med 2005;353(16);1685-93.
3. Pesenti A, Tagliabue P, Patroniti N, Fumagalli R. Computerized tomography scan imaging in acute respiratory distress syndrome. Intensive Care Med 2001;27:631-7.
4. Brochard L, Isabey D, Piquet J, Amaro P, Mancebo J, Messadi AA, et al. Reversal of acute exacerbations of chronic obstructive lung disease by inspiratory assistance with a face mask. N Engl J Med 1990;323(22):1523-30.
5. Plant PK, Owen JL, Elliott MW. Early use of noninvasive ventilation for acute exacerbations of chronic obstructive pulmonary disease on general respiratory wards: a multicentre randomised controlled trial. Lancet 2000;355(9219):1931-5.

6. Keenan SP, Sinuff T, Cook DJ, Hill NS. Which patients with acute exacerbation of chronic obstructive pulmonary disease benefit from noninvasive positive-pressure ventilation? A systematic review of the literature. Ann Intern Med 2003;138(11):861-70.

7. Masip J, Betbese AJ, Paez J, Vecilla F, Canizares R, Padro J, et al. Non-invasive pressure support ventilation versus conventional oxygen therapy in acute cardiogenic pulmonary oedema: a randomised trial. Lancet 2000;356(9248):2126-32.

8. Nava S, Carbone G, DiBattista N, Bellone A, Baiardi P, Cosentini R, et al. Noninvasive ventilation in cardiogenic pulmonary edema: a multicenter randomized trial. Am J Respir Crit Care Med 2003;168(12):1432-7.

9. L'Her E, Duquesne F, Girou E, de Rosiere XD, Le Conte P, Renault S, et al. Noninvasive continuous positive airway pressure in elderly cardiogenic pulmonary edema patients. Intensive Care Med 2004;30(5):882-8.

10. Nava S, Ambrosino N, Clini E, Prato M, Orlando G, Vitacca M, et al. Noninvasive mechanical ventilation in the weaning of patients with respiratory failure due to chronic obstructive pulmonary disease. A randomized, controlled trial. Ann Intern Med 1998;128(9):721-8.

11. Girault C, Daudenthun I, Chevron V, Tamion F, Leroy J, Bonmarchand G. Noninvasive ventilation as a systematic extubation and weaning technique in acute-on-chronic respiratory failure: a prospective, randomized controlled study. Am J Respir Crit Care Med 1999;160(1):86-92.

12. Evans TW. International Consensus Conferences in Intensive Care Medicine: noninvasive positive pressure ventilation in acute respiratory failure.Organised jointly by the American Thoracic Society, the European Respiratory Society, the European Society of Intensive Care Medicine, and the Societe de Reanimation de Langue Francaise, and approved by the ATS Board of Directors, December 2000. Intensive Care Med 2001;27(1):166-78.

13. Schettino G, Altobelli N, Kacmarek RM. Noninvasive positive-pressure ventilation in acute respiratory failure outside clinical trials: experience at the Massachusetts General Hospital. Crit Care Med 2008;36(2):441-7.

14. De Keulenaer BL, De Backer A, et al. Abdominal compartment syndrome related to noninvasive ventilation. Intensive Care Med 2003;29:1177-81.

15. Brower RG, Shanholtz CB, Fessler HE, et al. Prospective, randomized, controlled clinical trial comparing traditional versus reduced tidal volume ventilation in acute respiratory distress syndrome patients. Crit Care Med 1999;17:1492-98.

16. The Acute Respiratory Distress Syndrome Network. Ventilation with lower tidal volumes as compared with traditional Tidal volumes for acute lung injury and the acute respiratory distress syndrome. N Engl J Med 2000;342:1301-8.

17. Parsons PE, Eisner MD, Thompson BT, Matthay MA, Ancukiewicz M, Bernard GR, et al. Lower tidal volume ventilation and plasma cytokine markers of inflammation in patients with acute lung injury. Crit Care Med 2005;33:1-6.

18. Brower RG, Lanken PN, MacIntyre N, Matthay MA, Morris A, Ancukiewicz M, et al. Higher versus lower positive endexpiratory pressures in patients with the acute respiratory distress syndrome. N Engl J Med 2004;351:327-36.

19. MacIntyre NR, Cook DJ, Ely EW, Jr., Epstein SK, Fink JB, Heffner JE, et al. Evidence-based guidelines for weaning and discontinuing ventilatory support: a collective task force facilitated by the American College of Chest Physicians; the American Association for Respiratory Care; and the American College of Critical Care Medicine. Chest 2001;120:375S-95S.

20. Rivers E, Nguyen B, et al. Early goal-directed therapy in the treatment of severe sepsis and septic shock. N Engl J Med 2001;345(19):1368-77.

21. Dellinger RP, Levy MM, et al. Surviving Sepsis Campaign: International guidelines for management of severe sepsis and septic shock: 2008. Intensive Care Med 2008;34:17-60.

22. Trzeciak S, Dellinger RP, Chansky ME, Arnold RC, Schorr C, Milcarek B, et al. Serum lactate as a predictor of mortality in patients with infection. Intensive Care Med 2007;33:970-77.

23. Howell MD, Donnino M, Clardy P, Talmor D, Shapiro NI. Occult hypoperfusion and mortality in patients with suspected infection. Intensive Care Med 2007;33:1892-9.

24. Westphal M, et al. Anesthesiology 2009;111(1):187-202.

25. Levy B, et al. Comparison of norepinephrine and dobutamine to epinephrine for hemodynamics, lactate metabolism, and gastric tonometric variables in septic shock: a prospective, randomized study. Intensive Care Med 1997;23(3):282-7.

26. Malbrain ML, et al. Results of the international conference of experts on intra-abdominal hypertension and abdominal compartment syndrome. I. Definitions. Intensive Care Med 2006;32:1722-32.

27. Cheatham ML, et al. Results of the international conference of experts on intra-abdominal hypertension and abdominal compartment syndrome. I. Definitions. Intensive Care Med 2007;33:951-62.

28. Institute of Medicine. To err is human: Building a safer healthcare system. Washington DC. National Academy Press, 2000.

29. Institute of Medicine. Crossing the quality chasm: a new health system for the 21st century. Washington, DC. National Academy Press, 2001.

30. Reason J. Human Error: Models and management. BMJ 2000;320(7237):678-70.

31. Pronovost PJ, Goeschel CA, et al. Framework for patient safety research and improvement. Circulation 2009;119(2):330-7.

CHAPTER

5

Trauma: Utmost Attention Needed

Rajeev Gupta, Dinesh Vyas

INTRODUCTION/HISTORY

Trauma has been the most common cause of death for Indians/ Americans under the age of 45. It occupies close to one-third of critical care admissions the United States and western countries. There is no data from India, as development of the critical care setups is in early stage. There has been immense development in care of trauma patient, with incorporation of tele-communication, training and educational programs like Advance Trauma Life Support (ATLS). Courses for physicians, paramedics, and nurses and other specialists, specialized emergency care team, development of designated trauma centers and application of new tool and diagnostic equipments. These developments have been unevenly distributed across the globe. It can be attributed to economic condition of a particular country. There is a need of proper training and courses tailored for the paramedics, emergency physicians and surgeons. Stratifying trauma centers according to the resources and experts these help in better outcomes, as has been shown by Sampler et al.

India has a sorry story of trauma deaths, the survival percentage is abysmal, as compared to other countries and there is urgency for better care and results. There has been worsening trend in trauma mortality in India as compared to major western countries like the US. Mortality increased more than 100 percent in a short period of 5 years: road accidents increased in India from 40,000 in 1986 to 85,000 by 2001. There will definitely be a good number of unreported cases in these statistics. The age group of mortality stays the same across the globe, 66 percent younger than 44 years in India. Trauma system development is initiated in few states around 2005, but it is in its fetal phase and will take a long time to mature.

Trauma care system is a three pronged care: prehospital care (emergency), hospital (acute care), and posthospital (reha-bilitation) care. Development of this system has done wonders in trauma care, after its first incorporation of Advanced Trauma

Life Support Course by the American College of Surgeons and by development of first state-of-the-art trauma center at the Crowley Shock and Trauma System, by Maryland, US.

According to a recent publication from WHO 2004, there can be at least 15 to 30 percent reduction in mortality, even if there is a proper organization in places with minimal resources. The importance of golden hour was introduced by Trunkey (1983), as they noticed 50 percent death occurs within first hour, 30 percent within first day and 20 percent in first week.

Box of important points
• Prehospital care
• Field triage decision scheme
• Hospital care
• Primary survey
• Importance of airway control
• Identifying shock and treatment
• Emergency department thoracotomy
• Secondary survey
• Surgeon performed ultrasound and its relevance
• Head injury
• Neck injury
• Spine injury
• Chest injury
• Abdominal injury
• Pelvic injury
• Genitourinary trauma
• Extremity injury
• Pregnancy related injury
• Pediatric injury
• Geriatric injury
• Peripheral vascular injury
• Burn injury
• Trauma damage control
• Evaluation of trauma system

Appropriate and timely medical care can have better outcome only if medical personnel understands and realize the consequences of better care. Every step/action in the trauma care is generally necessary because any deviation from the protocol during training, will have potential of negative result, with profound implication, and this will be discussed in each part of this chapter. Thus attention and protocol driven training is extremely important in each stage of trauma care protocol. Trauma involves motor vehicle accident, industrial accident, home accident, terror activities, fall and others.

PREHOSPITAL CARE

Prehospital care is the most crucial aspect of trauma. The standard "Golden hour and now Platinum Ten Minutes" are the aspects of care that are very critical for survival and better prognosis. The Table 5.1 illustrate it in detail and will enable or structured care for the trauma patient.

1. Safety of the patient.
2. Status of other victims or accompanying passenger in motor vehicle crash.
3. Mechanism of injury and speed of vehicle.
4. Primary survey (ABCDE), for immediate necessary action.
5. Cervical spine stabilization (C-collar, although its hard to find in major setups in India). There are a large number of quadriplegics due to cervical spine injury as will be discussed in later part and these injuries are avoidable. If there is no cervical collar, there is a need for neck stabilization with the best possible resources.
6. Airway intubation in drowsy patient or unconscious patient, pressure over bleeding area.
7. IV fluid and temperature control.
8. Blood O negative, after 2 liters of crystalloid, till cross match available.
9. Whole body immobilization in patients who are complaining of back pain, unconscious, or hard to examine, till thoracolumbar spine scanned.
10. Transport to nearby major hospital, inform them with initial information to help them prepare for the situation.
11. Secondary survey and ascertain major medical problem, if possible full history.

Emergency Room and Trauma Team

Coordinated Care of Patient

Primary survey (A, B, C, D, E)
Secure airway, Breathing status, Circulation, Disability and Exposure)
(Check: Phonation, breath sounds, pulses, JVD, dyspnea, altered metal status)
(Imaging: CXR, Pelvic X-ray)
(Intervention: Cervical collars, intubate, chest tube, IV access, hemorrhage control) *Make sure these steps are done, before moving to secondary survey*

PRIMARY SURVEY

American College of Surgeons Committee on Trauma (ACSCOT) has developed and refined Advanced Trauma

Secondary survey (Head to toe examination)
1. Face and Head Examination   • Quick cranial nerve examination/Normal occlusion/Pain   • Following commands/Wounds/Lacerations/Facial instability   • CT scan (Head/Facial reconstruction) is preferred, but can perform facial X-ray. Important for intubation   • ICP, ICU care   • Ventriculostomy, Craniotomy
2. Spine Examination   • Spinal examination for tenderness, instability on log rolling   • Neurologic deficit   • Spine X-rays have a low sensitivity and hence CT scan recommended. For C2-5 injury CT angiogram to see carotid injury, to prevent stroke
3. Chest Examination   • Chest pain, subcutaneous air, flail chest (asymmetric breathing), crepts   • Decrease air entry, minimal air entry, vocal cord positioning   • Stat CXR or CT scan, if stable: You will never go wrong if you place chest tube in patient with any of the above findings
4. Abdomen/Pelvis   • Pain/Distension/Seat belt mark/Unexplained hypotension/Hematoma/Blood in urine   • Pelvis stability examination   • FAST (a very useful tool for trauma surgeon to decide for surgery)/pelvic X-ray   • If pelvic bleed suspected, needs intervention radiology to coil bleeding vessels
5. Extremity   • Pain/Bleeding/Crepitous   • Stabilization obvious fracture to prevent pain, and further vascular injury, pressure to control bleed   • X-ray, as appropriate   • Angiography in major vascular injury to prevent future vascular ischemia

Table 5.1: Triage scheme for transportation to trauma center

Measure vital signs and level of consciousness

Step One

Glasgow coma scale	<14 or
Systolic blood pressure	<90 or
Respiratory rate	<10 or >29 (<20 in infant < one year)

Yes   No

Take to a trauma center. Steps 1 and 2 attempt to identify
the most seriously injured patients.
These patients would be transported preferentially to the
highest level of care within the trauma system.

Assess anatomy of injury

Step Two
- All penetrating injuries to head, neck, torso, and extremities proximal to elbow and knee
- Flail chest
- Two or more proximal long-bone fractures
- Crush, degloved or mangled extremity
- Amputation proximal to wrist and ankle
- Pelvic fractures
- Open or depressed skull fracture
- Paralysis

Yes   No

Take a trauma center. Steps 1 and 2 attempt to identify the most   Assess mechanism of injury and evidence
seriously injured patients. These patients would be transported   of high-energy impact
preferentially to the highest level of care within the trauma system.

Step Three
- Falls
  - Adults: >20 ft. (one story is equal to 10 ft.)
  - Children: >10 ft. or 2-3 times the highest of the child
- High-risk auto crash
  - Intrusion: >12 in. occupant site; >18 in. any site
  - Ejection (partial or complete) from automobile
  - Death in same passenger compartment
  - Vehicle telemetry data consistent with high risk of injury
- Auto v. pedestrian/bicyclist thrown, run over, or with significant (>20 mph) impact
- Motorcycle crash >20 mph

Yes   No

Transport to closest appropriate trauma center which, depending   Assess special patient or system considerations
on the trauma system, need not be the highest level trauma center.

Step Four
- Age
  - Older Adults: Risk of injury death increases after age 55
  - Children: Should be triaged preferentially to pediatric-capable trauma centers
- *Patient with:*
- Anticoagulation and bleeding disorders
- Burns
  - Without other trauma mechanism: Triage to burn facility
  - With trauma mechanism: Triage to trauma center
- Time sensitive extremity injury
- End-stage renal disease requiring dialysis
- Pregnancy >20 weeks
- EMS provider judgment

Yes   No

Contact medical control and consider transport   Transport according to protocol
to trauma center or a specific resource hospital.

WHEN IN DOUBT, TRANSPORT TO A TRAUMA CENTER.

Life Support (ATLS) course over years and ATLS-recommended guidelines have become the "gold standard" for the first hour of hospital care for trauma patients around the world. ATLS uses the term initial assessment and management for the urgent evaluation and treatment of the trauma victim. The terms primary survey and secondary survey are used to differentiate between the rapid evaluation and treatment of the immediately life-threatening injuries (primary survey) and the more detailed evaluation, diagnosis, and treatment of the occult or nonimmediate threats to life (secondary survey). Both, the primary survey and the secondary survey, are parts of initial assessment and management of the injured patient.

The ultimate goal of initial assessment is to establish adequate oxygen delivery to the vital organs. This is accomplished by ABCs: airway control with cervical spine precautions, assisted breathing with ventilation, and empirical tube thoracostomy to relieve a pneumothorax if indicated. These maneuvers are carried out to maximize oxygen delivery to the alveoli. Support of the circulation (tamponade of external bleeding and fluid administration) is instituted to restore effective blood volume, thereby enhancing myocardial performance and thus oxygen delivery to the tissues.

The evaluation portion of the primary survey consists of the ABCDEs of trauma care:

- Airway maintenance with cervical spine protection
- Breathing and ventilation
- Circulation with hemorrhage control
- Disability; neurologic status
- Exposure/Environment (completely undress the patient and prevent hypothermia).

Adjuncts to the primary survey include administering oxygen, electrocardiogram (ECG) and pulse oximetry monitors, starting intravenous crystalloid administration with two large-bore cannulas, drawing blood for initial blood work, and visualizing the entire patient, front and back. The patient should be covered with a warm blanket as soon as possible to avoid hypothermia, also insertion of a gastric tube and urinary catheter when indicated. The primary survey and associated therapeutic interventions may need to be repeated several times depending upon the patient's response, even if it prevents the physician from proceeding to the secondary survey. Life-threatening injuries, such as cardiac tamponade, tension pneumothorax require definitive surgical therapy before even attempting a secondary survey. It may not be possible to complete the entire initial assessment, including both the primary and the secondary survey, until the postoperative period. Trauma patients should be reassessed at regular intervals so that the team can find and treat previously unidentified injuries and monitor the patient's response.

IMPORTANCE OF AIRWAY CONTROL

After blunt trauma, airway control should proceed on the assumption that an unstable cervical spine fracture exists; thus, hyperextension of the neck must be avoided. Evaluation begins by asking the patient a question such as "How are you?" A response given in a normal voice indicates that the airway is not in immediate jeopardy; a breathless, hoarse response or no response at all indicates that the airway may be compromised. Cervical spine protection is integral to airway management but should not be allowed to delay necessary interventions. Significant spinal cord injury without radiographic abnormalities (i.e., the SCIWORA syndrome) is a relatively rare event (0.5% of patients undergoing radiography). Even good-quality cross-table lateral cervical spine films may not detect 15 percent of unstable fractures. Therefore, in high-risk patients, a cervical collar is left in place until the cervical spine has been radiologically evaluated for bony and ligamentous integrity.

Airway obstruction and hypoventilation are the most likely causes of respiratory failure. The critical decision is whether active airway intervention is needed. The first maneuver is to clear the airway of debris and to suction secretions. In the obtunded patient, this procedure is followed by elevation of the angle of the mandible to alleviate pharyngeal obstruction and placement of an oropharyngeal or nasopharyngeal tube to maintain airway patency. Supplemental oxygen is given via a nasal cannula (6 L/min) or a nonrebreathing oxygen mask (12 L/min).

The best method of airway control depends on: (1) the presence of maxillofacial trauma, (2) possible cervical spine injury, (3) overall patient condition, and (4) the experience of the physician. Patients in respiratory distress with severe maxillofacial trauma warrant operative intervention. Cricothyrotomy is the preferred approach in adults and has virtually replaced tracheostomy in the ED; the rare exceptions are in patients with major laryngeal trauma or extensive tracheal disruption (these patients need intubation under vision with flexible bronchoscopy). In all other patients, the current standard approach is rapid sequence intubation (RSI) of the trachea orally with inline immobilization. In adults, a large (8 mm internal diameter) cuffed endotracheal tube is inserted to a distance of 23 cm from the incisors. In children, tube size is gauged to equal the diameter of the little finger. The proper depth (in centimeters) to which the tube is inserted can be estimated by multiplying the tube's internal diameter (in millimeters) by 3. A chest X-ray should be obtained as soon as possible to rule out the possibility of right mainstem intubation and patient should be monitored by pulse oximetry on high FiO_2.

IDENTIFYING SHOCK AND TREATMENT

Shock has been defined in many different ways but essentially **shock is suboptimal tissue perfusion**. Shock is best defined as inadequate delivery of oxygen and other nutrients that are required for normal cellular and organ function. There could be a variety of reasons leading to the same end result of impaired organ perfusion, and depending on these, the types of shock could be hypovolemic or hemorrhagic, cardiogenic, septic, neurogenic, or obstructive.

For a trauma patient, systematic approach is by simply dividing shock into two categories, hemorrhagic and nonhemorrhagic. The hemorrhagic category would consist of bleeding from any site including chest, abdomen, pelvis external, and long bones. The nonhemorrhagic category would include tension pneumothorax, cardiac tamponade, cardiac contusion, myocardial infarction, spinal cord injury (neurogenic), and rarely sepsis.

The most common cause of shock in trauma patients in hypovolemic or hemorrhagic. Hypovolemia from acute blood loss causes sympathetic stimulation leading to the release of epinephrine and norepinephrine, activation of the renin angiotensin system, and increased release of vasopressin, in addition decreased intravascular volume and tone cause change in signals from baroreceptors, chemoreceptors and atrial stretch receptors. That all leads to peripheral vasoconstriction in order to maintain perfusion to vital organs.

Hypovolemic shock has been classified into four levels based on amount of blood volume loss.

Class I hemorrhage (loss of 0-15%)—Usually, no changes in BP, pulse pressure, or respiratory rate occur, and in the absence of complications, only minimal tachycardia is seen. A delay in capillary refill of longer than 3 second corresponds to a volume loss of approximately 10 percent.

Class II hemorrhage (loss of 15-30%)—Clinical symptoms include tachycardia (rate >100 beats per minute) tachypnea, decrease in pulse pressure, cool, clammy skin, delayed capillary refill, and slight anxiety. Increased catecholamine

level causes an increase in peripheral vascular resistance and a subsequent increase in the diastolic blood pressure, reflecting as the decrease in pulse pressure.

Class III hemorrhage (loss of 30-40%)—Patient shows marked tachypnea and tachycardia, decreased systolic BP oliguria, and significant changes in mental status, such as confusion or agitation.

Class IV hemorrhage (loss of >40%)—All of the symptoms and vitals get worse, e.g. marked tachycardia, decreased systolic BP, narrowed pulse pressure (or immeasurable diastolic pressure), markedly decreased (or no) urinary output, **depressed mental status (or loss of consciousness), and cold and pale skin. This amount of hemorrhage is immediately life-threatening.**

Source of blood loss is obvious in profuse external bleeding from vascular injury, which should be managed with direct pressure initially. It is relatively simple to diagnose the source in penetrating injury, as potential bleeding source will be in the path of the injury; this most often requires operative intervention. Diagnosing the source of blood loss is challenging in blunt trauma patients or in with multiple injuries. Pelvic fracture, long bone fractures intrathoracic bleeding can cause large amount of concealed blood loss only to present as shock, and close attention is required. The most common source of acute blood loss causing shock in blunt trauma patients is intraperitoneal hemorrhage, clinically manifested as distended abdomen, generalized abdominal tenderness. Clinical findings are very unreliable or usually late to diagnose intraperitoneal blood loss, therefore, ultrasound focused assessment sonography in trauma (FAST) is used frequently in the resuscitation area to rapidly identify intraperitoneal blood namely in right upper quadrant, left upper quadrant pelvis and also in pericardium. Diagnostic peritoneal lavage is indicated in very few selected patients, but DLP can be a very handy tool in places with no ultrasound facility in the emergency department to expedite the care.

Major retroperitoneal hemorrhage from unstable pelvic fracture would need temporary pelvic stabilization interventional radiology embolization of bleeding vessel, followed by definitive immobilization.

EMERGENCY DEPARTMENT THORACOTOMY

Emergency department thoracotomy (EDT) is a life-saving procedure in a select group of patients, and can be an important part of early resuscitative scheme. Very few trauma centers see a sufficient number of patients who really fit into the strict patient selection criteria. An outcome of 5 to

10 percent has been reported in literature, but some centers claim to have a successful outcome in up to 60 percent of selected patients. Overall EDT is a controversial topic, but we will try to clarify some of the points.

There is no controversy about indication for EDT in patient with penetrating chest trauma who suffers cardiac arrest in emergency department. Other indications are given below.

Clear Indications

Penetrating Thoracic Injury

- Traumatic arrest with previously witnessed cardiac activity (prehospital or in-hospital)
- Unresponsive hypotension (BP <70 mm Hg)

Blunt Thoracic Injury

- Unresponsive hypotension (BP <70 mm Hg)
- Rapid exsanguination from chest tube (>1500 ml).

Relative Indications

Penetrating thoracic injury
- Traumatic arrest without previously witnessed cardiac activity

Penetrating nonthoracic injury
- Traumatic arrest with previously witnessed cardiac activity (prehospital or in-hospital)

Blunt thoracic injuries
- Traumatic arrest with previously witnessed cardiac activity (prehospital or in-hospital).

Contraindications

Blunt injuries
- Blunt thoracic injuries with no witnessed cardiac activity
- Multiple blunt traumas
- Severe head injury.

Operative Technique

In supine position, with patient's left arm extended parallel to head and neck, the entire area is rapidly prepped with sterile precautions and draped. A nasogastric tube is helpful in differentiating the aorta and esophagus. The standard approach is a left anterolateral thoracotomy incision in fourth or fifth intercostals space, just below the nipple in males or in inframammary fold in females. The curvilinear incision should start from the lateral border of left sternochondral junction to avoid injury to internal mammary vessels. The incision is deepened to the intercostals muscles and should

course the superior border or rib to protect intercostals neurovascular bundle. Then the rib retractor is used to gain entry into the chest cavity. If needed this incision can be extended to right thoracic cavity by cutting through sternum after ligating internal mammary artery.

The pericardium is incised anteriorly and opened longitudinally to avoid injury to left phrenic nerve. Any blood clots present should be removed and myocardium examined thoroughly, cardiac bleeding from small wounds should be controlled with direct pressure, inserting a Foley catheter subsequently inflating the balloon and using gentle traction. For larger injuries, sequentially stacked Allis clamps can be used for temporary control in all chambers of heart except the left ventricle. Cardiac wounds can be directly sutured using pledgeted nonabsorbable 3/0 sutures such as nylon. For aortic cross-clamping, the lung is elevated anteriorly and superiorly to expose descending thoracic aorta, then mediastinal pleura is dissected bluntly to separate esophagus from aorta. Nasogastric tube may help in differentiating the aorta from esophagus. With the left hand, aorta is encircled after separating the esophagus anteriorly and prevertebral fascia posteriorly, and a clamp is applied with the right hand. A clamp can be left in place for 20-30 minutes, but for most practical purposes, this time is not sufficient for the patient to take to operating room, perform the definitive repair of complex injury and resuscitate enough to compensate for the reperfusion injury on removal of the clamp.

For open cardiac massage, the clapping method is preferred with the wrists apposed and pressure applied with the flat of the fingers from the apex to the base of the heart. Care must be taken not to use fingertips for the fear of injuring the myocardium.

SECONDARY SURVEY

The secondary survey is second, rapid, more detailed, head to toe evaluation of the patient including digital rectal examination. Now, adjuncts to evaluation like urinary and gastric catheters should be considered, chest and pelvis X-ray done and focused assessment with sonogram in trauma (FAST) be performed to determine the cause of deterioration in patient's clinical status.

History

A simple mnemonic from ATLS can be used, the AMPLE method:

    Allergies
    Medications
    Past illnesses/Pregnancy

Last meal
Events/Environment related to injury.

Physical Examination

A thorough inspection of scalp, pupils, tympanic membrane and palpation of head, midface and mandible is done to identify any occult laceration or cephalohematoma, intracranial hypertension, midface or mandibular fracture respectively. Neck examination involves looking for any laceration, penetrating injury, distended neck veins from cardiac tamponade, deviated trachea from tension pneumothorax and shifted mediastinum, any neck hematoma should be serially evaluated to assess for expansion or ongoing blood loss. Back of neck is easier to examine during log roll. Chest exam is basically looking for any tenderness, crepitus over rib fractures, subcutaneous emphysema from decompressing pneumothorax or paradoxical movement of chest wall over flail chest, and any positive finding on CXR, also FAST if needed. Bilateral auscultation of breath sounds is although subjective and difficult in noisy trauma bay but can provide important information if decreased on one side.

The abdominal cavity stretches from fourth intercostal spaces to pelvis and the retroperitoneum. General palpation should reveal extreme tenderness and peritoneal signs warranting exploratory laparotomy, keeping in mind the confounding variables like rib and pelvic fractures. Unstable patient must have intra-abdominal hemorrhage ruled out by FAST or diagnostic peritoneal lavage (DPL). Stable patients can be evaluated by abdominal CT. Pelvis is assessed for any bony instability and tenderness, hip dislocation. Upper and lower extremities are examined for any deformities, laceration, neurological loss, and peripheral pulses examined bilaterally, ankle brachial index (ABI) can be performed as easy bedside tool to assess peripheral circulation in presence of injury to the extremity.

Back examination is performed as a team approach with at least three persons performing the log roll one to maintain inline immobilization, second person to turn the patient, and *third to do the examine* the back for any tenderness site deformity and performing the DRE at the same time as well.

HEAD INJURY

The core concept in management of head injuries is rapid evaluation of the extent of primary injury, stopping it progression of damage or herniation and most importantly preventing additional secondary injury mainly by maintaining intracranial pressure (ICP) to optimize cerebral blood flow.

Evaluation

While evaluating the patients for head injury, primary principles of trauma should not be forgotten and airway control with cervical spine stabilization must be ensured first. The neck should be immobilized with cervical collar until cervical spine is cleared by appropriate imaging and/or clinically. A lateral cervical spine film showing C1-T1 space should be obtained. The next thing to keep in mind is that in patients with head injury from nonpenetrating mechanism, likelihood of sustaining injuries to other organ system is very high.

The goal of the primary neurologic survey is a rapid, accurate categorization of the severity of the brain injury and search for clinical evidence of large intracerebral hematomas that could require immediate evacuation. Glasgow Coma Scale (GCS) is the main tool of primary neurological survey along with examination of pupillary responses, corneal responses, and gag response. GCS is a 3-component scoring system, involving the best response for eye opening, verbalization and motor response. Evaluation of a patient with GCS, is quick to perform and reproducible therefore can be used to follow patient's neurological status over time.

In any patient, the possible scores can range from 3 to 15 with points given to the better response in all the

Glasgow Coma Scale	
Parameters	Points
Eye opening:	
Spontaneous	4
To voice	3
To pain	2
None	1
Best verbal response:	
Oriented	5
Confused, disoriented	4
Inappropriate words	3
Incomprehensible sounds	2
None	1
Best motor response:	
Obeys	6
Localizes	5
Withdraws (flexion)	4
Abnormal flexion posturing	3
Extension posturing	2
None	1

categories. Intubated patients may be given a score of "T," or their verbal score may be estimated from other communicative efforts that they make. A score between 3 and 8 indicates severe traumatic brain injury, 9 to 12 indicates moderate brain injury, and 13 to 15 indicates mild closed head injury. Patients with score less than 8 need endotracheal intubation for airway protection, and a neurosurgical consult. Out of the three categories, the motor response is more predictive of patient's future outcome. Patients with a severe head injury, the noncontrast brain CT should be obtained as quickly as possible and should be evaluated for presence of blood extradural or intradural, any mass effect or midline shift, and presence or absence of cerebrospinal fluid in the basal cisterns. A patient with a mass lesion and a GCS score of 8 or less should undergo rapid surgical decompression.

Acute Subdural Hematoma

Subdural hematoma originates in the space between the dura and arachnoidal meningeal layer on the surface of the brain and is a result of injury to the bridging veins and the brain parenchyma beneath it, and occurs in approximately 20 to 40 percent of severely head-injured patients. As it layers on the surface of the brain it forms a crescent shape.

Epidural Hematoma

The dura adheres to the inner table of the skull like a laminate. The epidural space, the space between the dura, and the inner table is therefore a potential space, created only when something peels the dura off of the inner table. That is why epidural hematomas have a convex shape, created as the blood detaches the dura back, creating a space filled with blood trapped between the inner table and the dura, causing a mass effect.

Epidural hematomas are caused by injury to middle meningeal artery from temporal bone fracture, or injury to the dural sinuses or fractures through the diploic spaces, causing venous bleeding into the epidural space.

A lucid interval, phases of unconsciousness-consciousness, is classically associated with epidural hematoma, but it happens in only about 30 to 40 percent of patients with epidural hematoma, and is also not specific to it.

Intracerebral Hematoma/Contusion

Intracerebral hematoma can occur in the brain parenchyma—intraparenchymal or in the ventricles—intr-

aventricular both more common in hemorrhagic stroke but can also happen in trauma patients and account for about 20 to 30 percent of patients. Cerebral contusion are areas of bruised tissue in which the blood-brain barrier has lost its integrity, creating heterogeneous region of injured cerebral parenchyma mixed with extravasated blood. They evolve after injury and become more apparent on head CT, also can cause increased mass effect through cerebral edema in the injured brain and hemorrhage from injured smaller blood vessels.

Surgical Management

Acute Epidural Hematoma

All patients with an acute epidural hematoma, and a GCS of 8 or less should undergo craniotomy as soon as possible regardless of the size of the hematoma. All epidural hematomas with a volume > 30 cm^2 need to be evacuated regardless of the patient's GCS. The criteria for nonoperative management are a volume on CT <30 cm^2, a thickness of <15 mm and midline shift <0.5 mm in a patient with a GCS more than 8, and no focal deficit.

Acute Subdural Hematomas

All patients with subdural hematoma, with a thickness greater than 10 mm or a midline shift greater than 5 mm should be evacuated regardless of the patient's GCS. A patient with fixed and dilated or asymmetric pupils, an ICP >20 mm Hg, or a decline in GCS of two or more points from the time of injury to hospital admission should have craniotomy. All patients with a GCS <9 and an acute subdural hematoma should be monitored with an ICP monitor.

Nonsurgical Management

The goal is to maintain intracranial pressure at or around normal level to optimize cerebral blood flow and to prevent secondary brain injury. This applies to patients not needing surgery, pre- and postoperative patients. Although historically widely accepted, in the patients with severe head injuries, current standards of patient management recommend against the chronic prolonged hyperventilation therapy (PaCO$_2$ $\leq$ 25 mm Hg), use of glucocorticoids and prophylactic use of phenytoin, carbamazepine or phenobarbital.

The medical management centers on monitoring and treating elevated intracranial pressure. Current literature strongly supports:

1. ICP monitoring is indicated in the patient with:
   a. GCS score of 3 to 8 and an abnormal CT scan
   b. GCS score of 3 to 8 and normal head CT scans, if patients demonstrated two of three adverse features (age >40 years, unilateral or bilateral motor posturing, or systolic blood pressure <90 mm Hg).
2. ICP should be monitored by ventriculostomy, advantage being that drainage of the cerebrospinal fluid can be used to decrease ICP.
3. Mannitol can be used as a large bolus (1 g/kg) when ICP increases above a threshold such as 25 mm Hg, or it can be used as small boluses (0.25 g/kg) every few hours regardless of the ICP. Serum osmolarity should be followed closely and kept below 320 mOsm.
4. Hypertonic saline up to 7.5 percent can be used to obtain hyperosmolarity by raising serum sodium level to a goal of 155-160.
5. All patients requiring intravenous fluids should get normal saline.
6. All patients admitted with abnormal head CT scan following trauma should have a repeat head CT scan 2 hours after the trauma.

NECK INJURY

The mechanism of injuries to the neck could be penetrating or blunt trauma. The management of injuries to the neck that penetrate the platysma is dependent upon the anatomic level of injury. The neck is divided in 3 zones: Zone I also known as the thoracic outlet extends from the clavicles to the cricoid cartilage, Zone II extends from the cricoid cartilage to the angle of the mandible. This area includes the carotid arteries, jugular veins, vertebral vessels, larynx, trachea, esophagus, vagus nerves, recurrent laryngeal nerves, and spinal cord. Zone III includes a small area from the angle of the mandible to the base of the skull and is exceptionally difficult to access surgically. The central neck area (Zone II) can be accessed more expeditiously should an injury necessitate operative intervention unlike Zones I and III that are bounded by bony structures.

History and physical examination should focus on sign and symptoms arising from injury to respiratory, vascular or digestive tract. These include acute airway obstruction, tenderness in trachea, hoarseness, hemoptysis, dysphonia, subcutaneous emphysema from respiratory tract injury; pulsatile or expanding neck hematoma, loss of pulses, bruit from vascular, and hematemesis, odynophagia, dysphagia, subcutaneous emphysema, air bubbling from the wound and

from aerodigestive tract. Hard signs for vascular injuries include active bleeding, a large, pulsatile or expanding hematoma, a bruit or thrill, or presence of central neurologic deficit; all mandating surgical exploration.

Blunt cerebrovascular injury (BCVI) include a wide range of injuries cased by blunt trauma to the neck.

Sign/symptoms of BCVI

- Arterial hemorrhage
- Cervical bruit
- Expanding cervical hematoma
- Focal neurological deficit
- Neurologic examination incongruous with CAT scan findings
- Ischemic stroke on secondary CAT scan

Risk factors for BCVI

- High-energy transfer mechanism with Le Fort II or III fracture
- *Cervical spine fracture patterns*: Subluxation, fractures extending into the transverse foramen, fractures of C1-C3
- Basilar skull fracture with carotid canal involvement
- Diffuse axonal injury with GCS ≤ 6
- Near hanging with anoxic brain injury.

Penetrating and blunt neck wounds present serous challenges in diagnosis and management. Thorough physical examination with attention to the overt findings of vascular and aerodigestive injury (hard signs) is critical. Eastern Association for the Surgery of Trauma (EAST) recommended some clinical practice guidelines based on the level of evidence for the management of neck injuries.

EAST guidelines for penetrating neck injuries:
1. Operation vs selective nonoperative management
   Selective operative management and mandatory exploration of penetrating injuries to Zone II of the neck are equally justified and safe (Level 1).
2. Diagnosis of arterial injury
   a. Angiography or duplex ultrasonography can be used in lieu of arteriography to rule out an arterial injury in penetrating injuries to Zone II of the neck (Level 2).
   b. CT of the neck (even without CT angiography) can be used to rule out a significant vascular injury if it demonstrates that the trajectory of the penetrating object is remote from vital structures. With injuries in proximity to vascular structures, minor vascular injuries such as intimal flaps may be missed (Level 3).

3. Diagnosis of esophageal injury

Either contrast esophagography or esophagoscopy can be used to rule out an esophageal perforation that requires operative repair. Diagnostic workup should be expeditious because morbidity increases if repair is delayed by more than 24 hours (Level 2).

4. Value of the physical exam

Careful physical examination, including auscultation of the carotid arteries, is >95 percent sensitive for detecting arterial injuries that require repair. Given the potential morbidity of missed injuries, imaging is still recommended (Level 3).

5. Management of specific vascular injuries

a. Except for minimal intimal irregularities or small pseudoaneurysms without neurologic deficits, penetrating injuries to the internal carotid artery should be repaired, even when severe neurologic deficits are present (Level 2).

b. Angiographic approaches to the vertebral artery are preferred to operative approaches for patients with bleeding from vertebral artery injuries (Level 2).

c. Ligation of the jugular vein is appropriate for complex injuries or unstable patients (Level 2).

6. Cervical spine immobilization

Immobilization of the cervical spine is unnecessary unless there is overt neurologic deficit or an adequate physical examination can not be performed, e.g. the unconscious victim (Level 2).

SPINE INJURY

Cervical spine and the thoracolumbar junction are the most common sites of spinal injuries. Spinal cord injuries occur more commonly in young adults and in polytraumatized patients. The basic principles of spine injury management are avoidance of the progression of neurologic deficit, reduce unacceptable spinal deformity, maintain spinal alignment within a functional range throughout the course of treatment; and to achieve healing of the spine to permit return of physiologic loads through the spine. Spine injury represents a common, potentially devastating portion of the trauma patient population, by causing prolonged morbidity.

A detailed neurological examination of all extremities and documentation of the level of sensory and motor injury is essential not only to assess the needs of patient and plan the treatment but also for comparing the serial examinations to monitor the progress or deteriorating of the patient.

Screening

Early detection, proper initial emergency center management, and appropriate treatment can minimize many of the complications associated with spine injuries. Patients who have no cervical spine tenderness at posterior midline, no focal neurological deficit, a normal level of alertness, no distracting injury, not intoxicated do not require any imaging and their neck can be cleared clinically by confrontational exam.

Patients who have focal neurological deficit, cervical spine tenderness or those who cannot be assessed would require imaging to rule out spinal injury.

Initial Management

Airway should be assessed first, and should not be an issue in patients with spinal cord injury alone, unless high cervical injury as discussed below or accompanied by other injuries, and cervical spine should be immobilized and considered to be having injury in every patient unless proven otherwise. The effect of spinal cord injury on breathing is directly related to the level and completeness of injury. Higher lesions affect the respiratory function more severely. Injuries below C5 have lesser effect on respiration, as phrenic nerve (C3-C5) supplying the diaphragm is spared giving the patient a good chance to perform spontaneous breathing. Patient with injuries higher than C3 will require continuous ventilator support.

Spinal shock is loss of all spinal reflexes along with sympathetic activity below the level of complete spinal cord injury, usually seen in patients with injury at high neurologic level. Patients need adequate initial volume loading followed by pressor support if required, to compensate for the loss of sympathetic vascular tone. Foley catheter should be inserted to prevent from urinary retention, as bladder is often areflexic. Long-term Foley, suprapubic catheter, intermittent catheterization are options to be considered in future for bladder management.

Regarding the use of steroids in spinal cord injuries, methylprednisolone should be given to all patients with acute spinal cord injury secondary to blunt trauma, as per the recommendations of National Acute Spinal Cord Injury Studies (NASCIS). This is based on their findings that patients with acute SCI have improved recovery of neurologic function at 6 months after injury if treated with methylprednisolone within 8 hours of injury.

- The recommended dosage is a 30 mg/kg bolus followed by an infusion of 5.4 mg/kg/hr for 23 hours.
- Patients treated within 3 hours of injury should receive treatment for 24 hours.
- Patients treated within 3 to 8 hours of injury should receive treatment for 48 hours.
- There appears to be no benefit in starting the treatment more than 8 hours after injury.
- There is no role of steroids in spinal cord injury caused by penetrating trauma.

Deep venous thrombosis (DVT) and pulmonary embolism (PE) prophylaxis should be started with sequential compression devices in all patients. Pharmacologic prophylaxis with heparin, low molecular weight heparin, and later on change over to Coumadin should be initiated as soon as the bleeding risk is acceptable, ideally no longer than 72 hours after injury.

Management

Cervical spine fractures are more common than thoracolumbar spine fractures; most are treated non-operatively with external support, the operative management is aimed for appropriate alignment and stabilization by hardware and/or fusion. The atlanto-occipital junction is the articulation of the cranium onto C1, the serious injury to this area is the atlanto-occipital dislocation, which is uncommon and is almost always fatal. More common is unilateral, nondisplaced, occipital condyle fracture, which can be treated with a hard cervical collar for 6 weeks. Jefferson fracture is C1 fracture caused by traumatic axial load to the upper cervical spine and can be managed by halo immobilization until bony union is achieved, except in patients with greater than 7 mm of instability, who should considered for C1-2 arthrodesis.

Odontoid fractures can be of 3 types–Type I fractures consist of apical ligament avulsion injuries which are essentially stable and require limited support. Type II odontoid injuries occur at the waist of the odontoid, require anatomic reduction and maintenance of fracture stability. Type III fractures extending below the waist of the odontoid into the body of C2 and usually result in uneventful bony union Type III fractures of the waist (junction of the dens and body) can be treated with either a halo or preferentially surgical stabilization, especially if they are displaced. Thoracic spine injuries are not common but these fractures cause significant neurologic deficits. The type and stability of thoracic spine will dictate the management plan.

Thoracic and thoracolumbar spinal stability is analyzed using the Denis three-column theory. The anterior column comprises the anterior longitudinal ligament and the anterior half of the vertebral body and intervertebral disk. The middle column includes the posterior half of the vertebral body, the intervertebral disk, and the posterior longitudinal ligament. The posterior column consists of the spinous processes, interspinous ligaments, pedicles, lamina, ligamentum flavum, transverse processes, and intertransverse ligaments. Any injury that involves two of the three columns, bony vertebral compression with more than 50 percent loss of height, greater than 2.5 mm of sagittal displacement, or greater than 20 degrees of angulation in the sagittal plane is considered to be causing frank instability. Unstable fractures should be considered for operative alignment and fusion by anterior or posterior approach.

Compression fracture of thoracolumbar junction is common and can be managed with thoracolumbosacral orthotic (TLSO) bracing to maintain the alignment. Lower lumbar fractures do not case any neurologic compromise, but may result in chronic low back pain and difficulty in sitting.

Practice management guidelines for identification of cervical spine injuries following trauma–from the EAST Practice Management Guidelines Committee:

1. Cervical collars should be removed as soon as feasible after trauma (Level 3).
2. In the patient with penetrating trauma to the brain, immobilization in a cervical collar is not necessary, unless the trajectory suggests direct injury to the cervical spine (Level 3).
3. In awake, alert trauma patients without neurologic deficit or distracting injury, who have no neck pain or tenderness with full range of motion of the cervical spine, imaging is not necessary and the cervical collar may be removed (Level 2).
4. All other patients, in whom cervical spine injury is suspected, must have radiographic evaluation. This applies to patients with pain or tenderness, patients with neurologic deficit, patients with altered mental status, and patients with distracting injury.
5. The primary screening modality is axial computed tomography (CT) from the occiput to T1 with sagittal and coronal reconstructions (Level 2).
6. Plain radiographs contribute no additional information and should not be obtained (Level 2).
7. If CT of the cervical spine demonstrates injury, obtain spine consultation.

8. If there is neurologic deficit attributable to a cervical spine injury, obtain spine consultation and MRI.

9. For the neurologically-intact awake and alert patient complaining of neck pain with a negative CT, options are to continue cervical collar, or cervical collar may be removed after negative MRI (Level 3). Alternatively, cervical collar may be removed after negative and adequate flexion/extension films (Level 3).

10. For the obtunded patient with a negative CT and gross motor function of extremities:

    a. Flexion/extension radiography should not be performed (Level 2).

    b. The risk/benefit ratio of obtaining MR in addition to CT is not clear, and its use must be individualized in each institution (Level 3).

    c. Options are to continue cervical collar immobilization until a clinical exam can be performed, remove the cervical collar on the basis of CT alone, or obtain MRI and if MRI is negative, the cervical collar may be safely removed (Level 2).

APPLICATION IN YOUR SETUP

This chapter discussed the standard care, in the centers with state-of-the-art technology, but also discussed the methods to optimize care using the tools that are available in your center. The tools available in some centers might not be that sensitive, as the state-of-the-art equipment. To overcome this limitation, it must be understood the sensitivity of the available and nonavailable investigation, and its limitation. If patient's clinical situation suspicious for a certain injury, manage as if the patient has that particular injury. If the patient is managed in a small setup, plan how can that patient be safely transferred to a facility with better care, or what are the alternatives available at your disposal to investigate the patient.

Here are the tools available that can be safely employed in various setups, where state-of-the-art technology is not available.

Head and Neck

- Concussion patient/patient with GCS less than 13, or patient with memory loss, patient with depressed fracture of skull needs CT scan of head and if not available develop a protocol to transfer patient to the center with facilities once patient is stable.

- *Stability of patient is accessed from primary survey:* Airway must be secured. There are a lot of ways to secure airway as discussed above. Even with most limited sources, there is always an option of surgical airway/tracheostomy for any surgeon.

- All patients must have 2 large IV cannula.

- All sorts of hemorrhage should be controlled with external pressure where applicable. In case of internal bleeding, like pelvis stabilize pelvis, abdominal bleed after DPL, perform exploration.

- Prioritize the injuries, although at times it might be confusing, but protocol to prioritize is to see, the most grievous injury, that might kill a patient first and treat it, before transferring.

DETAILS OF FOLLOWING ARE COVERED IN TIPS AND TEASERS CHAPTER

Chest Injury
Abdominal Injury
Pelvic Injury
Genitourinary Trauma
Extremity Injury
Pregnancy Related Injury
Pediatric Injury
Geriatric Injury
Peripheral Vascular Injury
Burn Injury
Trauma Damage Control

BIBLIOGRAPHY

1. Trauma Practice Guidelines by EAST. www.east.org/research/treatment-guidelines.
2. Trauma: David V Feliciano, Kenneth L Mattox, Ernest Eugene Moore, 2008.

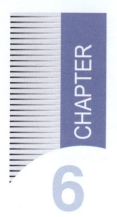

Hernia—Femoral and Inguinal, and Scrotal Diseases

Dinesh Vyas, K Kant

Scrotal pathology requires an urgent workup and treatment as the condition can have bad outcomes (e.g. testicular torsion, testicular cancer).

Testicular examination helps to evaluate the tunica vaginalis and the epididymis. The spermatic cord, which consists of the testicular vessels and the vas deferens, is another important anatomical structure easily palpated on routine exam, and changes from normal anatomy must be appreciated by the examiner to help diagnose the pathological condition.

A focused history helps in diagnosis and examination:
- Details of pain: Onset and severity, common etiologies: testicular torsion, torsion of testicular or epididymal appendages, and epididymitis
- Trauma
- Change in testicular or scrotal size
- Flank pain or hematuria
- Sexually active
- Onset of this change/diurnal variation/variation with position, or Valsalva maneuver (varicocele or hydrocele with and without hernia).

The examination should be preceded with a brief discussion regards examination procedure.

For most aspects of the examination, the patient should be in standing position. The examiner can sit or stand. The evaluation of patients with scrotal pain or swelling should include a detailed examination of the abdomen, inguinal region, and genitalia, including the testes, epididymis, spermatic cord, scrotal skin, penis, and cremasteric reflex.

GENITAL EXAMINATION

Inspection: Inspect the penis and groin area, when the patient is standing. The position and orientation of the testicles and left testicle is lower than the right testicle. Examine varicocele in both standing and lying position.

Palpation: Examine testis and epididymis

Cremasteric reflex: Limited clinical use, present between 2 to 12 years of age, but almost always absent in patients with testicular torsion.

Prehn sign: Not a reliable test to clinically differentiate between testicular torsion, epididymitis, and other testicular conditions. It involves elevation of the scrotal contents for symptomatic pain reduction in patients with epididymitis but has no effect on the pain in patients with testicular torsion.

Differential Diagnosis for Testicular Pain

Testicular torsion: Abrupt onset of severe pain
1. Doppler ultrasonography: Testis for torsion—this is a surgical emergency
2. Operative scrotal exploration: If proven torsion or equivocal imaging study

Incarcerated inguinal hernia

Torsion of the appendix testis also has abrupt onset of pain— less than in testicular torsion and localized to the region of the appendix testis

Epididymitis: Subacute pain with swelling of epididymis only

Scrotal trauma

Another surgical emergency: Fournier's gangrene (necrotizing fasciitis of the perineum).

PAINLESS TESTICULAR CONDITIONS

Hydrocele: Cystic scrotal fluid collection that trans-illuminates. They are 2 types—communicating and non-communicating, and differentiated by change in size with progression of day. Communicating increases in size as day progresses.

Varicoceles: The spermatic cord feel like a bag of worms, certain medical conditions have been historically attached with it.

Testicular cancer: Painless mass and approximately 20 percent of cancer in males—15 to 35 years old.

Common risk factors are:
1. Cryptorchidism
2. Family history of testicular cancer
3. Cancer of the other testicle.

Scrotal ultrasound is the first diagnostic test and histopathology is the definitive diagnostic test. Once radiology is concerning next step is blood tests for various tumor markers, and finally radical inguinal orchiectomy.

The inguinal canal is a fibromuscular tunnel of the abdominal wall through which the spermatic cord/round ligament passes from the abdomen. **It is very important to understand the anatomy of the tunnel, as it is helpful in the treatment of hernia.** The aponeurosis of the external oblique muscle (anteriorly) and the transversus abdominus muscle and the transversalis fascia (posteriorly) form this structure. Laparoscopic hernia repairs especially transabdominal preperitoneal approach (TAPP) gives the best view to understand it.

Hesselbach's triangle weakness increases the risk for direct hernia, as mentioned earlier and is bounded by the inferior epigastric vessels, the inguinal ligament, and the rectus sheath. The canal is barely present in infants, hence hernias are more common.

- The external inguinal ring defect in external oblique muscle—superior and lateral to the pubic tubercle
- The internal inguinal ring defect in transversalis fascia with muscular shutter of transversus abdominus and internal oblique muscles
- Indirect inguinal hernias—lateral to the deep epigastric vessels through the inguinal canal
- Direct inguinal hernias are medial and inferior to the deep epigastric vessels and do not go through the inguinal canal
- Femoral hernias, below the inguinal ligament and medial to the femoral artery.

INGUINAL AND FEMORAL HERNIAS—DIAGNOSIS

Repair of hernia is the commonest surgical procedure and hence utmost important topic to learn. Hernia involves a weakness in fibromuscular layer. It can be internal or external. Details of internal and external hernia will be discussed in detail and examples are inguinal, femoral, ventral and umbilical. Greater than 95 percent groin hernias are inguinal hernias with M:F—9:1. Lifetime risk of inguinal hernia is 25 to 30 percent. There is an ongoing debate for indications of inguinal hernia surgery, but all femoral hernias need surgery.

Indirect inguinal hernias: The most common groin hernias in men and women. Its origin is lateral to the inferior epigastric artery, in contrast to direct hernias which arise medial to the inferior epigastric vessels.

Direct inguinal hernias: Defect in the Hesselbach's triangle (inguinal ligament inferiorly, the rectus abdominus muscle medially, and the inferior epigastric vessels laterally). It can be due to either congenital weakness or weakness in fibers with age or a combination of both.

Femoral hernias: It is an uncommon hernia, more commonly seen in elderly females, due to less muscular mass and post-pregnancy anatomical changes. Close to 40 percent are emergencies such as incarceration or strangulation in the empty space at the medial aspect of the femoral canal. Femoral hernias are at times difficult to differentiate from inguinal hernias and at time imaging studies like CT scan and MRI can be handy in identifying anatomy. There is some financial cost attached to it, hence majority of time, clinical history and examination assist in making diagnosis, and then definitive intraoperative diagnosis is made. Of all the hernias, femoral hernia has higher percentage of bowel symptoms.

Additional risk factors: Collagen disease type I and III. Smoking and steroid use have also been implicated in weakening of collagen fiber and hence hernia occurrence. There is also good evidence of ventral hernia in patients with aortic aneurysm. These patients have some genetic disorders of metalloproteinase and elastase enzyme.

Patients with hernia have a spectrum of presentation from a small bulge or bubonocele to bowel gangrene and peritonitis from strangulated hernia. In most cases there is worsening pain at the end of day.

Pain out of proportions is a sign of incarceration or strangulation, and it follow sequence of venous and lymphatic congestion, leading to incarceration and subsequent arterial blockage leads to gangrene. Patients may also have obstructive symptoms before incarceration and it can be relieved with gentle reduction (taxis). There are also situations where preperitoneal fat or omentum get involved, and patients have pain from the ischemia or necrosis of fat.

These patients have nonobstructive abdominal presentation with fever and localized redness. Patients with incarcerated hernia should be treated with emergency surgery, to rescue bowel from becoming gangrenous, if the hernia is not reduced. In case, hernia is reduced, patient must be observed in the hospital to confirm the reduced bowel was not gangrenous. If so, patient will need emergency surgery to have bowel resection. Patients with emergency surgery may not get definitive hernia repair as there is high risk of mesh infection, which is discussed in detail, in the later part of this chapter.

Patient should be examined with patient facing to sideways, and examiner's eye level with patient's hernia. In small hernia examine with coughing, straining, or performing a Valsalva maneuver.

As mentioned before radiologic techniques have been successful in an unclear clinical diagnosis.

Herniography, not a very sensitive test, and similarly ultrasound still not commonly used, but MRI is a very good test, and high cost still prevent its common use.

Inguinal hernia: One to five percent of all newborns and 9 to 11 percent of those born prematurely, 33 percent kids who have birth weight less than 1000 gm have hernia.

MANAGEMENT OF INGUINAL HERNIA—SURGICAL REPAIR

Incarcerated hernia is a surgical emergency and must be reduced at the earliest using sedation, Trendelenburg position, ice packing and the most important taxis/manual reduction, to avoid strangulation of the contents of the hernia sac. Manual reduction is the treatment, if child is appearing healthy, and is contraindicated if the child appears extremely ill with peritonitis or septic from gangrenous bowel. Emergency surgery has more complications hence manual reduction is opted, and is successful in greater than 95 percent of patients. **Manual pressure can take upto half an hour for reduction. The technique for reduction is very specific and must be learned from an experienced surgeon.**

Surgical repair is different in children than in adults. We will discuss management in premature infants, infants, adults, open and laparoscopic surgery.

- High ligation—the procedure of choice in pediatric patient population
- Although hernia is less common in female children, but needs a thorough evaluation for reproductive structure being inadvertently ligated and excised
- Laparoscopic herniorrhaphy can be advised in recurring hernia in pediatric population

- Another strong indication of laparoscopic repair is a proven or suspected bilateral hernia
- Patient should be advised surgery in elective setting. If hernia is incarcerated and subsequently reduced, a delay of 5-7 days, may enable more successful surgery, as swelling at hernia site will subside enabling better repair and low recurrence
- Premature infant should be operated sooner, as there is more likelihood of incarceration
- Children less than one year, also need elective surgery at the earliest, even if they do not have any incarceration, as the chances of incarceration are high. There are few studies to this effect, and more studies with randomization needed
- Preterm infants with low birth weight have 33 percent chance of having hernia, and surgery should be done before discharge, only when patient is medically stable.
- There is an increasing trend to not operate the contralateral side for inguinal hernia if it is nonclinical. It is more likely patent processus vaginalis will obliterate, if left alone.
- Patients postsurgery can have seroma, hydrocele, and may take 3 weeks to 3 months for swelling to resolve. Patients have 1 percent risk of infection. There is 5 to 10 percent chance of testicular atrophy, and vas injury
- Female infants with incarcerated hernia need emergency surgery even after reduction, as there is risk of ovarian torsion and gangrene. The chance to salvage ovary is good, if surgery is performed in 2 hours.

Inguinal hernioplasty has seen changes in philosophy of the technique, with aim to reduce hernia recurrences. The main principle of hernia repair was aimed at strengthening, the floor of the inguinal canal and tighten the external inguinal ring, then came the principle of tension free repair, to reduce recurrences. Various techniques of tension free repair are releasing/relaxing incision of rectus, placement of mesh, and laparoscopic repair. As of 2010, there is no consensus over the superiority of open mesh and laparoscopic hernia repair. Each has its own weaknesses and strengths, as discussed in the later part.

It is very important to learn old time tested nonmesh technique, tissue approximation repairs—the Bassini or McVay repair, as they are the hernia repairs in infected and gangrenous hernia. Use of mesh is absolutely contraindicated in these situations.

Open approaches—the Lichtenstein, a plug and patch, or an open preperitoneal approach. They have recurrence from 1 to 5 percent depending on the surgeons experience.

It is the duty of a surgeon, to discuss the risks and benefits of surgery. A clear expectation of the patient must be determined. All potential complications must be discussed in light of all the benefits.

LICHTENSTEIN REPAIR

- Preoperative antibiotics given in all patients, subcutaneous heparin given in patients over 40, or patient's with medical problems.
- Surgery can be performed under local, spinal or general depending of patient's requirements, and surgeon's expertize.
- A nerve block of the ilioinguinal and iliohypogastric nerves helps in surgery with little tissue swelling.
- Polypropylene mesh or any synthetic mesh is used to cover inguinal area.
- The medial edge of the mesh should be at least an inch medial to pubic tubercle.
- Surgeons should feel comfortable to sacrifice nerves and embed in muscles of conjoint tendon, rather than entrap in suture to prevent chronic groin pain. Ilioinguinal nerve is commonly involved.
- Nerve pain is the most common and dreaded complication of the procedure.
- The lower edge of the mesh is sewn to the shelving edge of the inguinal ligament.
- The upper edge of the mesh is sewn to the rectus sheath and internal oblique muscle.
- A key hole defect in the mesh is used to pass the cord structure and helps prevent future recurrences.
- Scarring from mesh prevents long-term hernia recurrence, and tension during mesh placement is the common cause of hernia recurrence. **Always secure mesh tension free.**
- Tension free placement of mesh, is the objective of laparoscopic surgery, both TEP (totally extraperitoneal) and TAPP (transabdominal properitoneal patch)—discussed in detail in later part.
- TEP is technically challenging in females due to dense scar between sac and round ligament.
- Females are more likely to have obstetric or gynecological procedures, and this makes laparoscopic procedures more challenging.
- Preperitoneal repair makes future anterior prostate surgery challenging in males, so patients with questionable prostate issues are better off with Lichtenstein repair.
- Lichtenstein repair does not help in femoral hernia.

- If there is difficulty in finding inguinal hernia during repair, explore the femoral hernia, by opening transversalis fascia.
- Dual mesh system commonly used by some surgeons, is a Lichtenstein repair with preperitoneal mesh, it covers both femoral and inguinal hernia.
- Results of Dual mesh repair are almost same as Lichtenstein repair.
- Some quick steps of preperitoneal repair—transversalis fascia over Hesselbach's triangle is opened, in the same direction as inguinal incision.
- Fascia opened from the pubic tubercle to the deep epigastric vessels.
- The preperitoneal space is dissected, the peritoneum and preperitoneal fat is freed from the muscles above.
- The extension of dissection is from linea alba medially and the anterior superior iliac spine laterally.
- Extent of exposure posteriorly the symphysis pubis, Cooper's ligament, femoral ring, cord structures, psoas muscle, and external iliac vessels.

Shouldice repair: This is a nonmesh technique developed in Shouldice Institute, Canada. The institute does tissue approximation in layers, and has a long postoperative rehabilitation path. It claims the recurrence rate of 1 percent, not achieved by any study with any technique so far.

Bassini repair: Approximating the conjoined tendon to the inguinal ligament from the pubic tubercle medially to the area of the internal ring laterally, using suture and closing the hernia defect. This procedure is still advocated in infected situation where prosthetic mesh is contraindicated. Only **used for inguinal hernia, no use in femoral hernia.**

McVay repair: Used for the repair of femoral and inguinal hernias. It is most challenging inguinal surgery to understand, as the anatomical landmarks require meticulous dissection. The repair creates tension and requires a relaxing incision.
- Divide transversalis fascia (Hesselbach's triangle) and delineate pectineal ligament (Cooper's ligament), (extension of the lacunar ligament on the pectineal line), in the preperitoneal space.
- Suture conjoined tendon to Cooper's ligament from the pubic tubercle medially to the femoral vein laterally.
- Here on, place a suture including the conjoined tendon, Cooper's ligament, and the inguinal ligament.
- Remaining repair is done by approximating conjoint tendon to the inguinal ligament lateral to the internal ring.

- Relaxing incision involves exposing rectus sheath. Important thing to remember is to spare the external oblique aponeurosis in relaxing incision. Almost 2-3 inches of relaxation incision is required.
- This procedure has a painful postoperative course.
- Mesh plug has been successfully used for femoral hernia as well.
- Preperitoneal mesh placement covers all the hernia defects (femoral, direct and indirect inguinal) and this technique is used both open or laparoscopically.
- Femoral hernia must be suspected when an exploration of inguinal hernia reveals no sac with cord or in Hesselbach's triangle. This is achieved by open fascia transversalis and opening preperitoneal space.
- TAPP has an added advantage of visualizing all the defects in one view, and the same mesh covers all the three openings.
- Repair: Incarcerated or strangulated inguinal and femoral hernias—an open approach.
- Opening sac before reducing the content ensures it is viable.
- If during anesthesia induction contents are spontaneously reduced, the bowel should be retrieved through the defect and examined for viability.
- The laparoscopy is another tool of importance to quickly examine the viability of bowel.
- Incarcerated femoral hernia have some challenges: In difficult cases—the lacunar ligament incised to enlarge the femoral ring.
- In extremely difficult situations: the inguinal ligament is divided above the defect.
- Gangrenous bowel is resected, and if there is difficulty in delivering bowel, lower midline incision can also be used.
- Bassini repair with a relaxing incision for incarcerated and strangulated inguinal hernias.
- McVay repair for incarcerated and strangulated femoral hernias.
- Truss use was advised in earlier times, but has been proven to be of no benefit.
- Sliding hernias have bowel, reproductive structures as wall of hernia. Extra care should be taken while placing sutures, and in case of small hernia, open the sac to ensure the presence of sliding hernia. The standard term will be peritonealization of sac.
- Another challenging area in hernia surgery is recurrence. Chances of failure increases with each surgery. The rule of thumb:

1. Recurrence after open surgery: Laparoscopic repair a better option, depending on surgeons expertise
2. Recurrence after laparoscopic surgery: Open repair a better option.

- Most common area of recurrence after repair is next to pubic tubercle:
  1. Hernia recurrence in standard hands is less than 5 percent, with a target of 2 percent.
  2. Mesh infection, chronic testicular pain, and testicular ischemia are serious complications.
  3. Most bothersome and common complication is groin pain, 30 percent patients may complain of pins and needles for 1 month and close to 5-10 percent for 3 months or more.
  4. Seroma is a common finding after surgery and is normal, unless it is infected.

Conservative watchful waiting of hernia has been discussed looking at the complications mentioned above. The studies have still not definitely indicated the factors that may lead an asymptomatic hernia to incarcerated/strangulated hernia. The incarceration risk is highest soon after the hernia is noticed, and decreases with time and size. It is necessary to be aware of the WW trial, and after two years follow-up, it did not show difference between the two groups.

Laparoscopic Repair

1. The totally extraperitoneal (TEP) repair is performed in the preperitoneal space. Peritoneum is not violated. Three ports are placed in midline from umbilicus down and the space is developed. This is most common of all the three repairs.
2. The transabdominal properitoneal patch (TAPP) repair, as the name suggests involve entering and reducing the hernia from abdominal side, and then placing the mesh and covering it with peritoneum, to prevent adhesions. In this technique peritoneum flap is raised and the hernia sac is reduced after identifying the anatomy. Then mesh is placed covering all defects, including direct, indirect and femoral defects. The mesh is mainly secured to pubic bone.
3. The intra-abdominal properitoneal onlay mesh (IPOM) repair, the mesh is placed from peritoneal side to cover the defect exposing the mesh to the bowels. This technique is completely out of favor and rarely used now.

Laparoscopic surgery advantages and disadvantages— Some of the details have already been discussed and some are discussed here. Major advantages are reduced postoperative pain, examination of all hernia defects, especially if there is questionable another hernia during office visit examination, visualization and repair of bilateral hernia, simultaneous repair of bilateral hernia, evaluation of other intra-abdominal conditions. However, serious complications with laparoscopic surgery have also been reported, including major vascular injury, bowel obstruction, bladder injury and nerve injury.

A large section of surgical community still is not convinced with the advantages of laparoscopic repair. Its surgeon's preference and competence in repair and fixation can be good either way, as long as surgeon has expertise in his technique.

Laparoscopic repair enables heavy manual labor to work quicker.

Open repair helps an older and debilitated patient, as the surgery is done under local anesthesia.

Special considerations for femoral hernia: we have already discussed the common fixation technique:

1. The easier approach is anterior and caudal to the inguinal ligament. The hernia sac and its content identified and reduced and the defect repaired with mesh or direct suture.
2. If hernia and sac is large or if there is concern for bowel gangrene or viability, the best approach is the pre-peritoneal approach. The transversus abdominis and transversalis fascia are divided and any intra-abdominal contents are removed from the hernia. This enables as mentioned before reduce large incarcerated hernia with division of lacunar ligament and in rare cases inguinal ligament.

Patients with manual labor should refrain from heavy lifting in excess of 10 kg for approximately four weeks, and driving should be avoided, till patient is off of all pain medication and generally its 7-10 days.

Surgical Complications Hernia Repair

1. Pain and neuralgia: This is the most common complication early and delayed. The ilioinguinal and genitofemoral nerves are commonly involved in open surgery. Prophylactic ilioinguinal neurectomy at the time of surgery has lower incidence of chronic groin pain at six months, about 60 percent less and no difference in sensory loss, than patients with preserved nerve.

The lateral femoral nerve of the thigh involved in laparoscopic repair.
2. Seroma and bruising
3. Early recurrence: Seen in cases of infection, undue tension, obese patients, smoking, questionable steroid therapy and tissues devascularization.
4. Infection: This is very dreaded and frightening complication especially in cases where mesh is infected. The risks have been documented from 2 to 10 percent in various studies. The risk of infection reduction with preoperative antibiotic use decreases from 4 to 3 percent (in one large RCT), and this reduction is not statistically significant, to make a case for mandatory preoperative antibiotics.
5. Patients with mesh repair have an increased wound infection. There is evidence in mesh repair, of reduction in mesh infection with preoperative antibiotics; again this is a meta-analysis.
6. Patients with large hernia, especially after laparoscopic hernia may complain of swelling in the groin, which can be fluid in the sac left behind. This is at times called pseudohernia. If on examination no impulse on coughing wait and watch is a reasonable option, or perform CT scan to ensure no recurrence, again each test has its limitations.

Recurrent hernia: Hernia recurrences is studied in three time frames:
- Immediate: Can be technical, missed hernia or biomaterial breakdown or patient's noncompliance
- Six months to five years: Generally technical
- Late recurrences later than 5 years: Patients tissues and body physiology.

BIBLIOGRAPHY

1. Nyhus and Condon's hernia, Oct 1, 2001.

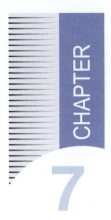

Pediatric Surgery

Tarun Kumar, Pankaj Dangle

PHYSIOLOGY

Pediatric patients necessitate a unique surgical intervention due to the distinctive physiologic and anatomic causes for variety of illness.

- The management of prepubertal patients is immensely different than in adult.

PHYSIOLOGICAL ASPECT OF CHILDREN

Metabolism/Nutrition

1. During the growth phase the metabolic requirements in children's are geared towards different goals compared to adults.
2. Both the neonatal and juvenile age group necessitates substantially higher energy requirements as compared to adults with:
   - higher basal metabolic rate
   - majority of energy substrates being utilized for growth. In neonatal age group the birth weight is twofold by 5 months, three times by 1 year and 4 times by 3 years with subsequent decline till puberty.
3. Due to the higher energy requirements children are at higher risk to switch to catabolic state during periods of stress.

   In the pediatric population the pattern on the "Growth Curve" is unique and substantially well defined. With which, any deviation in the normal growth is a preliminary evidence of a pathological process.

   In many instances, starvation and/or a stress response are the primary initiators of a catabolic metabolism.

   During starvation metabolism, the energy source for most vital organs is via ketogenesis.

While with any stress response such as surgery and/ or any acute illness, the pathway of ketogenesis is inhibited making tissue glucose requirements critically important.

4. Energy consumption
   - The baseline resting energy expenditure in neonates is twofold (45-50 kcal/kg/day) as compared to adolescents and adults (20-25 kcal/kg/day).

Age in years	Kcal/kg/day
0-1	90-120
1-7	75-90
7-12	60-75
12-18	30-60

- Glucose is the major source of energy in the neonatal age group.
  - At birth, subsequent to the separation of the placenta, glycogenolysis is the vital source of glucose until feeding is commenced.
  - Since the major source of glycogen stores is produced 36-40 weeks of gestation, preterm infants are at increased risk for starvation metabolism.
  - **In premature infants** the skeletal muscle and fat represent only 1 percent of body weight compared to term infants (15%) making trivial reserve for both lipolysis and gluconeogenesis to provide alternative source of energy supply.
  - When enteral feeding cannot be initiated or tolerated, alternative forms of energy in the form of total parenteral nutrition should be commenced.
- During fasting-neonate and young children tolerate 1 week without nutritional support, whereas old children and adolescent comparable to adults can go up to 1-3 weeks without nutrition.

- Enteral nutrition
  - First year of life at least 100-120 kcal/kg/day are required to meet baseline resting energy requirements to fulfill the growth
  - Both the breast milk and formula contains 0.67 kcal/ml (20 kcal/oz)
  - To calculate 3 hours oral requirements based on gastric emptying = weight in kg × 22.5 (where 22.5 is a coefficient derived from energy requirements and kcal density of standard formula; for continuous feedings via feeding tubes, the coefficient is 7.3 (i.e. 22/3).

Renal Physiology and Fluids/Electrolytes

1. Deficient homeostatic mechanism and even a trivial derangement in chemistry can lead to significant changes and response in both the neonates and small children.
2. In neonates the majority (75-80%) of the total body weight is due to water.
3. Immediate post delivery, the decreased vascular resistance leads to increased renal blood flow and thereby giving 3 distinct phases of fluid management:

Phase	Duration	Amount of urine produced
Prediuretic	Initial 24 hrs of life	1 ml/kg/hr
Diuretic	24 hrs -4th day of life	5-10 ml/kg/hr
Postdiuretic	2nd week to 1-2 years	Slow decline to adult level of renal blood flow and glomerular filtration rate

Thus it is important to be aware of the weight loss in first week of life is a normal phenomenon related to the diuretic phase even in preterm infants.

4. Renal concentrating capacity (RCC)
   - The serum osmolality in children especially in infants as is lower roughly 600-700 mOsm/L compared to adults (1200-1400 mOsm/L)
   - Despite lower GFR, the lower concentrating capacity of kidney makes handling of large water load is uncomplicated.
   - As compared to adults (70-100 mOsm/L), infants are able to make diluted urine upto dilute as 50 mOsm/L.
5. Urine output is the most reliable indicator of fluid balance in all age groups.
   - Renal solute excretion is maintained at a rate of 0.5 ml/kg/hr

- Pediatric patients require elevated fluid turnover secondary to the augmented metabolic demand with growth.
  - Premature infants—4 ml/kg/hr
  - Infants—2 ml/kg/hr
  - Toddlers—1 ml/kg/hr

In pediatric patients maintenance fluid requirements per hour could be roughly calculated as given below:

Weight	Maintenance fluid per hour
First 10 kg	4 ml/kg/hr
Next 10 kg	2 ml/kg/hr
Additional kg BW	1 ml/kg/hr

6. Physiological handling of sodium
   - In term infants and young children the per day sodium requirements are approximately 2-3 mEq/kg/day.
   - Whereas premature infants are "salt-wasters" and require relatively higher levels of sodium replacement.
   - In healthy young children (D10 ¼NS) whereas in preterm infants (D10 ½ NS) will meet the required sodium requirements.
   - Both the third space losses and electrolyte shifts requiring a change in fluid administration are paramount importance in postsurgical patients. The preferred fluids for managing these patients are:

Age	Type of solution	Rate for initial 12 hrs
<6 months	D10 ½ NS	1.5 times maintenance
>6 months	D10 Lactated Ringer's	1.5 times maintenance

Pulmonary Physiology

1. There are 5 phases of pulmonary development:
   - Embryonic (Gestation week 3)
   - Pseudoglandular (week 7-16)
   - Canalicular (week 17-24)
   - Terminal saccular (week 24-40)
   - Alveolar (birth to 8 years).
2. The type II pneumocytes responsible for surfactant production develop in the canalicular phase, i.e. phase 3. The canalicular phase is critical in preterm babies as this is the earliest time at which functional gas exchange occurs and is the earliest survivable gestational age at birth which is currently 22-24 weeks gestation.
3. The term infants are born with roughly 20 million alveolar units as compared to the adult level of 300 million during the alveolar phase.

4. Total lung capacity (TLC) = inspiratory reserve volume (IRV) + tidal volume (TV) + expiratory reserve volume (ERV) + and residual volume (RV)

   The 2 critical measures within the combined spectrum of the ERV and RV are the functional residual capacity (FRC) and closing capacity (CC)
   - FRC is the volume of air at the end of a tidal breath
   - CC is the volume at which alveolar units begin to collapse.
5. Role of surfactant
   - Produced by type II pneumocytes during the terminal saccular phase and reduces the surface tension in the alveoli. The surfactant reduces the surface tension and thereby the CC based on the Laplace relationship of P = 2T / R (P = pressure, T = wall tension, R = radius): Due to the direct relationship reducing T, reduces the pressure at which low radius alveoli must be maintained to resist elastic recoil and collapse and thus the CC reduced.
   - Respiratory distress syndrome (RDS) of newborn with resultant alveolar collapse secondary to insufficient surfactant is seen in neonates born during the late canalicular to early terminal saccular phase of development.

Cardiac Physiology

- Transition from placental to postnatal circulation is the critical difference between pediatric and adult cardiac physiology.
- The intrauterine phase, two physiologic shunts allow the oxygenated blood from the placenta to pass directly into the systemic circulation
  - Foramen ovale: Window between the right and left atria.
  - Ductus arteriosus: Vascular connection between the pulmonary artery and the aorta letting diversion of right heart blood away from the unexpanded fetal lungs.
  - The right and left flow are in parallel rather in series.
- Changes in circulation after birth
  - Compression in birth canal amniotic fluid is expelled from the lungs.
  - The lungs expand and pulmonary vascular resistance drops with the first breath.
  - Low vascular resistance leads to increased blood flow into the lungs with increased preload to the left atrium.
  - The flap over forman ovale closes secondary to higher pressures in the left atrium, closing the first of the two shunts.

- Patent foramen ovale-failure of closure leads to a common defect called atrial septal defect. Patent doramen of ovale generally remains asymtomatic but can be symptomatic ossasionally.
- Ductus arteriosus closes mostly within 24 hrs of birth due to decreasing circulating placental prostaglandins and an increasing oxygen.
  - Patent ductus arteriosus (PDA) is common in preterm babies and based on the pressure difference between pulmonary artery and aorta, it can lead to right to left shunt leading to pulmonary hypertension and congestive heart failure or left to right shunt causing hypoxia.
  - The stasis the ductus venosus/umbilical vein shuts as well as the flow through the umbilical arteries.
  - In extreme circumstances the umbilical vein may be kept open via catheterization and used as venous access.

Differences in Pediatric and Adult Cardiac Physiology

Cardiac output is determined by preload/heart rate and contractility/afterload:
- **Preload**
  - The main determining factor is venous return, increasing myocardial stretch with increased blood volume at end-diastole. The neonatal heart is less compliant than the adult heart.
  - The neonatal myocardium characteristically fills maximally at diastole with consequential maximum stretch at baseline.
- **Contractility**
  - The neonatal myocardium has decreased contractility secondary to lesser contractile fibers than adult.
  - Neonate myocardium is more sensitive to negative ionotropic stimuli secondary to an immature sympathetic innervation resulting in a dominant parasympathetic system.
  - Whereas neonatal myocardium is more resistant to negative effects of hypoxia and acidosis as compared to adults.
- **Afterload**
  - Following the first breath resultant low vascular resistance decreases right heart afterload whereas the shunt closure on left simultaneously increases the left afterload.
  - Increased systemic afterload during the initial 2-3 years of life, leads to left heart hypertrophy.

– Neonatal myocardium in early life is exquisitely sensitive to high afterload such as seen with aortic stenosis or coarctation of aorta.
- Neonate has lower cardiac reserve and is rate-dependent for cardiac output; secondary to immature myocardium it is unable to adjust preload, contractility, and afterload effectively as compared to adults.

TORTICOLLIS

Congenital

A congenital shortening of the sternocleidomastoid muscle and term is derived from Latin word "toquere" for twisted and "collum" for neck.

It could be secondary to two possible causes:
1. Fixed position in uterus leads to shortening and tightening of one sternocleidomastoid muscle.
2. Trauma during passage through the birth canal due large baby or abnormal presentation.

Acquired

Acquired type which is due to a variety of causes:
   i. Atlantoaxial subluxation
  ii. Brainstem tumors
 iii. Infectious causes like tonsillitis, retropharyngeal abscess and cervical lymphadenopathy.

Physical examination: Head is tilted toward the involved side with the chin slightly rotated away from the involved muscle.

Management

Physiotherapy for gentle stretching of the neck muscle. If condition does not improve with physiotherapy, then surgical intervention may require (**division of the involved sternocleidomastoid**).

Cystic Hygroma

A benign multiloculated lymphatic malformation from due failure of fusion of lymphatics with the venous system, and resulting in a malformed collection of blind ending lymphatics form causing a hygroma.

Embryology: Lymphatics begin to develop from mesenchymal clefts in the 6th gestational week.

Incidence: Approximately 60 to 70 percent present at birth, the remainder present within the first two years of life and mostly in the neck or axilla, but they may occur anywhere in the body.

Presentation

a. Mostly asymptomatic.
b. It can be symptomatic with various presentations:
   - Respiratory distress due to airways obstruction or due huge size of hygroma, it could be life-threatening
   - Infectious and presents with erythema, fever, pain and leading to septicemia, if not treated with antibiotics in infective stage
   - Hemorrhage can occur in 10 to 15 percent of cases and presents with rapidly enlarging, painful mass.

Management

Imaging studies may require CT or MRI scanning depending on the availability, and preferably MRI is better to delineate the lesion and its relation to adjacent vital structures.

Treatment

Medical treatment: Injection of sclerosing agents (Bleomycin, ethanol and OK-432, a derivative of penicillin and *Streptococcus pyogenes*, is a trial drug that has been effective in large, cystic lesions and less effective in multicystic lesions.

Surgical resection is the treatment of choice.

If mass is asymptomatic and increasing in size, surgery may be delayed until 6 to 12 months. Immediate surgery is indicated, if there is airway obstruction. The complications include persistent leak of lymph or fistula formation, chylothorax, hemorrhage.

BRANCHIAL CLEFT REMNANTS

A congenital anomaly of the neck due to persistence of the fetal branchial clefts.

Embryology

The branchial clefts form in the 4th to 8th week of gestation and four pairs of branchial arches form in the cervicofacial region of the embryo with clefts expressed externally and pouches expressed internally.
- Cleft I becomes the Eustachian tube and a portion of the external auditory canal
- Cleft II is obliterated without a distinct adult counterpart
- Cleft III migrates inferiorly to form the inferior parathyroid glands and the thymus
- Cleft IV migrates inferiorly, but stops above the final level of cleft III, and forms the superior parathyroid glands and thyroid C-cells.

Pathophysiology

Incomplete obliteration of the clefts as the fetal neck develops.

It may form cysts, sinuses, fistulas, and cartilaginous remnants and cleft remnants.
- Cleft I remnants occur along the angle of the mandible and sinuses/fistulas may extend to the external auditory canal.
- Cleft II remnants occur along the anterior border of the sternocleidomastoid muscle and may communicate with the tonsillar fossa (the most common form)
- Cleft III and IV remnants are rare and communicate between the piriform sinus and the glands they form or the neck lower than 2nd cleft remnants.

Management

Diagnosis

Clinical presentation may be discharging sinus or cystic mass and location of the lesion as mentioned above.
- **Cleft I** remnants may present as sinuses or fistulas draining along the angle of the mandible with history of recurrent watery discharge with or without infection.
- **Cleft II** remnants are by far the most common and present as fistulas or sinuses along the anterior border of the sternocleidomastoid (**Fistulous tracts cross the bifurcation of the carotid artery between the internal and external carotid arteries and it may ends in the tonsillar fossa**).
- **Cleft III** and IV remnants typically present as thyroid lobe abscesses at later age in childhood and CT scan may be helpful.

Treatment

Complete surgical excision is the treatment of choice after treating the infection.

Thyroglossal Duct Cysts

Cyst formed from thyroglossal duct remnant, the path of downward migration of the thyroid gland from the base of the tongue to its adult location.

It is found in the midline and may contain of thyroid tissue or only thyroid tissue in the body.

Pathophysiology

It develops when the thyroglossal duct fails to obliterate following migration of the thyroid gland from the foramen cecum on the base of the tongue to the neck. It may occur anywhere along the path of the thyroglossal duct. The ectopic thyroid tissue along the duct may develop into papillary adenocarcinoma. The duct passes through the central portion of the hyoid bone during its descent. It could be the patient's only functional thyroid tissue in rare cases.

Management

Diagnosis

Clinical presentation of a mass in the midline between the submental region and the superior aspect of the trachea and may present as a midline abscess in the neck if there is communication with the base of the tongue with resultant contamination.

Non-infected cysts are soft, smooth, and non-tender and cysts may move with swallowing or protrusion of the tongue.

Treatment

The surgical excision is the treatment of choice. It should include the cyst, tract, and the entire central portion of the hyoid bone and carried up the foramen cecum at the base of the tongue.

If thyroid tissue is present in the resected specimen, thyroid function tests should be performed to rule out iatrogenic hypothyroidism. If it left untreated or inadequately treated, recurrence or the possibility of ectopic thyroid carcinoma is the possibility.

THORAX

Chest Wall Anomalies

It represents deformity in development of the supportive architecture of the chest and the functional impairment.

Embryology

The ribs are formed by segmental somites that advance ventrally toward the sternum, which develops from two mesoderm bands that eventually fuse in the center. The costal cartilages link the developing ribs to the sternum.

Types

1. Pectus excavatum
2. Pectus carinatum
3. Sternal cleft.

Pectus Excavatum

The most common chest wall deformity, present in 1/300-400 live births. It can be unilateral or bilateral, but typically involves 3 or more ribs on the affected side, and degree of deformity can vary due to abnormal growth regulation of the costal cartilages. It rarely affects cardiopulmonary function and it may leads to psychosocial impairment due to cosmetic look.

Mostly it is asymptomatic. It could be symptomatic depending on the severity of deformity and compromising the cardiopulmonary functions.

Management

X-ray chest and CT scan may be helpful.

Treatment

Surgical correction is in late childhood or adolescence as earlier correction can lead to thoracic dystrophy. The surgical techniques, as described by Ravitch, involve resection of costal cartilages, elevation of the sternum off of mediastinal and muscular structures, osteotomy of the sternum and reinforcement of the sternum with a strut.

Nuss procedure is a minimally invasive technique in which a metal bar is advanced under the sternum, which is then left in place to push the defect back into normal position. The bar is removed usually after 2 years.

Pectus Carinatum

A protrusive appearance with outward displacement of the sternum and it becomes more pronounced in adolescence and disfiguring.

Management

Nonoperative Treatment

Brass application is effective way for correcting the deformity.

Operative Treatment

Surgical correction is purely cosmetic as no physiologic deficit occurs with pectus carinatum and includes osteotomies that flatten the sternum.

Sternal Cleft

It occurs when the sternal bars of mesoderm fail to completely fuse during development.

It usually occurs as the part of the pentalogy of Cantrell: sternal cleft, omphalocele, diaphragmatic defect, pericardial defect, and intracardiac defect.

Surgical Correction

Reapproximation of the cleft in the midline is curative and if it is incomplete, the cleft must be divided completely for adequate healing.

Pulmonary Sequestration

It is an abnormal lung tissue that develops without normal communication with the trachea or a bronchus with an aberrant blood supply. It is more common in male (M: F 4:1).

Blood supply: Arterial supply from the aorta and venous drainage is either the pulmonary or systemic circulation.

Types: Intralobar vs extralobar

	Intralobar	Extralobar
Location	Within chest/medial aspect of lower lobes	Chest/diaphragm or retroperitoneum
Covering	Visceral pleura	No pleura
Blood supply	Mostly vessel from infradiaphragmatic aorta	Mostly vessel from infradiaphragmatic aorta

a. *Intralobar sequestrations* are essentially within the chest and are invested by visceral pleura and are located in medial or posterior segments of the lower lobes. With majority are fed by vessels arising from the infra-diaphragmatic aorta running through the inferior pulmonary ligament.
b. *Extralobar sequestrations* are not invested by pulmonary pleura and may occur within the chest, diaphragm, or the retroperitoneum.

Most often incidentally detected and is frequently associated with other congenital anomalies. Left side is more commonly affected with rarely a communication with foregut.

Pathogenesis: Not completely understood with possible origin from either accessory lung bud or primitive foregut with angiogenesis occurring from the aorta.

In intralobar variant there is no distinctive bronchus present, but usually has microcommunications with the airways leading to infection of the lung sequestration.

Most common presentation is recurrent lung infection in early childhood.

Diagnosis

Chest X-ray reveals an inferiorly located consolidation with aeration.

Recently contrast CT scan and MRI has replaced the need for angiography.

The extralobar variety is diagnosed during an evaluation for a different congenital anomaly. It is rarely associated with aeration unless has a communication with foregut.

Treatment

Intralobar: In symptomatic cases surgical resection is the standard of care. Due to inability to distinguish between the sequestration segments from surrounding pulmonary lobe, frequently a completion lobectomy is required.

Extralobar: Typically observed unless communication with foregut with resultant infection or an extrinsic compression on GI tract.

Esophageal Atresia/Tracheoesophageal Fistula

Esophageal atresia is defined as a congenital disruption of esophageal development resulting in blind ending esophagus with obstruction.

Tracheoesophageal (TE) fistula is defined as an abnormal fistulous communication between the trachea and esophagus that often occurs in conjunction with esophageal atresia.

Anatomical variants of esophageal atresia/TE fistula
1. Blind ending proximal and distal pouches without TE fistula (6%)
2. Proximal TE fistula with distal blind pouch (2%)
3. Proximal blind pouch with distal TE fistula (85%)
4. Proximal and distal pouches with TE fistula (1%)
5. Pure TE fistula without esophageal atresia (2%).

Both esophageal atresia and TE fistula is frequently seen with a constellation of multiple anomalies known as the **VACTERL syndrome.**

[V = Vertebral Anomalies, A = Anorectal Malformation, C = Cardiac Abnormalities, TE = Tracheoesophageal Fistula, R = Renal Anomalies, L = Limb Deformity]

In a patient either one, multiple or all anomalies may be present together.

Pathogenesis

During 4th week of gestation, the laryngotracheal tube, a common embryologic source for both the trachea and esophagus, forms. A tracheoesophageal septum formed by lateral invagination divides the tube into trachea and esophagus.

A defect in the formation of septum or the division of the results in esophageal atresia and TE fistula.

Diagnosis is established at birth with excessive secretion and inability to pass nasogastric tube.

Once the primary diagnosis is established, imaging to rule out associated VACTERL anomalies should be performed.
- Imaging of the chest and spine
- Echocardiogram
- Renal ultrasonography
- Examination of anus and limbs
- Genetic work-up.

Treatment is surgical with division of TE fistula and anastomosis of the esophageal ends.
- *Short gap atresia* (defined as < 2 ½ vertebral body height) –single stage repair
- *Long gap atresia:* Staged procedure based on the length and type of defect, also requires feeding gastrostomy prior to anastomosis.
  - stretching of both pouches by serial dilation
  - surgical fistulization and suture placement at both the ends
  - Circular esophagomyotomy with primary anastomosis
  - Cervical spit fistula of proximal end with sequential lengthening down the neck.

Congenital Diaphragmatic Hernia

Congenital diaphragmatic hernia (CDH) is defined as congenital defect in the development of the diaphragm that allows migration of peritoneal contents into the chest cavity leading to pulmonary hypoplasia.

Two distinct types:
a. Bochdalek: Most common type, with defect in the posterolateral location.
b. Morgagni: Rare anteromedial defect located behind the sternum.

Pathophysiology

The muscular diaphragm is formed by combination of inward growth of lateral body musculature and the primordial diaphragm formed by the pleuroperitoneal membranes. Failure of closure the pleuroperitoneal membranes lead to CDH. The right sided defects are less common due to earlier closure of the right pleuroperitoneal membrane and the protective mass effect of the liver. The overall mortality rate is about 30 to 40 percent.

Occasionally, CDH is difficult to differentiate from eventration of the diaphragm, either congenital or the acquired from paralysis of the phrenic nerve.

Diagnosis: Classically diagnosed on prenatal ultrasound by polyhydramnios (80%) and at birth the neonates present with cyanosis and respiratory distress.

Mild cases may remain asymptomatic or present with chronic respiratory infections, pneumonia, feeding difficulty or bowel obstruction.

Most cases are usually confirmed with the chest X-ray.

Treatment

In utero fetal surgery in select centers (EXIT procedure).

Postnatal
- Treatments in neonatal intensive care unit with pulmonary support
- Extracorporeal membrane oxygenation (ECMO)
- High oscillation ventilation
- Partial liquid ventilation
- Inhaled nitric oxide and exogenous surfactant.
  Mainstay of treatment: **Surgical repair** with reduction of the abdominal contents.

In spite of improve diagnosis surgical care and postnatal care survival is significantly dependent on the degree of the pulmonary hypoplasia.

Abnormalities of Abdominal Wall

Gastroschisis

Gastroschisis or "split stomach" is a misnomer. The condition is secondary to defect of the anterior abdominal wall musculature.

Presentation

Always presents with intestine protruding through the abdominal wall defect into the amniotic cavity. More common in males, with defect being exclusively on right side and umbilicus is always spared. These subgroups of patients have low risk of congenital or genetic anomalies.

Pathogenesis

There are no well-defined etiological causes known, but the proposed etiological agents are as follows:
- More frequent with maternal age < 20 years of age

- Increase use of cigarette, alcohol, and recreational drug
- Increase use of aspirin, ibuprofen, and pseudoephedrine.

The intestine is typically shortened, thickened, and matted or adherent together, occasionally 15 percent cases present with intestinal atresia.

Diagnosis

Routinely detected on prenatal ultrasound, once diagnosed should be managed at a facility with neonatal intensive care, pediatric surgery, and high-risk obstetrics coverage.

Management

The immediate post-delivery care includes:
- Covering the intestine in a moist, sterile dressing
- Nasogastric tube decompression
- Intravenous access with hydration and broad antibiotic coverage.

Definitive Treatment

Abdominal contents are easily reducible—**primary closure**.

Unable to reduce: **Application of silo bag** with sequential tightening until intestines reduce back and abdominal wall closure without much tension.

Postoperative course is prolonged with inevitable postoperative ileus. The patients are managed with parenteral nutrition with frequent monitoring of liver function test.

Omphalocele

Definition

Abdominal wall defect in which viscera extrude through the umbilicus and are covered by a peritoneal and amniotic sac.

High association with genetic and congenital abnormalities:
- Trisomy 13, 18, and 21
- Cardiac, musculoskeletal, and gastrointestinal anomalies are common
- Beckwith-Wiedemann syndrome: Exomphalos (omphalocele), macroglossia, gigantism and hyperinsulinemia, hypoglycemia
- 1:5000 live births have omphalocele with herniation of intestine
- 1:10,000 live births have omphalocele with herniation of intestine and solid organs.

Pathogenesis

- Between the 6th and 10th week of normal gestation, the abdominal contents herniate into the umbilicus and undergo a series of coordinated rotations before returning to the peritoneal cavity after which the abdominal wall closes.
- Omphalocele occurs when the intestine fails to return to the abdominal cavity. The inner lining of the omphalocele sac is peritoneum; the outer covering is epithelium of the umbilical cord, derived from the amniotic sac.

Diagnosis and Treatment

- Typically diagnosed by prenatal ultrasound
- Pre- and postnatal care is essentially the same for omphalocele as for gastroschisis
- Work-up for associated anomalies should be undertaken.

Exstrophy of the Bladder

Definition

- Defect in the infraumbilical abdominal wall with failure of the median inferior portion to close, resulting in exposure and protrusion of the posterior wall of the urinary bladder through the defect
- In males, almost uniformly associated with epispadias
- In females, almost uniformly associated with bifid clitoris
- Occurs 1 in every 10,000 to 40,000 live births.

Pathophysiology

- During the 4th week of gestation, mesenchymal cells migrate into the space between the cloaca and ectoderm of the primitive abdomen
- Failure of this migration leads to no development of abdominal musculature in this position
- Eventually the thin epidermis and anterior wall of the bladder rupture allowing wide exposure of the mucous membrane of the bladder.

Diagnosis and Treatment

- Diagnosis is clinical by inspection
- Surgical correction consists of closure of the bladder plate and concurrent repair of epispadias in boys
- Surgical repair should proceed within 72 hours of birth.

Umbilical Hernia

Definition

- A defect in the connective tissue around the umbilicus present at birth
- The most common abdominal wall defect in the newborn
- Tends to occur more commonly in African-American infants than in Caucasian infants.

Pathophysiology

- Failure of complete closure of the linea alba at the umbilicus
- The umbilicus is reinforced by the paired umbilical ligaments (umbilical artery remnants), the round ligament (umbilical vein remnant), the urachus (remnant of the primitive allantois), and the transversalis fascia
- Weakness or failure of any of the reinforcing structures can predispose to umbilical hernia.

Diagnosis and Treatment

- Diagnosis is clinical by inspection and palpation
- In most cases of congenital umbilical hernia, the defect with close spontaneously during the first 3 years of life
- If the hernia persists at five years of age, surgical closure is indicated.

Congenital Inguinal Hernia/Hydrocele

Definition

- *Inguinal hernia*: Due failure of processus vaginalis to close and allowing herniation of abdominal contents into the inguinal ring and possibly the scrotum
- *Hydrocele*: A collection of fluid around the testicle within tunica vaginalis
- Predisposing factors include prematurity
- Represents the most common indication for surgery in the infant population.

Pathophysiology

- The testes develop intra-abdominally and migrate along a path created by the gubernaculum
- The testis descends into the scrotum through the processus vaginalis, a canal which protrudes through the abdominal wall into the inguinal canal

- After descent of the testis, the processus vaginalis closes and is obliterated
- Failure of the processus vaginalis to close, allowing herniation of intra-abdominal contents results in a congenital inguinal hernia
- Partial closure of the processus vaginalis with resultant collection of fluid results in hydrocele
- Hydrocele may be *communicating*, in which a small opening in the proximal processus vaginalis remains open, that allows fluid passage but not herniation; or *noncommunicating* in which proximal closure of the processus vaginalis occurs with distal fluid collection.

Diagnosis and Treatment

- Diagnosis is clinical
  - Typical history of a groin bulge that enlarges with crying or straining with hernias or a stable scrotal or groin swelling for hydrocele
  - Most reduce spontaneously or with gentle pressure
  - Hydrocele will transilluminate on exam
- Surgical treatment is indicated at the time of diagnosis for inguinal hernias and communicating hydrocele, which have a tendency to develop into true hernias
- Noncommunicating hydrocele may be observed as they tend to resolve spontaneously during first 2 years of life.

Common Cystic Lesion in the Abdominal Cavity

- *Mesenteric cyst*
  - Cystic intra-abdominal mass
  - Pain and emesis
  - Mostly located at the mesenteric side of the intestine
- *Duplication cyst*
  - Anywhere along the gastrointestinal tract
  - All three layers of intestine present in the cyst
  - Types
    - Tubular (communicating)
    - Cystic (noncommunicating)
  - Diagnosis
    - Physical findings
    - X-ray abdomen
    - Ultrasonography and CT abdomen
  - Surgery
    - Excision of cyst with or without bowel resection depending on extent of lesions
- *Omental cyst*
  - Cyst filled with lymphatic fluid
  - Palpable mass, tenderness

- Treatment: Laparoscopic or open exploratory laparotomy
- *Hepatic cyst (single or multiple)*
  - Congenital
  - Acquired
  - Clinical features
    - Abdominal pain
    - Jaundice, if big enough to cause pressure over the biliary tree
  - Imaging
    - US abdomen
    - CT scan of the abdomen
    - If complicated cyst MRCP or MRI abdomen is useful.
    - HIDA scan to rule out biliary connectors
  - Surgery
    - Noncommunicating cyst
      - Laparoscopic or open marsupalization
    - Communicating cyst
      - Roux-en-Y drainage
- *Choledochal cyst*
  - Cystic malformation of biliary tree (types)
    - Saccular or diffuse dilatation of extrahepatic bile duct
    - Diverticulum of extrahepatic bile duct
    - Choledochocele
    - Multiple cysts of extra- or intrahepatic bile duct
    - Single or multiple intrahepatic bile duct
  - Clinical features
    - Palpable mass and pain abdomen (cholangitis)
    - Cholestatic jaundice (obstructive)
    - Clay colored stools (alcoholic)
  - Diagnosis
    - Conjugated hyperbilirubinemia
    - Ultrasound abdomen
    - CT abdomen
    - MRCP is superior than CT abdomen
    - HIDA scan
    - ERCP may be useful in late presentation as kids are grown up
  - Treatment
    - Cystectomy with Roux-en-Y end to side hepatico-jejunostomy
- *Lymphangioma*
  - Abnormal cystic collection of lymph, mostly in the retroperitoneum
  - Clinical features
    - Palpable mass
    - Pain

- Laparoscopic or open operation
  • Marsupialization of cystic area with drainage
  • Total excision, if possible.
• *Urachal remnant*
  - Lower abdomen mass, mostly in midline along the course of urachus
  - Presents with discharging umbilicus
  - Diagnosis
    • Ultrasound abdomen and pelvis
    • Cystourethrogram
  - Treatment
    • Excision of urachus remnant with repair of urinary bladder, if it is involved.

GASTROINTESTINAL TRACT

Hypertrophic Pyloric Stenosis

• Definition: Gastric outlet obstruction due to hypertrophy of the pyloric muscle, resulting in narrowing of the pyloric lumen.
• Incidence: More common in males than females
• Pathophysiology:
  - It is not clear, few theories are proposed and most commonly accepted theory is deficiency of nitric oxide synthase in the pylorus resulting in inability of pyloric muscle to relax resulting in muscular hypertrophy
  - The maximum thickness occurs between the 4th and 8th week of age
• Diagnosis:
  - Projectile, non-bilious emesis beginning in the 2nd to 4th week of life
  - Palpable abdominal mass or "olive" in the epigastrium
  - Hypokalemic-hypochloremic alkalosis on blood work-up
  - Diagnostic procedure of choice is pyloric ultrasonography that shows a thickened pyloric muscle (4 mm or more) and pyloric channel length (17 mm or more)
  - Contrast upper GI series is required, when physical examination and USG abdomen are not conclusive.
• Treatment:
  - Preoperatively fluid resuscitation-IV hydration and serum electrolyte correction
  - Surgical pyloromyotomy (Laparoscopic or open Ramstedt) in which all layers except mucosa are divided along the entire hypertrophied segment.

Duodenal Atresia/Stenosis/Web

• Obliteration of a segment of duodenum during development that results in a stricture or blind-ending obstruction (atresia)
• Narrowing of duodenal lumen secondary to annular pancreas (stenosis)
• Diaphragm with or without hole blocking the duodenal lumen (web)
  - Three types:
    • Type 1 (92%): Intraluminal web or diaphragm with intact mesentery and intact seromuscular layers in the involved intestinal segment
    • Type 2 (1%): Fibromuscular cord replaces intestinal segment on an intact mesentery
    • Type 3 (7%): Complete atretic segment with mesenteric gap, and proximal/distal blind-ending intestinal pouches
• Incidence: 1 in 6,000 to 10,000
• Pathophysiology:
  - Failure to recanalization
  - Atresia occur with vascular disruptions during development
  - Annular pancreas
• Diagnosis:
  - Maternal history: Polyhydramnios
  - Birth history: Prematurity
  - Epigastric fullness
  - Bilious emesis
  - Double-bubble sign on X-ray abdomen
• Treatment:
  - IV fluid, antibiotic and naso- or orogastric tube
  - Surgery
    • Duodenoduodenostomy
    • Duodenojejunostomy.

Intestinal Atresia/Stenosis

• Definition:
  - Obliteration of a segment of intestine during development that results in a stricture or blind-ending obstruction of the intestine
  - 4 types:
    • Type I: Intraluminal web or diaphragm with intact mesentery and intact seromuscular layers in the involved intestinal segment
    • Type II: Fibromuscular cord replaces intestinal segment on an intact mesentery

– Type III: Two subtypes:
  • 3a: Complete atretic segment with mesenteric gap, and proximal/distal blind-ending intestinal pouches
  • 3b: Complete atretic segment with mesenteric gap, with distal pouch corkscrewed around a single mesenteric vessel (*Apple Peel* or *Christmas Tree*)
– Type IV: Multiple atretic segments in succession with mesenteric gaps and also known as *string of sausages*
• Incidence: 1 in 500 to 1 in 1500 live births and in about 15 percent of gastroschisis cases
• Pathophysiology:
  – Fetal intestine develops from the midgut and undergoes a sequence of elongation, herniation from the coelomic cavity, rotation, return to the coelomic cavity, and fixation to the posterior abdominal wall
  – Blood supply is derived from the superior mesenteric artery that arises off of the dorsal aorta during development
  – Atresia occur with vascular disruptions during development
  – The greater the vascular insult, the more severe the atresia type
• Diagnosis:
  – Maternal history: Polyhydramnios
  – Birth history: Prematurity
  – Bilious emesis
  – Abdominal distension
  – Failure to pass meconium
  – Plain abdominal films, which show a dilated proximal intestine and a decompressed distal intestine/colon
  – Barium enema: Microcolon
• Treatment
  – Nasogastric suction should be initiated upon diagnosis of atresia
  – Correction of any fluid or electrolyte imbalances should be undertaken before surgery
  – Surgery may be performed semielectively after stabilization
    • Tapering jejunoplasty and end-to-back anastomosis.

Necrotizing Enterocolitis (NEC)

• Intestinal ischemic injury that begins in the mucosa, but may progress to full-thickness necrosis of segments of small bowel and/or colon
• Occurs most commonly in premature infants
• Associated with the initiation of enteral feeding
• Incidence is increasing as neonatal intensive care advances allowing younger gestational age infants to survive past delivery

• Pathophysiology:
  – Etiology is multifactorial
    • Decreased perfusion leading to hypoxia in the intestine
      – Cardiac defects with shunting
      – Respiratory failure
      – Hypotension
    • Infectious etiology
      – Tends to occur in clusters (group)
      – *Clostridium, Pseudomonas, Klebsiella, Enterobacter,* and *Staphylococcus* species
    • Immunologic factors
      – Host inflammatory response and free radical damage play a role
      – May help to propagate and worsen an existing case of NEC
• Diagnosis:
  – Clinical features: Abdominal distention, bloody stools, bilious emesis, and intolerance of feedings
  – Physical examination: Findings include abdominal distention with tenderness, decreased bowel sounds, blood per rectum, and/or abdominal wall erythema
  – Lab values may show thrombocytopenia, neutropenia, elevated PT/PTT, metabolic acidosis, and/or hyponatremia
  – Imaging may reveal diffuse bowel distention/ileus, pneumotosis intestinalis, fixed loops on serial X-rays, and/or portal venous air/free air
• Treatment:
  – *Medical management* is the mainstay treatment
  – Nasogastric decompression
  – Total parenteral nutrition
  – Broadspectrum intravenous antibiotics
  – Close monitoring and correction of fluid and electrolyte abnormalities
  – Proper ventilation/avoidance of hypoxemia
  – Surgical intervention:
    • Surgery is indicated in any case of bowel perforation/necrosis with pneumoperitoneum
    • Abdominal compartment syndrome and failure of medical management
    • Goal of surgery is to resect necrotic segments while maintaining as much viable bowel as possible to avoid short bowel syndrome
    • Standard surgical approach is to create an ostomy rather than primary anastomosis as the disease process may still progress.

Meconium Ileus

- The distal ileum is obstructed in newborn infants with cystic fibrosis due to inspissated meconium
- The presenting symptom of cystic fibrosis in 10 to 20 percent of patients with the disease
- Pathophysiology:
  - Cystic fibrosis is a disorder of chloride channels caused by a single base deletion in the cystic fibrosis transmembrane conductance regulator (CFTR) gene
  - GI and pulmonary secretions are abnormally thick due to diminished volume of secretions and increased reabsorption of sodium chloride via normal sodium-potassium pump function leading to further dehydration of the secretions
  - Pancreatic and GI secretions are abnormally thick and patients will usually require pancreatic enzyme replacement
  - Death typically occurs by age 30 due to progressive pulmonary disease
- Diagnosis:
  - Clinical features: Failure to pass meconium, abdominal distention, and bilious emesis
  - X-ray abdomen shows dilated loops of small bowel and soap bubble sign (ground-glass appearance due to meconium mixed with air)
  - Enema study: Microcolon
  - A family history of cystic fibrosis
- Treatment:
  - Conservative treatment (effective in up to 70% cases)
    - Saline enemas/irrigation
    - Gastrograffin enemas
    - Dilute N-Acetylcysteine enemas
  - Failed medical management—surgery is indicated
    - Exploratory laparotomy with enterotomy and manual removal meconium
    - Simple enterotomy with primary closure
    - Doubtful bowel viability, intestinal resection ostomy (proximal and mucus fistula)
    - T-tube placement into terminal ileum for continued irrigation may also be used
  - Postoperatively, the continued irrigation of the bowel with dilute N-Acetylcysteine via nasogastric tube or enema may be helpful for the passage of meconium.

Malrotation

- Abnormal anatomic position of the bowel due to aberrant or absent embryologic rotation of the gut (5th to 10th weeks of gestation), results in shortened intestine with abnormal attachments to the peritoneal wall
  - The dense attachments between the body wall and cecum in incomplete rotation are known as Ladd bands, pass anterior to the small intestine, and may serve as a point of obstruction
- Three variations
  - Nonrotation: Very shortened small intestine on the right, duodenum does not cross midline, cecum at midline, and colon on left
  - Incomplete rotation: Small intestine mostly on the right, colon on the left with cecum in the left upper quadrant densely affixed to the right posterior body wall
  - Mesocolic hernia: Incomplete rotation resulting in essentially normal length of bowel, but with non-fixation of the right or left colon allowing for potential space for internal herniation of bowel to occur.
- Pathophysiology:
  - Normal midgut rotation occurs along the axis of the superior mesenteric artery (SMA) with a 270° counterclockwise rotation resulting in an anteriorly located colon and posteriorly located small intestine
  - Rotation occurs during physiology herniation outside of the coelomic cavity between weeks 5 and 10 of normal gestation and is associated with a significant lengthening of the jejunoileal segment during this time
  - The failure or cessation of rotation and fixation due to unknown causes is the source of malrotation.
- Diagnosis:
  - Bilious emesis
  - Volvulus due to non-fixation and narrow base of mesentery
  - Many patients will remain asymptomatic and may be discovered incidentally due to studies performed for other reasons
  - Diagnostic study of choice is upper GI series with small bowel follow-through.
    - Duodenum does not crosses the midline
    - The most of small bowel loops are on right side
- Treatment:
  - Exploratory laparotomy and repair even in asymptomatic patients
  - Ladd's procedure
    - Detorsion of the midgut
    - Division of Ladd bands
    - Placement of the cecum in the left upper quadrant, and placement of the duodenum and right upper quadrant

- Passage of a catheter through the duodenum to rule out associated duodenal obstruction
- Widening of the base of mesentery
- Appendectomy to prevent future misdiagnosis.

Hirschsprung's Disease

- Definition:
  - It is a functional, rather than mechanical obstruction of the colon due to failure of ganglion development in a segment of the colon
  - Leads to failure of colonic peristalsis and obstruction.
- Pathophysiology:
  - From 5th to 7th gestational weeks, neural crest cells migrate (craniocaudal migration) into the wall of the colon forming Auerbach's myenteric plexus and Meissner's submucosal plexus
  - Failure of the migration of neural crest cells into the colon wall or subsequent failure of microenvironmental support
  - Genetic theory- several genes, including the RET proto-oncogene; Endothelin 3 gene, and endothelin B receptor gene have been possible culprit
  - Aganglionosis occur in distal to proximal.
- Diagnosis:
  - Bilious emesis
  - Abdominal distention
  - Infrequent bowel movements/constipation
  - Failure to thrive
  - In neonates, a delayed passage of meconium (>24 hours)
  - Anorectal exam to rule out anorectal anomaly
  - Abdominal X-ray to rule out other sources of obstruction and absence of gas in pelvis
  - Barium enema to identify the transition zone
  - Anorectal manometery
  - Biopsy.
    - Rectal suction biopsy-absence of ganglion cells confirms the diagnosis and hypertrophic nerve bundle is supportive finding
    - Full thickness rectal biopsy (FTRB) required if suction biopsy is inconclusive
    - AChE staining
- Treatment:
  - Surgical correction is curative
    - Primary pull through with or without ostomy
    - Staged repair
      - Requires temporary colostomy proximal to the transition zone

- Pull through (Duhamel/Soave/Swenson)
- Closure of ostomy (either colostomy or ileostomy depending on the length of diseased segment)
- Definitive procedure is performed at age 6 to 12 months.
  - *Duhamel-Martin procedure*: Resection of aganglionic segment with colorectal anastomosis of normal colon posteriorly to aganglionic remnant of rectum anteriorly (retrorectal colonic pull trough)
  - *Soave procedure*: Division of the colon at the transition point with transanal mucosal proctectomy and transrectal pull-through (endorectal pull through) excision of aganglionic segment, and colorectal anastomosis
  - Laparoscopic assisted pull through.

Intussusception

- Definition:
  - Invagination or "telescoping" of a segment of bowel into itself causing mechanical obstruction
  - May occur in any segment of intestine, but ileocolic intussusception is the most common type
  - Intussusception is more common in infants and young children
  - It can happen in adults too
- Pathophysiology:
  - Mostly it occurs due to a "lead point" at which the intussusceptum initiates and peristalsis propagates
  - Lead points may be lymphoid hyperplasia due to viral infections, Meckel's diverticulum, polyps, lymphoma or other space occupying lesions in the gastrointestinal tract.
- Diagnosis:
  - Young child with colicky abdominal pain (severe alternating with periods of pain free interval)
  - Bilious vomiting, abdominal distention with a sausage-shaped right lower quadrant mass
  - Rectal exam- "currant jelly stools" (stool mixed with blood and mucus).
  - Guaiac positive stools occur in 90 to 95 percent of cases.
  - Diagnostic procedure of choice is contrast enema, which is also therapeutic in roughly 80 to 90 percent of cases (dependening on the experience of radiologist).
- Treatment:
  - Hydrostatic reduction with contrast enema is the initial therapeutic procedure

– Pneumatic reduction with air-contrast enema
  • Pressures are 80 mm Hg for infants and 120 mm Hg for young children and successful in up to 80 to 90 percent of patients, again results depends on the duration of disease
  • Surgery is indicated for peritonitis/shock or with failure of nonoperative means
  • Manual reduction on exploratory laparotomy (open or laparoscopic) is usually sufficient in uncomplicated cases
  • Resection may be required if bowel necrosis or a lead point suspected for malignancy
  • Most surgeons will perform an appendectomy to prevent future misdiagnosis
– Patients should be kept in the hospital post-reduction as approximately 10 percent of intussusceptions may recur
  • Mostly recur within 24 hours
  • After 6 months of first episode, incidence is equal to the rest of population.
– Recurrent intussusceptions in older children warrant exploratory surgery to rule out tumors as a causative lead point.

Imperforate Anus

• Definition: Absence of the anorectal orifice to develop
  – Associated with the VACTERL syndrome
  – Types:
    a. Low: Located distal to the puborectalis muscle
      i. Does not require colostomy
      ii. Frequently presents with perineal meconium fistula
    b. High: Located above the puborectalis muscle
      i. Requires colostomy
      ii. Mostly with fistulization to urethra, bladder, or vagina
• Pathophysiology:
  – Abnormal development of the urorectal septum, which results in incomplete division of the fetal cloaca into urogenital and anorectal portions
  – Abnormal connection between the rectum and urogenital systems anywhere *in the pelvis.*
• Diagnosis:
  – Clinical examination
  – Plain-ray of the pelvis (pronogram) 24 hours after birth (to allow distal passage of swallowed air) with the infant held upside down or placed in prone position helps to assess l the level of involvement.

• Treatment:
  – *Low type:* Primary repair with perineal approach (cut back anoplasty) or limited PSARP
  – *High type:*
    • Colostomy in infancy followed by posterior sagittal anorectoplasty (PSARP) at age 4-8 months
    • Laparoscopic-assisted anorectoplasty (LARP).

Biliary Atresia

• Definition:
  – Obliteration of the biliary tract in infants resulting in neonatal cholestatic jaundice
  – Classified as
    • Intrahepatic: Biliary hypoplasia, a rare condition has patent but underdeveloped biliary system
    • Extrahepatic: It is more common form and has atrophied extrahepatic bile ducts and gallbladder
      – Type I: Obliteration of the common bile duct
      – Type II: Obliteration of the proper hepatic duct with cystic dilation of the porta hepatis
      – Type III: Atresia of the left and right hepatic ducts extending up to the level of the porta hepatic – the most common type
• Pathophysiology:
  – Mostly idiopathic etiology
  – Possible causes includes inflammatory process in the biliary ductal system after birth
  – Viral (CMV) infection or toxin exposure in the ductal system may play a role
    • Rare in premature
    • If left untreated, will progress to cirrhosis and hepatic failure
• Diagnosis:
  – Neonatal jaundice lasting more than 2 to 4 weeks, dark colored urine, and alcoholic, clay-colored stools suggestive.
  – Elevated direct bilirubin suggestive of diagnosis.
  – α1-antitrypsin with Pi typing to rule out deficiency of this enzyme, and sweat chloride test to rule out cystic fibrosis as sources for cholestasis
• Imaging studies
  – HIDA scan showing rapid liver uptake with no excretion of radiotracer into bowel
  – Liver ultrasound showing increased liver echogenicity and biliary dilation with a small, shrunken or atrophied gallbladder
    • Liver biopsy
      – The most important diagnostic and prognostic test

- High sensitivity in a suggestive clinical picture
- Intraoperative cholangiogram via gallbladder cannulation at time of surgery
- Treatment:
  - Intrahepatic form requires orthotropic *liver transplant.*
  - Extrahepatic form can be treated with *porto-enterostomy*
    - Kasai procedure
      - Involves resection of the atretic biliary ductal system and anastomosis of a Roux-en-Y limb to the porta hepatic
      - Level of resection determined by frozen section to assess duct diameter
- Complications:
  - Cholangitis is a frequent postoperative complication
  - Twenty five to thirty five percent of patients will have a 10 year survival without liver transplant, the remaining two-thirds eventually will need liver transplant.

Oncology

The leukemia and lymphoma represent the most common cancer diagnoses in children and the most common solid tumors of infancy and childhood, where general pediatric surgical therapy is a mainstay of treatment.

Neuroblastoma

- Incidence is 1 in 8000 to 10000
  - Ten percent of childhood tumors
  - More than 50 percent present within 2 years of life
- Locations:
  - Adrenal gland (50%)
  - Paraspinal (25%)
  - Mediastinum (20%)
  - Cervical (5%)
  - Pelvis (<5%) pelvic organ of Zuckerkandl
- Definition:
  - A solid tumor arising from primitive neural crest cells and locations tend to be in the distribution of derivatives of neural crest cells
  - Represents the most common extracranial solid tumor in children
- Pathophysiology:
  - Genetics
    - Association with the N-myc oncogene
    - Abnormalities of deletions on the p arm of chromosome 1 and gain of DNA on the q arm of chromosome 17, both of which confer a worse prognosis

- High cellularity, uniform tumor with varying degrees of stroma within the tumor
- Graded on the Shimada scale
  - Favorable factors are tumor rich in stroma, young age, and a low mitosis/karyorrhexis index (MKI)
  - Unfavorable factors are nodular pattern, greater age at diagnosis, poor differentiation, and high MKI
  - MKI assesses the number of mitoses and karyorrhexis per 5,000 cells in the tumor
- Clinical presentation:
  - Typically present as a cervical, abdominal, or pelvic solid mass
    - Cervical
      - Occasionally airway obstruction, depending on the size
      - Origin from the cervical sympathetic chain and can cause Horner's syndrome on the involved side
      - Rarely metastasis and lymph node involvement
    - Abdominal
      - Mostly present as hard mass in the abdomen arising from the adrenal medulla or midline sympathetic chain and the lymph node involvement along the aorta
    - Pelvic
      - Intestinal or ureteral obstruction
      - Sacral nerves involvement affecting the motor function of lower extremity and anal sphincter tone
  - Other signs/symptoms
    - Periorbital ecchymosis due to venous congestion/rupture with metastasis to the eyes
    - Myoclonus due to anti-tumor antibody cross-reaction with purkinje fibers in the cerebellum
    - Secretory diarrhea syndrome due to secretion of vasoactive intestinal peptide (VIPOMA)
- Diagnosis:
  - Imaging with contrasted CT or MRI will show tumor extent
  - MIBG scan
  - Serum and urinary marker (Increased level of serum and urinary catecholamine and by products)
  - Biopsy is the mainstay of diagnosis and staging.
- Staging:
  - 1: Tumor localized to site of origin with no nodal or distant metastasis
  - 2A: Unilateral tumor with incomplete gross excision without metastasis

- 2B: Unilateral tumor with ipsilateral positive nodes, no contralateral nodal or distant metastasis
- 3: Unilateral tumor with bilateral nodal involvement or tumor that crosses midline
- 4: Distant metastasis to nodes, bone marrow, bone, or liver
- Stage 4S: Localized primary tumor as for stage 1 and 2 with dissemination limited to liver/skin (limited to infants < 1 year of age)
- Treatment:
  - Low-risk tumor can be treated with resection alone
  - High-risk tumor should be treated with resection and central venous access device placement for chemotherapy and radiation.

Nephroblastoma (Wilms' Tumor)

- Definition:
  - A tumor of primitive metanephric blastema cells
  - The most common pediatric renal tumor and the 5th most common pediatric cancer
- Pathophysiology:
  - Sporadic form results from two allele loss in a specific tumor suppressor gene
  - WT1, an oncogene located on chromosome 11 involved in development of Wilms tumor
  - Association with other clinical syndromes
    - Denys-Drash syndrome: Wilm's tumor, pseudohermaphroditism, glomerulonephropathy
    - WAGR syndrome: Wilm's tumor, Aniridia, Genitourinary malformation, mental Retardation
    - Beckwith-Wiedemann syndrome
    - Hemihypertrophy
- Diagnosis:
  - Palpable abdominal or flank mass, with or without abdominal pain.
  - Hematuria, hypertension
  - Fever
  - Imaging
    - Renal ultrasound to assess renal mass and renal vascular involvement
    - CT of the chest, abdomen and pelvis allows assessment of tumor, differentiation from Neuroblastoma of the adrenal, assessment of the opposite kidney, and nodal or distant metastasis
  - Staging
    - I: Tumor confined to kidney and completely resected

- II: Tumor completely excised, but with extension beyond renal capsule, or biopsy of confined tumor with local spillage
- III: Tumor incompletely excised, positive lymph nodes, or peritoneal seeding, or intra abdominal tumor spillage
- IV: Hematogenous or lymph node metastasis beyond the abdominal cavity
- V: Simultaneous bilateral involvement
- Treatment
  - Surgical resection is required for treatment and staging
  - Chemotherapy is required for all Wilm's tumor diagnoses and consists typically of Doxorubicin, Dactinomycin, and Vincristine
  - Radiation therapy is used for stage 3-5 disease
  - Inoperable by CT scanning, neoadjuvant cytoreductive chemotherapy should be given.

Hepatoblastoma

- Definition:
  - The most common liver cancer in the pediatric age group is the Hepatoblastoma
  - Incidence of 1 in 1 million
  - 6 months to 3 years of age
- Pathologic features:
  - Epithelial
    - Fetal (31%)
    - Embryonic (19%)
    - Macrotrabecular (3%
    - Anaplastic (3%)
  - Mixed epithelial/mesenchymal (44%)
- Associated with Beckwith-Wiedemann syndrome and familial adenomatous polyposis (FAP)
- Diagnosis:
  - Palpable abdominal mass with or without abdominal swelling, pain, irritability, gastrointestinal disturbances, fever, pallor, and/or failure to thrive
  - Alpha-Fetoprotein (AFP) levels are significantly elevated with hepatoblastoma (>90%)
  - Imaging
    - Abdominal X-ray may show hepatomegaly
    - CT reveals a heterogeneous mass and is the imaging procedure of choice to assess metastasis, but is less sensitive than MRI for primary diagnosis
    - MRI is the imaging of choice
  - Staging
    - I: Complete surgical resection

- II: Microscopic positive margins without regional spread, confined to one lobe of the liver
  - III: Partially resected tumor, spillage of tumor at time of surgery, involving two lobes of the liver positive lymph nodes
  - IV: Distant metastasis
- Treatment
  - Neoadjuvant chemotherapy with doxorubicin and cisplatin prior to surgical resection
  - After reducing the tumor load, surgical resection with hepatic lobectomy is the procedure of choice, though in rare instances, a wedge resection may be used for small, peripherally located tumors
  - Liver transplantation (up to 5-7% of patients).

Testicular Tumors

- Mostly common in age group from 2 to 4 years old
- Diagnosis:
  - Nontender, solid scrotal mass
  - Imaging
    - USG of scrotum
    - CT scan of abdomen and pelvis
  - Tumor markers
    - Increased alfa feto protein (Yolk sac tumors)
    - Increased B-hCG (Seminoma and choriocarcinoma)
- Treatment:
  - Radical orchiectomy
  - If needed, retroperitoneal lymph node dissection (RPLND).

Pediatric Urology

Posterior urethral valve (PUV):
- Thin mucosal folds that look like membrane causing varying degree of obstruction during the act of urination.
- Only in males, leading to urethral obstruction in infants or newborns
- Incidence—1 in 8000 to 15000 live births
- 1/3rd progresses to end stage renal disease and children who undergo renal transplant 10 to 15 percent have PUV.

Types

- Young's classification
  - I-abnormally high insertion and fusion (95%)
  - II-hypertrophy of plicae colliculi
  - III- septum at the junction of anterior and posterior urethra

Clinical Symptoms

- Various degrees of obstruction (mild/moderate/severe)
- Poor, intermittent, dribbling stream
- Urinary infection, sepsis
- Severe obstruction associated with abdominal mass, distended midline bladder
- Failure to thrive.

Laboratory Findings

- Azotemia and poor concentrating ability of kidney
- Chronic anemia

Diagnostic Test

- *Voiding cystourethrogram (VCUG)* showing the most common type (I), associated reflux, elongation and dilation of posterior urethra with prominent bladder neck
- *Excretory urogram:* Hydroureter and hydronephrosis in severe cases
- *Ultrasonogram:* Can detect prenatally as early as 28 weeks of gestation
- *Cystoscopy:* Confirms the diagnosis, shows vesical trabeculation, diverticuli, bladder neck and trigone hypertrophy.

Treatment

Treatment depends on degree of obstruction and health of the child.
- Mild to moderate obstruction–with minimal azotemia- transurethral fulguration of the valve
- Severe: Require individualized approach.
- Treatment of sepsis: Drainage of bladder
- Correction of fluid and electrolyte imbalance
- Vesicostomy or percutaneous urostomy

Prognosis: Depends on azotemia and degree of sepsis and age of presentation.

Hypospadias

- Condition in which the urethral opening is seen on the ventral aspect of the penis
- Incidence: 1 in 250 male births, more common in white with 7 percent familial rate.

Pathophysiology

- Sexual and urethral development begins at 8 weeks and completed at 15 weeks. Failure of canalization of ectodermal cord that has grown through the urethral folds results in hypospadias.

Etiology

- Genetic: Eight fold increase, polygenic inheritance with 8 to 14 percent history in brother and father
- Endocrine: Decrease in available androgen or inability to use available androgen
- Environmental: Endocrine disruption by environmental factors
- Combination theory: Two or more causes together.

Types

Types based on the location of the urethral meatus:
- Glandular: Opening is proximal to glans penis (most common)
- Coronal: At coronal sulcus (most common)
- Penile shaft (Proximal, mid or distal)
- Penoscrotal
- Perineal.

Clinical Symptoms

- Abnormal opening at different sites
- Associated curvature (Chordee) of the penis: Ventral bending
- Association: Undescended testis
- In more proximal (Penoscrotal, scrotal) hypospadias it is essential to rule out ambiguous genitalia by buccal smear and karyotyping.

Treatment

- Aim of surgical repair: Orthoplasty (straight penis), urethroplasty (meatus at tip of penis), glansplasty (conical glans)
- Timing of surgery: Essential to repair hypospadias before the school age, for psychological reason (generally between 1 and 2 yrs)
- Technique: Multiple techniques are described; repair depends on type of hypospadias.
  - Most common is tabularized incised plate (TIP) urethroplasty where the urethral plate is incised in the midline to increase the width of the urethra for the tubularization.
  Single stage repair-
  - Duckett's procedure: Preputial flap
  - Koyanagi and modified Koyanagi repair: Using preputial flap with variation in divison of the flap by

either dividing at 12 o'clock or through a buttonhole procedure
- Denise-Brown technique: With burial of skin strip with spontaneous re-epithelialization.

Ureterocele

- Terminal dilatation, sacculation of terminal portion of the ureter.
- **Types**—based on the number of renal units and location of the opening
  - Single-system ureterocele
  - Duplex system ureterocele
  - Orthotopic (within bladder)
  - Ectopic.

Other classification is based on features of affected ureter:
- Stenotic
- Sphincteric
- Sphincterostenotic
- Cecoureterocele.

Incidence: 1 in 4000 live births, more in white females than in males.

Etiology: Precise etiology unknown:
- Most accepted theory is ureteral orifice obstruction with incomplete dissolution of Chwalla membrane
- Chwalla membrane is a primitive thin membrane separating ureteral bud from urogenital sinus.

Clinical Presentation

- Urinary tract infection, urosepsis
- Obstructive voiding symptoms
- Urinary retention
- Failure to thrive
- Ureteral calculus
- Hematuria.

Diagnosis

- Ultrasound: Cyst in cyst sign fluid filled cystic cavity in bladder, associated hydronephrosis, duplication of renal units
- Voiding cystourethrography (VCUG): To rule out lower urinary tract anomalies
- Nuclear renal scan: To assess the split renal function
- Intravenous urogram (IVU)
- Dropping lily sign: Hydronephrotic upper pole displacing lower moiety, Cobra head extension in bladder
- CT scan: In equivocal cases.

Treatment

Surgery is mainstay of treatment.

Aims
- Control infection
- Preserve renal function
- Protect ipsilateral and contralateral renal units
- Maintaining urinary continence.

Surgical approach depends on:
- Site of ureterocele
- Clinical situation
- Renal anomalies and size.

Surgical techniques are:
- Endoscopic incision
- Transurethral unroofing
- Upper pole heminephrectomy and partial ureterectomy
- Ureteropyelostomy
- Excision of ureterocele and ureteral reimplantation
- Nephrectomy.

Congenital Ureteropelvic Junction (UPJ) Obstruction

- It is most common cause of upper urinary tract obstruction in children and is secondary to functional impairment of transport of urine from pelvis to the ureter.
- Incidence: 1 in 500-700 pregnancies presents with hydronephrosis of which 40 to 50 percent are secondary to UPJ obstruction.

Pathophysiology

- Intrinsic narrowing of the lumen at UPJ secondary to aperistaltic segment
- Abnormal recanalization of the ureter
- Extrinsic—aberrant or supernumerary vessel.

Presentation

- Asymptomatic detected prenatally or incidentally
- Symptomatic:
  - Episodic flank pain
  - Flank mass
  - UTI
  - Nausea, vomiting
  - Failure to thrive
  - Hematuria secondary to blunt abdominal trauma.

Diagnosis

- Prenatal ultrasound: Criteria AP diameter of renal pelvis
  - 4 mm in less than 33 weeks of gestation
  - >7 mm in greater than 33 weeks of gestation
- Incidentally detected: On intravenous urogram, CT scan or MRI performed for other reasons.
- Nuclear renal scan: To assess the renal function.

Treatment

Surgery is the mainstay treatment, based on the etiology.
- Pyeloplasty: Open/minimally invasive (Endoscopic/laparoscopic/robotic)
- Principles of surgery: Formation of a tunnel at ureteropelvic anastomosis
  - Dependent drainage
  - Watertight anastomosis
  - Tension free anastomosis
- Rescue surgery: In failed primary surgery perform either ureterocalicostomy or place an interventional radiology assisted drain/nephrostomy.

Vesicoureteral Reflux (VUR)

- An abnormal movement of urine from bladder to ureter or kidneys
- Incidence: Unknown as most children are asymptomatic
  - Higher in children with UTI (urinary tract infection) 15 to 70 percent
  - Siblings of children with VUR have a 25 to 33 percent risk of also having VUR
  - More common in white.

Presentation

Two groups based on time of diagnosis:
- Prenatally detected: Progress through diagnosis and treatment
- Symptomatic: With UTI, failure to thrive, abdominal pain, pyelonephritis, sterile reflux with episodic abdominal pain, reflux nephropathy
- Etiology: For primary reflux is unknown
- Possible theories
  - Genetic predisposition
  - Urinary tract infection
  - Congenital bladder obstruction
  - Dysfunctional voiding.

Diagnosis: Standard test include ultrasound and VCUG (Voiding cystourethrogram).

Indication

- Evaluation with UTI in all children <5 years or any age with febrile UTI
- Boys with UTI any age.

Classification

Based on VCUG:
- Grade I: Reflux into nondilated ureter
- Grade II: Reflux into renal pelvis and calyces without dilation
- Grade III: Reflux with mild-to-moderate dilation and minimal blunting of fornices
- Grade IV: Reflux with moderate ureteral tortuosity and dilation of pelvis and calyces
- Grade V: Reflux with gross dilation of ureter, pelvis, and calyces, loss of papillary impressions, and ureteral tortuosity.

Treatment

- Aims: To prevent renal infection, damage and complications of renal damage
- Newly diagnosed UTI: Antibiotic therapy with prophylaxis till imaging reveals reflux
- All newly diagnosed grades I-IV and some grade V reflux are treated with antibiotics.

Surgical: Indications are as follows:
- Breakthrough UTI despite antibiotics, severe (grade V or bilateral IV reflux), mild to moderate reflux in pubertal females, poor compliance with medications and poor renal growth
- Approach : Endoscopic reflux procedure,
              Open intravesical/extravesical.

Undescended Testis

- Absence of one or both testicle from the scrotum at birth.
- Incidence: Three percent in full-term and 30 percent in premature infants.
- More common in
  - Premature, low birth weight
  - Environmental chemical as endocrine disruptor
  - Familial with h/o cryptorchidism 4 percent in father and 6 to 10 percent in brothers
  - Congenital malformation syndrome
    - Prader-Willi syndrome
    - Noonan syndrome
    - Cloacal extrophy.

- Diagnosis: Clinical, empty scrotum or palpable in inguinal canal.
- Imaging is limited value, diagnostic laparoscopy can be used in cases where testis is not palpable on imaging.
- Treatment: Surgery
  - To increase likelihood of fertility
  - Self-examination
  - Psychological effects of empty scrotum
  - Correction of associated hernia
  - Prevention of torsion.

Surgical approach is based on whether the testis is palpable or non-palpable with inguinal, extended inguinal/abdominal approach, or laparoscopy.

Renal ectopia is due to failure of ascent of the kidney during embryogenesis.

Types: Simple, crossed without fusion/fusion.

Problems: Associated abnormal vasculature from local tissue. Predilection for infection and obstruction.

Diagnosis: Clinically palpable, confirmed with imaging, incidentally detected for other issues.

Treatment: Not required for ectopia, but for associated complications of obstruction and infection.

Renal agenesis: Extremely rare, less than 400 cases are reported, condition is not compatible with life.

Absence of one renal unit is seen in 1 in 500 to 1000 live births.

Prenatally suspected in patients with oligohydramnios, associated pulmonary hypoplasia and facial deformities (Potter's syndrome) may be seen.

Autosomal Recessive Polycystic Renal Disease

Seen in 1 in 10,000 live births, cyst on both renal units, liver with varying presentations based on degree of renal/liver failure.

Many present with palpable masses, renal failure and portal hypertension secondary to fibrosis.

Many neonates may die in 1st few weeks of life secondary to pulmonary hypoplasia and insufficiency. If they survive, most present with renal and hepatic failure.

Treatment is based on presentation, either with replacement therapy, renal and/or liver transplantation.

Horseshoe Kidney

Most common fusion anomaly, result due to fusion of part of both the kidneys, most commonly lower pole.

Other sites of fusion: Isthmus, upper pole.

The horseshoe kidney is commonly located at L4 vertebra as inferior epigastric artery impedes the ascent of the kidney.

Presentation: Lump in the abdomen, infection, renal stones, ureteropelvic obstruction.

Diagnosis: Ultrasound, CT scan, intravenous urogram for diagnosis.

Functional imaging is done by nuclear imaging study.

Treatment: Based on the mode of presentation, either by open or laparoscopic route.

Other Types of Fusion

- Crossed fused renal ectopia
- Fused pelvic kidney (pancake kidney).

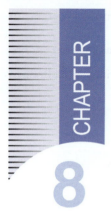

Benign Breast Diseases

Neelima Rehil, Vijay Mittal

INTRODUCTION

Many women will experience benign breast diseases during their lifetime. It is important to properly work-up these patients to differentiate benign and malignant diseases and reduce anxiety. The breast consists of different types of tissue which can produce benign lesions that often appear suspicious for malignant disease until properly diagnosed. In the following section, we will discuss various types of benign lesions of the breast and the work-up needed to properly diagnose such lesions. The work-up for a palpable breast lesion is discribed in (Fig. 8.1)

SCREENING

Detection of breast masses and abnormalities is essential in the proper diagnosis and treatment of both malignant and benign diseases. Screening is an invaluable tool in identifying both benign and malignant breast lesions and should begin at the level of the patient. Early detection of breast cancer is imperative in order to achieve the best outcomes with treatment, as well as early detection and diagnosis of benign lesions. The breast self-examination (BSE) is an examination that should be performed by patients in the comfort of their own home. The exam consists of palpation of the breasts and axillae to detect for irregularities. It is recommended that women perform such an exam monthly to assess for any changes in the breast that may occur with their menstrual cycles, as well as any new lesions or abnormalities.

In addition to the breast self-examination, female patients should have an annual breast exam in a clinical setting by their primary care provider. Patients with a known history of breast cancer or other breast lesion, who have undergone lumpectomy or excision should follow-up regularly with their surgeon in the clinical setting for examination. Patients over

the age of 40 should also undergo an annual mammogram to evaluate for microcalcifications or other abnormalities.[2]

IMAGING

Many imaging modalities have been found useful in identifying both benign and malignant lesions of the breast, including mammography, ultrasound, magnetic resonance imaging and computed tomography. Among these, the most commonly used imaging for both screening and diagnostic purposes are mammography and ultrasound.

Mammography

The only breast imaging modality which has been proven to reduce breast cancer mortality is mammography which makes it an invaluable tool. Mammography can be used both for screening and diagnostic purposes. Screening mammography is used to detect for early clinically occult lesions in asymptomatic patients. Due to the limitations of screening mammography in younger patients with more dense breast tissue, annual screening is not recommended to begin until the age of 40. In women with a higher risk of breast cancer, such as those with a strong family history, annual screening mammography can be started at an earlier age. Though no upper age limit for screening mammography has been established, patients older than 70 years with comorbidities reducing life expectancy to less than 10 years are no longer recommended to undergo screening.

Diagnostic mammography is used in patients who have a clinical complaint such as a palpable mass, discharge or focal pain, or patients whose screening mammography was abnormal. Diagnostic mammography for an abnormal screening mammogram is conducted by the radiologist and involves spot and roll views, with or without magnification

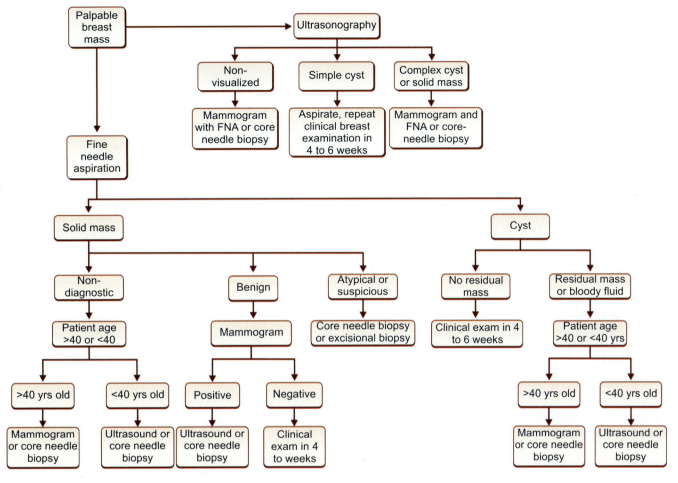

FIGURE 8.1: Algorithmic work-up of palpable breast mass

which help to determine whether or not the lesion on the initial exam was real or due to overlapping of normal breast tissue. If lesions are confirmed on diagnostic mammography, they are assigned a breast imaging reporting and data system (BI-RADS) score which will determine the need for patient follow-up and possible surgical intervention (Table 8.1).

Breast Ultrasound

High frequency ultrasonography is usually used in conjunction with mammography in the diagnosis of breast lesions and as an important follow-up modality. The main role of ultrasound in breast imaging is to aid in diagnosis after a screening mammogram returns an abnormal result. Breast ultrasound is useful when trying to distinguish between solid and cystic lesions, in diagnosing breast lesions

in younger patients because of the limitations of mammography in dense breast tissue, and for tissue diagnosis.

In solid breast lesions, or patients with BI-RADS scores of 4 or 5, it is important to obtain a tissue sample in order to properly diagnose a lesion. Ultrasound-guided core needle biopsy is a beneficial modality to use when a mass is visualized sonographically, as it is relatively inexpensive and requires no exposure to harmful radiation.

MRI

Magnetic resonance imaging uses strong magnetic fields to create cross-sectional images and requires a specific coil in addition to peripheral intravenous administration of gadolinium-based contrast medium to detect breast masses. MRI is useful in detecting both *in situ* and invasive breast

Category	Assessment	Recommendation
0	Additional imaging required	Additional imaging recommended
1	Negative finding	Routine screening recommended
2	Benign finding	Routine screening recommended
3	Probably benign finding	Short interval follow-up suggested for stability
4	Suspicious abnormality	Probability of malignancy, biopsy should be considered
5	Abnormality highly suggestive of malignancy	High probability of cancer, appropriate action should be taken

Table 8.1: American College of Breast Imaging Reporting and Data Collections (BI-RADS) classification of diagnostic mammography findings

carcinomas, as it is highly sensitive for both. MRI has also been noted to be useful in detecting mammographically occult lesions in the ipsilateral breast.

Due to its sensitivity, MRI was initially thought to be an invaluable tool during initial diagnosis of breast lesions and in identifying recurring lesions. Though MRI is still used in imaging of breast lesions, recent literature has questioned its benefits and costs in comparison to mammography and ultrasound imaging. A study published in the Journal of Clinical Oncology in January 2008, involved 756 patients who were diagnosed with early stage invasive breast carcinoma or carcinoma in situ and underwent breast conservation therapy. Of the 756 patients, 215 women had an MRI study in addition to mammography and ultrasound. In the 5-year follow-up, it was noted that there were no significant difference in failure rate or overall survival in the patients that had an initial MRI and those patients that did not.[11]

The same trends in magnetic resonance imaging have been noted in patients in which recurring lesions were identified and required reoperation. A randomized controlled trial published in February 2010 from the United Kingdom demonstrated that the addition of MRI to conventional imaging such as mammography and ultrasound was not associated with reduced rate of reoperation and was therefore an unnecessary expense.[12] As studies into the efficacy and cost of MRI will continue, magnetic resonance imaging used in addition to conventional mammography and ultrasound still remains an option for breast imaging and is most commonly used at the discretion of the surgeon.

BENIGN BREAST LESIONS

Benign breast disease can be classified into nonproliferative, proliferative, atypical hyperplastic and miscellaneous lesions. These different categories are defined based on the degree of atypia and cellular proliferation of a lesion as well as it propensity for developing into breast cancer. Non-

proliferative lesions are common and almost never increase the risk of developing breast cancer. Proliferative lesions without atypia are the most common type of benign breast lesions and are associated with a small increase in breast cancer risk. Atypical hyperplasia is associated with a moderate to high risk of the development of breast cancer, especially when patients present with a strong family history of breast cancer.[3] Miscellaneous lesions range from simple lipomas to more complex lesions which can mimic malignancy, but they generally have no association with increased risk of breast cancer.

NONPROLIFERATIVE BREAST LESIONS

Nonproliferative breast lesions are epithelial lesions that have very little to no association with the development of breast cancer. Some common nonproliferative lesions include breast cysts, fibrocystic disease, chronic cystic mastitis, and mammary dysplasia.

BREAST CYSTS

Cysts are the most common type of nonproliferative breast lesion. These lesions are round or ovoid fluid-filled masses noted most commonly during physical exam or as a mammographic anomaly. Cysts occur mostly in patients between 35 and 50 years of age and may cause sudden onset of severe, localized pain if they become enlarged acutely. Generally, breast cysts are divided into three categories: simple cysts, complicated cysts and complex cysts.

Simple Cysts

Simple breast cysts are non-fixed, round masses, generally non-painful and benign by definition. Cysts are very common in women of all ages and can present as multiple cysts in the ipsilateral or contralateral breast. Diagnosis of simple cysts is usually made by ultrasonography, especially in younger patients. They are easily identified on ultrasound of the breast as anechoic, circumscribed lesions with posterior acoustic enhancement and an absence of solid components (Figs 8.2A and B).[3]

In patients who have no discomfort or pain caused by the cyst, no intervention is necessary. Symptomatic patients should have resolution of the cyst and symptoms with simple fine needle aspiration. Generally, fluid from simple cysts consists of clear or serous, nonpurulent, nonbloody fluid. In cases where bloody or purulent fluid is obtained, the specimen should be sent for culture and cytology. Simple cysts do recur and a second attempt at aspiration to reduce the cyst can be performed. If the cyst continues to recur, surgical excision is the next option for the patient, and is recommended when the reoccurring lesion is associated with pain.

Complicated Cysts

Complicated cysts most commonly present as non-painful lumps or masses in the breast and, like simple cysts, are easily identified on ultrasound of the breast. Complicated cysts are defined by their appearance on breast ultrasound, having homogenous low level internal echoes due to echogenic debris, lacking solid components, thick walls and vascular flow (Fig. 8.3). Complicated cysts are sometimes visualized on mammography as well as ultrasound.[10]

These lesions are rarely malignant, but should be followed up with imaging and clinical examination. A repeat mammogram, ultrasound and clinical exam should be performed every six months for the first two years after diagnosis to establish the stability of the lesion. Aspiration of a complicated cyst for diagnosis is indicated if the lesion resembles differentials including abscess, hematoma, galactocele, or fat necrosis. Fine needle aspiration or biopsy is also indicated if a lesion changes on follow-up imaging, including increased size, new and different characteristics or the potential for a solid component cannot be ruled out.

Complex Cysts

Complex cysts are lesions with cystic and solid components as well as thick walls, or septa, measuring greater than 0.5 cm. On ultrasound, they demonstrate both anechoic and echogenic components. Inflamed or ruptured cysts, abscesses, hematomas and fat necrosis often present as complex cysts, but malignancy cannot be ruled out in complex cysts and biopsy of the lesion is imperative in diagnosis.

Fine needle aspiration can be performed if a lesion is thought to be a simple cyst, however, if a lesion has an obvious solid component, core needle biopsy under ultrasound guidance is a safe and accurate technique for diagnosis. A metal clip should be left in the biopsy site as a marker for follow-up and potential surgical excision.

FIBROCYSTIC CONDITION

Fibrocystic disease, more recently referred to as fibrocystic condition, is the most common benign breast lesion. It commonly occurs in women between 30 and 50 years of age, but is also known to occur in postmenopausal women not taking hormone replacement therapy. Women who drink alcohol, especially those between 18 and 22 years of age also have an increased risk of developing this condition. Estrogen is thought to be a cause of the development of fibrocystic condition.

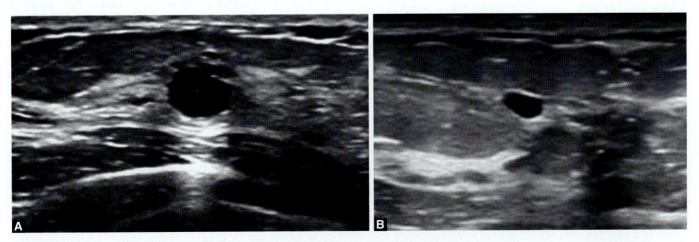

FIGURES 8.2A and B: Ultrasound images of simple cysts

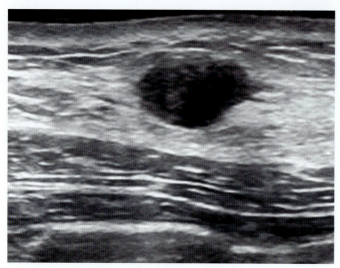

FIGURE 8.3: Ultrasound image of a complicated cyst with echogenic debris

Clinically, patients often present with one or more painful, palpable masses found bilaterally. Breast tissue in patients with fibrocystic change are often described as lumpy or having a cobblestone texture. The masses or lumps are smooth with well-defined edges and are most often non-fixed or free moving masses. Masses are most often found in the upper outer quadrant of the breast. Patients with fibrocystic change complain of persistent or intermittent pain that occurs most often in conjunction with their menstrual cycle. However, in some patients the masses may be asymptomatic and are only detected by screening in the office or at home.

Treatment for fibrocystic change is observation. This is a common condition among women and due to the alteration in size of the cysts with hormone fluctuation and minimal breast cancer risk associated with this condition, no aggressive treatment is required. Sudden increase in size or consistency of lesions warrants further imaging and investigation.

Proliferative Lesions without Atypia Fibroadenoma

Fibroadenomas are benign tumors showing evidence of both epithelial proliferation and proliferation of connective tissue. Clinically, they present as well-circumscribed rubbery, mobile, smooth masses. In 10 to 15 percent of patients, fibroadenomas present as multiple masses in the ipsilateral breast or bilaterally. Fibroadenomas are the most common cause of a new palpable breast mass in female patients under the age of 25. These benign tumors are considered to be an aberration of normal development resulting in hyperplasia or proliferation a single terminal duct unit. About 10 percent of fibroadenomas spontaneously disappear each year and of those that do not, most only grow to be about 2-3 centimeters large.[8]

Imaging modality depends on patient factors including patient age at presentation. Ultrasonography is useful in diagnosis of fibroadenoma in patients younger than 30 years of age, patients with palpable masses or patients who are pregnant. Breast ultrasound of a fibroadenoma will demonstrate a hypoechoic mass with smooth, partially lobulated margins typical of a fibroadenoma. Mammography is generally useful in patient older than 30 and demonstrates well-circumscribed round or oval masses which often have course calcifications.[10] Magnetic resonance imaging is also useful in breast tissue to identify fibroadenomas and can be used to distinguish them from carcinomas. MRI reveals smooth masses which have high signal intensity on T2-weighted images and enhance with gadolinium-based contrast.[11]

Treatment of fibroadenomas ranges from conservative to invasive, depending on the certainty of diagnosis on imaging. Monitoring of the lesions with mammography and clinical exam does not expose patients to unnecessary risk, therefore, it is common practice. In patients with rapidly growing fibroadenomas, lesions that cannot be distinguished from carcinoma, or suspicion for phyllodes tumor, more invasive treatment becomes necessary. Core needle biopsy can produce a definitive diagnosis and rule out phyllodes tumor, as well as carcinoma. If excisional biopsy is performed, a small margin of normal breast tissue is excised as well, in case the biopsy comes back for carcinoma or more commonly phyllodes tumor.[8]

Cryoablation is a relatively new treatment modality which is effective and less invasive than open surgical excision. In order for accurate results, the American Society of Breast Surgeons recommends that the fibroadenoma being treated should be less than 4 centimeters in diameter, sonographically visible and confirmed to be fibroadenomas on histology (Figs 8.4A and B). The procedure is convenient for patients as it takes little time and can be performed in an office setting. An ultrasound is used to allow for image guided insertion of the cryoablation probe which is inserted through a small 3 millimeter incision. Once inside, the probe reaches extremely cold temperatures of less than –40 degrees Centigrade and destroys the fibroadenoma and a small margin of surrounding tissue. After removing the probe, the skin is dressed and patients are able to go home.[9] Cryoablation can be used on multiple fibroadenomas in the same setting with enough allotted time to treat each lesion.

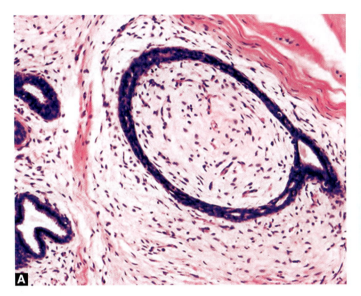
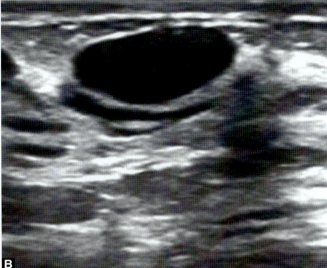

FIGURES 8.4A and B: Histological and ultrasonographic appearance of a fibroadenoma

Juvenile Fibroadenoma

Juvenile fibroadenomas are fibroadenomas which occur in a young patient population, usually in females under the age of 18. They tend to grow more aggressively than fibroadenomas in adults and in some cases result in deformity of the breast. Juvenile fibroadenomas are often referred to as giant fibroadenomas or giant juvenile adenomas due to their size and growth, and are on occasion mistaken for phyllodes tumors. Histologically, juvenile fibroadenomas are not different from common fibroadenomas. They are composed of stromal and epithelial hyperplastic tissue and lack the leaf-like growth pattern and stromal atypia of phyllodes tumors.[8] Ultrasonogram demonstrates a hypoechoic mass with smooth, partially lobulated margins typical of a fibroadenoma.

Due to the size and rapid growth of juvenile fibroadenomas, surgical excision is the best choice of treatment. Patients are young and deformities of the breast tissue can be easily reduced with resection of the mass. The nature of the juvenile adenoma to mimic phyllodes tumor is also an indication for excision so proper diagnosis can be made in pathology. The tumor should be excised with small margins to reduce chances of recurrence if the specimen does reveal phyllodes tumor.

ATYPICAL HYPERPLASIA

Atypical hyperplasia is usually an incidental finding discovered after biopsy of a radiographic abnormality on mammogram or ultrasound. Hyperplasia can be divided into proliferative lesions affecting the ducts or atypical ductal hyperplasia and lesions affecting the lobules, or atypical lobular hyperplasia. Atypical hyperplasia is associated with an increased risk of developing breast cancer. In most cases where advancement to breast cancer occurs, the ipsilateral breast is involved, however disease has been known to occur in the contralateral breast as well. Once diagnosis is made with core-needle biopsy, areas of atypical hyperplasia in the breast should be surgically excised and examined more closely. In almost half of these lesions, pathological examination of excisional biopsy results in diagnosis of ductal carcinoma in situ or microinvasive cancer.

Women diagnosed with atypical hyperplasia should be counseled on breast cancer risk reduction strategies. Surveillance with annual mammography and breast exams every 6 months is essential for early detection of abnormal tissues suspicious for breast cancer. Patients with atypical hyperplasia who are taking oral contraceptive pills or other types of hormone therapy should stop using them immediately. Women with additional factors for developing breast cancer may be candidates for breast cancer risk reduction therapies including tamoxifen and raloxifene, however, must be informed of potential side effects.

MISCELLANEOUS BREAST LESIONS

Phyllodes Tumor

Phyllodes tumor, also known as cystosarcoma phylloides, a term derived from the Greek for 'leaf-like fleshy tumor' is a predominantly benign breast tumor found in females. Grossly, phyllodes tumors resemble malignant sarcoma, however when it is sectioned it displays a unique leaf-like appearance and histologically it consists of epithelial cyst-like spaces (Fig. 8.5). The tumors have a smooth, well-demarcated texture, are freely mobile and tend to recur. Size varies from case to case, with the average tumors being 5 cm or smaller, however due to aggressive growth, some phyllodes tumors have been documented to reach substantially larger sizes of close to 30 cm.

Phyllodes tumor[4] is the most commonly occurring nonepithelial breast tumor, but is still a rare tumor as it only makes up 1 percent of all breast tumors. They occur almost exclusively in females, with no predilection for race. Though phyllodes tumors can occur in patients of all ages, they most often occur in the fifth decade of life. Patients present with a firm, well-circumscribed mass. The masses are usually nontender and mobile. Patients will commonly report a history of a small mass that rapidly changed size in a few weeks time. Phyllodes tumors occur more in the left breast than in the right breast, however, the cause for this is unknown.

Though almost 90 percent of phyllodes tumors are benign, they are grossly indistinguishable from their malignant counterparts. Malignant phyllodes tumors metastasize through hematogenous spread, with the lungs being the most susceptible organ affected. The skeleton, heart and liver are other organs where malignant phyllodes tumors tend to metastasize. Patients with metastasis of malignant disease present with symptoms of dyspnea, fatigue and bone pain.

Imaging such as mammogram and ultrasonography is not reliable in the diagnosis of phyllodes tumor due to its propensity to look like malignant sarcoma, therefore, a more invasive approach is required.[5] Although needle biopsy and core needle biopsy are options, they are usually inadequate for diagnosis and a more definitive approach involves surgical biopsy. In small lesions, excisional biopsy with margins is both diagnostic and therapeutic, while in large lesions, incisional biopsy is indicated until the diagnosis is confirmed histologically.[6,13]

Phyllodes tumors have a stromal and fibrous component and can appear similar to fibroadenomas, except for the clefts found in the walls of the tissue. Benign phyllodes tumors will demonstrate a large number of fusiform fibroblasts in the stromal tissue, and occasionally anaplastic cells with myxoid changes. Malignant phyllodes tumors will demonstrate a high degree of cellular atypia with increased mitotic count and increased stromal cellularity.

Treatment for phyllodes tumor is wide excisional biopsy with margins of normal tissue. Though defined margins have not been established for phyllodes tumor, a general rule is to take a two centimeter margin for small lesions, usually less than five centimeters, and a margin of 5 centimeters for larger lesions. It is important to remove the tumor and its wall without shelling out the lesions, as recurrence is much more likely when components of the phyllodes tumor are left behind. In cases where the breast is markedly distorted, a mastectomy can be performed with reconstruction, however, in most cases of phyllodes tumor, a minimal resection is recommended.[6]

BREAST ABSCESS

Breast abscesses are painful benign masses with surrounding erythema which arise spontaneously and have a sudden onset. Breast abscesses often have an area of fluctuance or are found to be draining pus and are usually localized to the lower half of the breast. These lesions tend to occur more often in patients who have large breasts, are overweight or have poor personal hygiene. These patients may have a long history of similar abscesses in the breast, or other areas of the body. Diabetic patients with poor sugar control are also at higher risk for developing abscesses and should be treated aggressively.

Abscesses are caused by bacterial colonizing in either in the central breast or in the periphery resulting in an inflammatory reaction and collection of neutrophils, white blood cells and bacteria in a localized area of the breast resulting in a painful mass. Diagnosis of breast abscess is

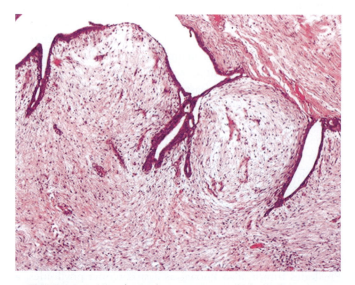

FIGURE 8.5: Histological appearance of phyllodes tumor

based on the history of the lesion and clinical examination. Patients present with a sudden onset of painful, growing mass that may be associated with fever and drainage of pus. The lesions usually present with a central area of fluctuance with surrounding erythema and induration and may have a history of purulent drainage.

Treatment of a breast abscess is similar to treatment of any abscess. In large lesions, those lacking a specific area of fluctuance or lesions in which a deep abscess cavity is suspected and ultrasound is indicated before definitive treatment. Nipple discharge consisting of pus or blood is concerning and also requires a breast ultrasound to evaluate the abscess cavity as well as follow-up with a surgeon to further work-up the lesion and rule out breast carcinoma as a cause. Once the diagnosis of abscess is made definitively, the lesion should be incised and drained under local anesthetic and left open. Wound cultures should be taken at the time of incision and followed for culture and sensitivity so the appropriate antibiotic can be administered.[7] If the abscess cavity is small and the patient shows no signs of systemic effect or increase in white blood cell count, empiric antibiotics may be given orally to the patient with instructions to follow-up as an outpatient. In cases where the white cell count is elevated above normal limits, or the areas of erythema and cellulitis are extensive, the patient should be admitted for intravenous antibiotics, fluid hydration and pain control.

MASTITIS

Postpartum mastitis is a localized cellulitis that is caused by an irritated or fissurized nipple resulting in bacterial invasion into the lactiferous sinuses and milk ducts. Patients generally present with a history of abrasion, trauma from breast feeding or a dry cracked nipple. Postpartum mastitis occurs in 2 to 3 percent of lactating women and most commonly occurs after the second postpartum week. Milk stasis plays a role in bacterial colonization as nutrients and temperature creates an ideal growth medium for bacteria once introduced. Stasis occurs when one breast is favored for breast feeding due to positioning or infant preference.

The most common organism involved in postpartum mastitis is *Staphylococcus aureus*, however, *Staphylococcus epidermidis* and streptococci are occasionally isolated as well. Treatment involves drainage of the affected segment by milking the breast or using a breast pump. Antibiotics that are effective on *Staphylococcus* species are prescribed as well. Warm compresses can be applied to the affected breast to reduce pain and aid in emptying of breast.[3] Lactating women

should be encouraged to alternate breasts when feeding or pumping milk to avoid milk stasis.

Mastitis unassociated with lactation can be divided into periareolar lesions and peripheral lesions. Periductal mastitis is a condition in which nondilated subareolar breast ducts become inflamed and occurs more commonly than peripheral nonlactating breast abscesses. Peripheral lesions are associated with conditions such as diabetes, rheumatoid arthritis, trauma and in patients who are being treated with steroids.[7] Patients present with localized erythema, warmth and pain in addition to fever and chills. Ultrasound should be used to rule out an abscess or cystic mass. Treatment involves antistaphylococcal antibiotics, followed by warm compresses and NSAIDs such as ibuprofen for control of pain and inflammation.[3]

FAT NECROSIS

Fat necrosis is a condition of the breast that can easily mimic breast cancer and was first differentiated from breast carcinoma as early as 1924.[1] Fat necrosis of the breast is a result of enzymatic breakdown of the subcutaneous fatty tissue into fatty acids. It usually occurs secondary to trauma to the breast tissue, but can occur spontaneously or less often as a result of diagnostic or therapeutic modalities involving the breast. Patients present with a painless, hard, indurated, fixed mass which has evolved over weeks to months after a traumatic event. The hard or firm nature of the mass and the appearance of fixation to the skin is due to the growth of new connective tissue in place of the lost subcutaneous fat. The masses often seem attached to deeper tissues as well, which is likely due to the inflammatory process involved in the necrosis. On occasion, the breakdown of subcutaneous fat can lead to the formation of an oil cyst, or a sac-like collection of greasy fluid composed of triglycerides and fatty acids.

Imaging used to evaluate lesions suspicious for fat necrosis includes ultrasonography (Fig. 8.6) and mammogram. Ultrasonography reveals solid masses which may be complex or cystic with ill-defined or discrete borders, and posterior shadowing. On mammogram, the appearance of fat necrosis ranges from lesions which are radiographically benign to those which are suspicious for malignancy. Radiographically benign lesions present as radiolucent masses with thin, well-defined capsules, while those suspicious for malignancy are complex masses with ill-defined borders.[10]

Fine needle aspiration should be performed for lesions suspicious for carcinoma of the breast, if radiological imaging

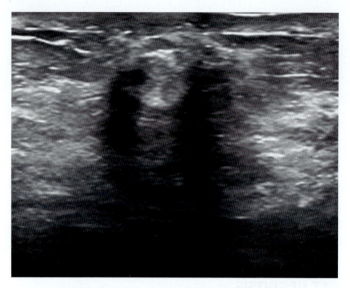

FIGURE 8.6: Ultrasound image of fat necrosis

is not definitive for breast necrosis. Histologically these lesions will demonstrate anuclear fat cells, unlike the atypia and increase in mitotic cells found in breast carcinoma. In radiographically benign lesions with areas of fluctuance, or oil cysts, aspiration can be therapeutic. Small masses, when left alone, tend to spontaneously resolve on their own over several months, where large lesions may require surgical excision of the area of necrosis, depending on patient preference and location of the lesion.

HAMARTOMA

Breast hamartomas are often refered to as fibroadenolipoma, lipofibroadenoma or adenolipomas. They consist of normal breast parenchyma including glandular tissue, adipose tissue and fibrous tissue, organized in a haphazard or unorganized fashion. Hamartomas of the breast are commonly discovered as an incidental finding on imaging but can also present in patients as discrete, painless and encapsulated masses. Though these lesions are benign, coincidental malignancy can occur in the region of growth of a hamartoma, therefore excision is recommended to rule out malignancy on pathological specimen.

GALACTOCELE

Galactoceles, also known as milk retention cysts, are collections of fluid consisting of breast milk which occur secondary to an obstruction of a milk duct. Patients present with a soft, round, mobile cystic mass and a history of breastfeeding. Galactoceles usually occur when a patient ceases breastfeeding or a significant change occurs in breastfeeding pattern and can occur weeks to months after cessation. The masses tend to be located centrally, just behind the nipple. Treatment is needle aspiration which will reveal a thick, creamy material. On occasion the aspirate is tinged brown or green, giving it the appearance of purulence, however this fluid is usually sterile, and aspiration alone is sufficient. In cases where an infection is present, showing signs of erythema, tenderness and possibly an elevated white blood cell count, or when a galactocele can not be aspirated, excisional biopsy is indicated.

REFERENCES

1. Adair FE, Burton JL. Traumatic fat necrosis of the female breast and its differentiation from carcinoma. Ann Surg 1924;80(5): 670–91.
2. American Cancer Society. Breast Cancer Facts and Figures 2007-2008. Available at http://www.cancer.org/downloads/STT/BCFF-Final.pdf. Accessed 06/04/2010.
3. Brennan M, Houssami N, French J. Management of benign breast conditions. Part 3—Other breast problems. Aust Fam Physician 2005;34(5): 353-5.
4. Brooks HL, Priolo S, Waxman. Cystosarcoma phylloides: a case report of an 11-year survival and review of surgical experience. Contemp Surg 1998;53:169-72.
5. Cole-Beuglet C, Soriano R, Kurtz AB. Ultrasound, X-ray mammography, and histopathology of cystosarcoma phylloides. Radiology 1983;146(2):481-6.
6. Chen WH, Cheng SP, Tzen CY, et al. Surgical treatment of phyllodes tumors of the breast: retrospective review of 172 cases. J Surg Oncol 2005;91(3):185-94.
7. Dixon JM. Outpatient treatment of non-lactational breast abscesses. Br J Surg 1992;79(1):56-7.
8. Greenberg R, Skornick Y, Kaplan O. Management of breast fibroadenomas. J Gen Intern Med 1998;13(9): 640-5.
9. Kaufman CS, Littrup PJ, Freeman-Gibb LA. Office-based cryoablation of breast fibroadenomas with long-term follow-up. Breast J 2005;11(5): 344-50.
10. Kerlikowske K, Smith-Bindman R, Ljung BM, et al. Evaluation of abnormal mammography results and palpable breast abnormalities. Ann Intern Med 2003;139(4):274-84.
11. Solin LJ, Orel SG, Hwang WT, Harris EE, Schnall MD. Relationship of breast magnetic resonance imaging to outcome after breast-conservation treatment with radiation for women with early-stage invasive breast carcinoma or ductal carcinoma in situ. Journal of Clinical Oncology 2008;26(3):386-91.
12. Turnbull L, Brown S, Harvey I, Olivier C, et al. Comparative effectiveness of MRI in breast cancer (COMICE) trial; a randomized controlled trial. Lancet 2010;(9714):563-71.
13. Wurdinger S, Herzog AB, Fischer DR. Differentiation of phyllodes breast tumors from fibroadenomas on MRI. AJR Am J Roentgenol 2005;185(5):1317-21.

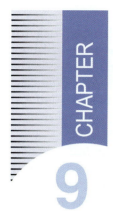

CHAPTER

9

Malignant Breast Diseases

Megan Hill, Vijay Mittal

Risk Factors

Factors that increase the duration or quantity of exposure to estrogen, increase the likelihood of developing breast cancer. Early menarche, late menopause, and nulliparity all result in a higher number of menstrual periods, which is associated with a greater risk of breast cancer.[1,2] Obesity, alcohol use, and hormone replacement therapy all increase the amount of estrogen exposure. Patients who undergo their first pregnancy after the age of 35 also are at increased risk.[3]

Nonhormonal factors have also been implicated. Radiation therapy predisposes women to development of breast cancer. First-degree relatives with breast cancer, a personal history or prior breast cancer, and certain genes substantially increase the risk for breast cancer.[4] Additionally, the presence of lobular carcinoma *in situ* or atypical hyperplasia increases the relative risk of breast cancer development fourfold.[5]

The average US female has a 12 percent risk of developing breast cancer over the course of her life. As noted above, the risk for each woman is multifactorial. Several risk assessment models have been developed to assess individual risk.[6] The most commonly implemented model is the Gail Model, first developed by Gail and associates in the 1970s. The Claus model is another commonly used risk assessment tool that places heavier emphasis on family history.[7] Neither the Gail nor Claus model takes into account specific genetic abnormalities, a risk factor that is gaining significance as further research is undertaken.

Based on the risk assessed, several medical decisions may be affected. Postmenopausal women at high-risk for breast cancer may elect to abstain from hormone replacement therapy (HRT) for control of vasomotor symptoms that could otherwise be ameliorated with estrogen replacement. The Women's Health Initiative was a large-scale phase III trial that evaluated the effect of HRT on cardiovascular disease, bone health and breast cancer. Based on results published in 2002, there were minimal protective cardiovascular effects of HRT, but a concerning three-fold increase risk of breast cancer when taken for greater than 4 years.[8]

Screening mammography is a noninvasive, cost-effective method for breast cancer detection. While recent recommendations have raised the age of screening mammography to 50 years, the American College of Surgeons continues to recommend screening mammography yearly for women greater than 40 years of age. The case for waiting to begin screening after the age of 50 years stems from an increased number of false-positive findings in women younger than 50 years as well as difficulty in reading the studies based on increased breast density in younger women.[9]

Tamoxifen, a selective estrogen receptor modulator is currently recommended for women with a Gail relative risk greater than 1.70. In the Breast Cancer prevention Trial (NSABP P-01) that looked at over 13000 women with a Gail score greater than 1.7, breast cancer development was reduced by 49 percent in those women who received tamoxifen as compared to placebo. Tamoxifen has been found to increase the risk of endometrial cancer development by 2.5 percent. Due to this adverse effect, raloxifene, another selective estrogen receptor modulator, was compared to tamoxifen with hopes of finding the same preventative effect on breast cancer but with a better side effect profile. In the STAR trial, 19000 postmenopausal women at high-risk for breast cancer were randomly assigned to treatment with tamoxifen or raloxifene. Both drugs were found to reduce the risk of breast cancer by half, but Raloxifene in fact was not associated with as high a risk of developing endometrial cancer.[10-12]

Genetic Mutations

Genetic mutations such as BRCA1 and BRCA2 are associated with 5-10 percent of all breast cancers. These are autosomal dominant mutations that display varying penetrance. Both genes function as tumor suppressors, and loss of both alleles is necessary for cancer initiation. These genes are involved in transcription, cell-cycle control and DNA damage repair. BRCA1 mutations have been implicated in 45 percent of hereditary breast cancers, and carry an associated lifetime risk of 40 percent for ovarian cancer development as well. Breast cancer secondary to BRCA1 mutations are associated with earlier onset, higher propensity for bilateral breast cancer, and the presence of other malignancies, especially ovarian, colon, and prostate cancers.[13-16] Two specific mutations of the BRCA1 gene have been found in Jewish populations, specifically Ashkenazi Jews. One percent of Ashkenazi Jews carry the 185delAG mutation, sometimes in conjunction with the 5382insC mutation, and these have been implicated in almost all BRCA1 mutations in this particular population.[17]

BRCA2 is also a DNA damage repair gene found on chromosome arm 13q, made up of 70 kb. It is believed to be co-regulated with BRCA1. Over 250 mutations of BRCA2 have been identified. BRCA2 infers a lifetime risk of breast cancer development of 85 percent and is also associated with ovarian breast cancer. BRCA2 is of particular importance in male carriers, as it is associated with a 100-fold increase in breast cancer development compared to that of the general male population (6% risk). BRCA2 is associated with a higher incidence of invasive ductal carcinomas. Like BRCA1, carriers of BRCA2 are more likely to develop breast cancer at a young age, develop bilateral breast cancer. It is linked to a greater variety of associated cancers: ovarian, colon, prostate, pancreatic, gallbladder, stomach, and melanoma. It is found with increased incidence in Ashkenazi Jewish and Finnish populations.[13-14]

BRCA mutation testing should be considered in women diagnosed with breast cancer before the age of 50, those who have concurrent breast and ovarian cancer, male breast cancer at any age, and those with a history of hereditary breast and ovarian cancer. Detailed family history should be obtained.

The decision to proceed with genetic testing requires informed consent and must be precluded by appropriate counseling. The affected individual is tested via a panel of mutations, and once the mutation is identified, other family members may be tested specifically for the identified mutation. A positive test is one which finds a BRCA mutation

that affects translation or transcription. If no mutation is identified, the woman carries an identical risk for developing breast cancer as that of the general population, and her children need not be tested for the mutation. The possibility of an unidentified genetic mutation remains. The Health Insurance Portability and Accountability Act (HIPAA) made it illegal for genetic information to be taken into account by insurance plans to deny coverage.[18-21]

Once a BRCA mutation has been identified, there are several options for risk management. These include prophylactic mastectomy with reconstruction, prophylactic oophorectomy with HRT, intensive surveillance for breast and ovarian cancer, and chemoprevention. Prophylactic mastectomy greatly reduces the risk for breast cancer, though any remaining breast tissue still is at risk. If intense surveillance is chosen, annual mammography should begin at age 25 years. MRI is more sensitive for identifying masses in dense breasts of these younger patients, but also leads to more identification of benign masses and subsequent false negatives. Tamoxifen has been suggested but has not been reliably found to decrease incidence of breast cancer in BRCA mutations. Tamoxifen is most effective on those cancers that are estrogen receptor (ER) positive, and most breast cancers associated with BRCA mutations are ER negative.

The American College of Obstetrics and Gynecology recommends that BRCA1 or BRCA2 carriers consider a prophylactic oophorectomy after childbearing. In those who defer or delay oophorectomy, the Cancer Genetics Studies Consortium recommends yearly transvaginal ultrasound and annual serum cancer antigen 125 screens beginning at age 25 years.

Hereditary breast cancer is also associated with Cowdens disease and Li-Fraumeni syndrome.[18-22]

EPIDEMIOLOGY

Breast cancer is the most common cancer in women, and is the leading cause of cancer death in women aged 20 to 59 years. Overall, it is surpassed only by lung cancer as the most frequent cause of death from cancer in all women. The probability of a woman in the United States developing breast cancer is now 1 in 8, increased from 1 in 13 in the 1970s. While the incidence of overall breast cancer has increased, in part due to greater detection via mammograms, the incidence of local metastasis and mortality from breast cancer has declined. In the 1960s, survival rates from Caucasian and African American women were 63 and 46 percent, respectively, while in the late 1980s, they were 85 and 71 percent respectively.

Breast cancer around the world varies greatly in incidence, from 29.6 per 100,000 in Cyprus to 2.0 per 100,000 in Haiti. The United States sits in the middle with 19.6 per 100,000. The incidence of breast cancer is higher in more industrialized nations. Atypically high incidences include Ashkenazi Jews (due to higher incidence of BRCA mutations) and nuns (due to nulliparity and resultant increased estrogen exposure). Though the rates of breast cancer rose throughout the 1990s in the United States, the incidence has since leveled off and now declined. The rise was attributed to the increase in number of women taking HRT, which has since declined. The variations in breast cancer incidence stem from cultural reductions in risk factors: in less developed countries, the women often begin childbearing at younger ages. However, due to less access to mammography, the breast cancer is often more advanced at time of presentation. In the United States, there exists disparity based on socioeconomic status. Lack of access to screening leads to delayed presentation in minorities and the poor. Additionally follow-up, systemic treatment, and reconstruction all are less common in lower socioeconomic groups. Notably, African American women have the highest incidence of breast cancer under the age of 45 years, as well as to have ER positive breast cancer.[23-26]

PRIMARY BREAST CANCER

Breast cancer begins with fibrosis that involves the stroma and epithelial tissue of the breast. When cancer invades into surrounding tissue, a desmoplastic reaction develops that entraps the Coopers ligaments and results in a classic retraction of the skin. When this spreads to involve the lymph flow, *peau d'orange* develops: thickened, dimpled skin. This progresses to invasion of the skin, areas of ulceration and satellite nodules.

The most important prognostic component is axillary metastasis. Breast cancer usually spreads first to the low axillary lymph nodes (Level I: lateral to the pectoralis minor), then to the middle nodes (Level II: posterior to pectoralis minor) and then the apical nodes (Level III, medial to the pectoralis minor). At first the nodes are soft and mobile, but as the cancer progresses, they become firm and fixed.

Distant metastasis occurs after breast cancers receive their own blood supply from neovascularization, which occurs after the 20th cell division. Distant metastasis is especially likely to occur after the 27th cell division, at which point the lesion has usually grown to greater than 5 millimeters. Metastasis is the leading cause of cancer-related death for up to 10 years after treatment of the original focus.[27]

PATHOLOGY

Breast cancer is first divided into two subtypes: noninvasive and invasive. A cancer is deemed invasive after it invades through the basement membrane, a characteristic seen on microscopic examination.

Noninvasive Breast Cancer

Noninvasive malignancies include lobular carcinoma *in situ* (LCIS) and ductal carcinoma in situ (DCIS). While previously considered a separate, malignant neoplasm, LCIS has recently been classified as a risk factor for breast cancer rather than a separate malignant subtype. LCIS is indistinguishable from normal breast tissue on gross examination: it appears the same as normal anatomic lobular breast tissue.[28] LCIS develops from the terminal duct lobular units. It is characterized by mucoid cytoplasmic globules. It may be associated with nearby calcifications. It most frequently occurs in women younger than 45 years. The average age at diagnosis is 44 years. Five percent of the time, a concurrent invasive breast cancer will be found (in either breast). LCIS is currently regarded as a marker for future development of breast cancer, usually ductal in origin. Prior to the use of screening mammography, LCIS was the most frequently diagnosed *in situ* lesion, but now DCIS is diagnosed by a ratio of >2:1. LCIS occurs bilaterally in 50-70 percent of cases.[29]

DCIS is regarded as a malignant lesion. It is present in 5 percent of male breast cancers. It is often classified as intraductal, which carries a higher risk for development into invasive cancer. Papillary growths project into the minor duct lumen on a histological level. Initially they are difficult to distinguish from benign lesions because of their lack of atypia. As the lesion progresses, it fills the lumen and develops pleomorphic and highly mitotic characteristics. DCIS is further subdivided into four histologic types: papillary, cribriform, solid, and comedo. DCIS lesions consist of discrete areas of malignant tissue contained within basement membrane. Solid and comedo histotypes are more aggressive, progressing more quickly to invasive malignancy than cribriform and papillary lesions. Often, however, more than one subtype is found in a single lesion.[28] DCIS is bilateral less than 20 percent of cases.[30] The presence or history of DCIS places women at a fivefold increased risk for invasive breast cancer, usually in the same quadrant of the same breast.

Calcifications may be the first detectable sign of malignancy, identified on mammograms. The blood supply is from outside the basement membrane and as a result, the lesions develop central necrosis and subsequent central calcification. It is not well understood what causes transformation into invasive cancer, but the lesions usually retain their morphologic structures (papillary DCIS develops into papillary invasive cancer, etc.). Counter-intuitively, histologic grade does not progress when the lesion becomes invasive: high grade DCIS becomes high grade invasive cancer, and likewise for low grade.[28] Multifocal lesions refer to the presence of more than one breast cancer within the same quadrant as the primary. Multicentricity refers to more than one cancer within the same breast, but within different quadrants.

INVASIVE BREAST CANCER

Invasive breast cancers differ from noninvasive primarily due to their lack of basement membrane, and as a result lack of containment of malignant cells. Like noninvasive breast cancer, invasive is divided into lobular and ductal histologic origin. Lobular malignancies extend in a linear nature which makes it more difficult to detect until the lesion has grown to be quite large. Ductal, on the other hand invades in a haphazard direction, creating a discrete mass that is picked up earlier on both mammography and physical exam.

Fifty to seventy percent of invasive breast cancer is invasive (infiltrating) ductal cancer. Ten to fifteen percent of breast cancer is lobular carcinoma. Invasive ductal cancer often has no specific identifying features, and is then known as infiltrating ductal carcinoma, not otherwise specified (NOS). When there is further differentiation, the lesions are named according to their identifying features.[28]

Invasive breast cancer can be divided into special type cancers, which require 90 percent of the histologic features of the lesion to be made up of one defining type, or no special type (NST), which carries a worse prognosis. Dr Foote and Stewart proposed the following classifications of special type breast cancer:[31]
- Paget's disease of the nipple
- Invasive ductal carcinoma
- Adenocarcinoma with productive fibrosis, 80 percent
- Medullary carcinoma, 4 percent
- Mucinous (colloid) carcinoma, 2 percent
- Papillary carcinoma, 2 percent
- Tubular carcinoma, 2 percent
- Invasive lobular carcinoma, 10 percent
- Rare cancers, including adenoid cystic, squamous cell, apocrine.

Paget's disease presents as a chronic scaly eczematous lesion that may progress to ulceration. It is often confused with superficial melanoma and can be distinguished using S-100 antigen immunostaining (positive in melanoma) and carcinoembryonic antigen (CEA, positive in Paget's disease). Paget's disease is diagnosed by a nipple biopsy which reveals Paget's cells: large pale, vacuolated cells and is often associated with underlying DCIS or invasive breast cancer. Treatment depends on the extent of the underlying lesion and may range from lumpectomy to mastectomy.

Invasive ductal carcinoma with productive fibrosis makes up 80 percent of invasive lesions. In up to two-third of cases, micro- or macroscopic axillary lymph node metastases are present at the time of diagnosis. Invasive ductal carcinoma usually presents in 50-60-year-old women as a firm, discrete mass. On mammography it displays stellate calcifications, and often involves several clusters of cancer cells. Within this classification there is a broad variety of cellular and nuclear grades.[31]

Medullary carcinoma is associated with BRCA1 hereditary breast cancer and presents as a large soft mass deep in the breast. It is associated with a favorable 5-year survival rate. Necrosis with hemorrhage may occur and result in a rapid increase in size. Histologically, medullary carcinoma has dense lymphoreticular infiltration with lymphocytes and plasma cells, large poorly differentiated pleomorphic nuclei, and a sheet-like growth pattern without ductal differentiation. DCIS is present along the borders of medullary carcinoma lesions in half of these cases. Due to the fact that medullary breast carcinoma carries with it an intrinsic involvement of lymph nodes that is usually simply benign or hyperplastic, this particular special-type cancer is often clinically staged incorrectly.[32]

Mucinous or colloid carcinoma presents in the elderly as a bulky mass. Extracellular mucin pools surround low-grade cancer cells. On gross exam, it is gelatinous, shiny, and firm. Two-third of these cancers carry hormone receptors. One-third have lymphatic involvement. Histologically, these carcinomas require many sections for diagnosis as the mucinous cells displace the few cancer cells.

Papillary carcinoma occurs in non-white females over the age of 70. These are small tumors, less than 3 cm in diameter with papillae that have fibrovascular stromal epithelium. They rarely involve lymph nodes.

Tubular carcinoma occurs usually in perimenopausal women and is found via mammography. It is characterized by a random array of tubular components. One-tenth of these women present with level 1 axillary node involvement.

Invasive lobular carcinoma makes up one-tenth of all breast cancer. The presentation of this particular type of cancer varies from clinically non-detectable to entire breast replacement. It can be multifocal, multicentric, and bilateral at time of presentation. Histologically invasive lobular carcinoma has rounded nuclei with minimal cytoplasm. Using special staining, intracytoplasmic mucin may be identified as signet-ring cells. Invasive lobular carcinoma grows slowly and displays subtle findings on mammography, leading to delayed diagnosis.[32]

Diagnosis

Despite the push for breast self-examination, only one-third of all breast cancers are first discovered as a palpable mass noted by the woman herself. More frequently, women present with complaints of breast enlargement or asymmetry, changes in the appearance of a nipple or associated discharge, erythema, axillary masses, or rarely, pain.

Inspection

First, the woman should be examined with her arms by her side, then with arms extended upward, then with her hands on her hips. Breast should be visually examined during this time for symmetry, size, edema, nipple retraction, or any skin changes. When the woman leans forward, this should exaggerate any underlying skin retraction. Once proper visual inspection has been performed, the physician should move to physical examination.

With the patient laying supine with her ipsilateral arm at her side, all quadrants of the breast should be palpated, from sternal border medially, to the edge of the latissimus dorsi laterally, and from the clavicle superiorly to the inframammary fold inferiorly. The three axillary levels of lymph nodes should then be palpated with the arm held in a relaxed position so the axilla may be palpated deeply. Attention should also be paid to the presence of parasternal nodes.

Mammography first came into use in the 1960s, but has gained more frequent use as technology has improved. It is especially useful as a screening tool in order to detect unexpected lesions. If a palpable mass is felt, two-view chest radiography may be employed. This utilizes a craniocaudal (CC) and a mediolateral oblique (MLO) view. The MLO view is useful for examining the greatest amount of breast tissue. However, the CC view is more efficacious in examining the medial aspect of the breast. Spot compression improves definition and decreases the radiation dose required. Magnification may also be used to better examine microcalcifications.[33]

Suspicious findings on X-ray include the following: solid masses, especially with stellate characteristics, thickened breast tissues, and areas of microcalcifications. Multiple pinpoint calcifications are highly suspicious and occurs in half of nonpalpable malignancies. This is particularly important in early cancer detection in young women.

Mammography may be performed as part of routine screening examination or as further investigation of a clinical abnormality. Mammography looks for density abnormalities as well as microcalcifications as findings suspicious for underlying malignancy. The findings are classified according to the Breast Imaging Reporting and Data System (BI-RADS).[34]

Nonpalpable abnormalities identified on mammography may be density lesions, microcalcifications, or a combination of both. Stellate dense lesions with associated microcalcifications are the most suspicious for breast cancer. All suspicious lesions should undergo biopsy. BI-RADS 1-3 may be monitored with interval mammography (annually for BI-RADS 1-2, Bi-annually for BI-RADS 3) (Table 9.1). A diagnostic mammogram may be used to further investigate a concerning, palpable lesion. According to two reports, a striking 10 to 22 percent of palpable lesions were not visualized on screening mammography.[35-36] In such cases, a marker may be placed on the area of concern to guide the study to focus on that area.[35] Additionally, ultrasound may

BI-RADS category	Description	Likelihood of malignancy	Recommendation
	Table 9.1: Breast cancer treatment (PDQ): Health professional version, National Cancer Institute		
0	Need more information	2-10%	Further imaging studies
1	Normal	0.05-0.1%	Routine screening mammography
2	Benign	0.05-0.1%	Routine screening mammography
3	Probably benign	0.3-1.8%	Short-term follow-up (5 months)
4	Highly suspicious	10-55%	Biopsy
5	Malignant	60-100%	Biopsy
6	Known cancer	100%	Treat malignancy

be employed as an alternate investigation for those palpable, concerning areas not visualized on mammogram.[36]

Ductography

If nipple discharge is the presenting symptom, a ductogram can be performed. This involves dilation of the suspicious duct with subsequent injection of radio-opaque dye while the patient is in the supine position. CC and MLO views are then obtained and the duct is outlined with the dye. It is examined for areas of obstruction or filling defects, which are suggestive of tumoral involvement.

Ultrasound

Ultrasound is of particular use in breast examination. Two major advantages are its noninvasiveness and its availability: most breast surgeons have this easily on-hand at their offices. Ultrasound is useful in examining cystic masses as well as further investigating echogenic qualities of abnormalities. Qualities that are suspicious for malignancy are ill-defined, irregular borders, stellate shapes, and strong internal echoes. Ultrasound can be used to guide needle aspiration and core biopsy. Ultrasound is of limited use in lesions less than one centimeter in diameter.[22,33,37] Ultrasound used in conjunction with mammography increases sensitivity and accuracy, and has a higher negative predictive value. Additionally, ultrasound may be more helpful in younger women as the density of their breasts makes mammography more difficult.[5]

MRI

Magnetic resonance imaging (MRI) is rapidly gaining utility in breast cancer workup. It is even more sensitive than mammography and can be used to further examine abnormalities found on mammography. In a study of 426 women with known cancer, MRI identified additional abnormalities in one quarter of these patients. Almost 2/3 of those sampled were found to have additional occult cancer foci.[38] This study has been used in arguments that suggest these patients would benefit from mastectomy instead of breast conserving therapy, though there have been no studies further evaluating outcomes of women with additional malignancy identified on MRI treated with BCT versus mastectomy. There has been increasing discussion of using MRI to screen women, especially young women at high-risk for developing breast cancer. Due to the presence of naturally dense breast tissue in younger women, mammography often is less effective in identifying small lesions. MRI potentially has an advantage in early detection in these young

patients.[22,33,37] Downsides to the utilization of MRI include high cost, lack of standard procedure, and difficulty in biopsying lesions identified on MRI.[5] MRI has also been suggested to be of use in identifying ruptured implants, locating primaries in women presenting with axillary adenopathy, as well as in assessing tumor response to neoadjuvant chemotherapy.

BIOPSY

While ultrasound can be used to guide biopsies in palpable lesions, stereotactic techniques must be utilized when the lesions are nonpalpable, such as in the case of microcalcifications. The combination of diagnostic mammography, ultrasound or stereotactic localization and subsequent fine-needle aspiration is almost 100 percent accurate in successfully diagnosing breast cancer via cytology. Open breast biopsy must be undertaken in order to analyze breast tissue architecture and grade. For nonpalpable lesions, core biopsy as an initial step is preferred not only because of cosmesis, but also it allows definitive surgery to be achieved with a single, better-planned surgery. This has the added benefit of lower overall cost to the patient as well.

For palpable lesions, intra-office fine-needle aspiration (FNA) is ideal. Under ultrasound guidance a 1.5 inch 22-gauge needle is advanced into the lesion. The needle is gently moved within the breast to create cellular debris. Once this is performed the cells are aspirated and then deposited on microscope slides. The slides are fixed and then sent for analysis. In palpable breast masses, the sensitivity and specificity of FNA is almost 100 percent. Core needle biopsy using a 14 gauge Tru-Cut needle is an alternative diagnostic modality. The downside to core needle biopsy is that a specimen that does not show malignant cells cannot completely rule out breast cancer.[28] Small, fibrotic tumors, or those with histology consistent with infiltrating lobular, tubular, and cribriform are associated with higher false-negative results.[5] As always, if radiologic findings are suspicious, despite a negative core biopsy or FNA, open biopsy should be undertaken. A working flowchart for management of breast cancer is attached, and it is important to understand the rapid changes in the breast care. The breast management is one of the disease that has seen most rapid changes in workup, and management in last 20 years (Fig. 9.1).

BREAST CANCER STAGING AND BIOMARKERS

Although there are multiple ways of staging breast cancer, the most frequently used is TNM (Tumor, Node, Metastasis)

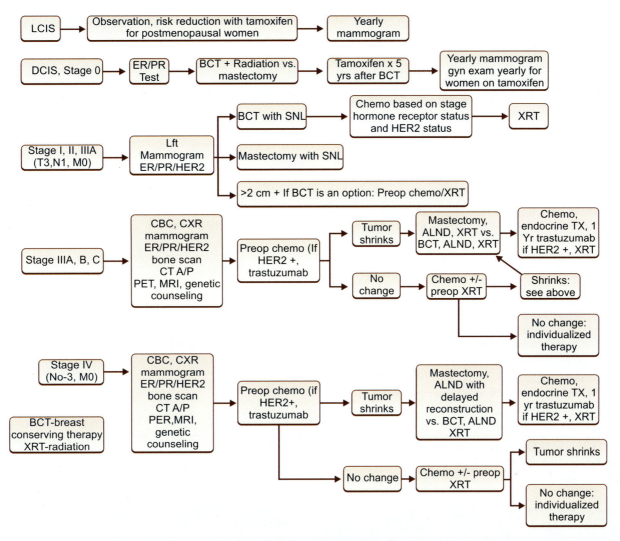

FIGURE 9.1: An algorithm for management of breast cancer

created by The American Joint Committee on Cancer (Tables 9.2 and 9.3). While there is correlation between tumor size, axillary lymph node metastasis and disease free survival, the single greatest predictor of 10 and 20-year survival is the presence and extent of axillary lymph node metastasis.

PROGNOSIS

The five-year survival for stage I breast cancer is 94 percent, for stage IIA 85 percent, for stage IIB 70 percent. Once a stage III cancer is diagnosed, the survival at five years is significantly impacted, dropping to 52 percent for stage IIIA and 48 percent for stage IIIB. Stage IV breast cancer has a dismal 18 percent five-year survival rate (Table 9.4).

However, breast cancer survival rates continue to increase as early detection improves and treatment modalities are advanced.

CHEMOPREVENTION

For those breast cancers that are found to be estrogen-receptor (ER) positive, tamoxifen, an estrogen antagonist, has been found to reduce breast cancer risk, as well as decrease the risk of contralateral breast cancer development when provided to women with known ER positive cancer. The Early Breast Cancer Trialists' Collaborative Group (EBCTCG) found a reduction of contralateral breast cancer development in women treated with tamoxifen (47%). This was met with mixed results in four subsequent studies,

Table 9.2: Breast cancer T, N and M categories

Primary tumor (T)

TX : Primary tumor cannot be assessed

T0: No evidence of primary tumor

Tis: Carcinoma *in situ* (DCIS, LCIS, or Pager's disease of the nipple with no tumor mass)

T1: Tumor is ≤ 2 cm

T2: Tumor is >2 cm but <5 cm

T3: Tumor is >5 cm

T4: Tumor of any size growing into the chest wall or skin

Lymph node status (N)

NX: Nearby lymph nodes cannot be assessed

N0: Cancer has not spread to nearby lymph nodes

N1: Cancer has spread to 1 to 3 axillary lymph nodes, and/or tiny amounts of cancer are found in internal mammary lymph nodes on sentinel lymph node biopsy

N2: Cancer has spread to 4 to 9 axillary lymph nodes under the arm, or cancer has enlarged the internal mammary lymph nodes

N3: One of the following applies:
- Cancer has spread to 10 or more axillary lymph nodes
- Cancer has spread to the lymph nodes under the clavicle
- Cancer has spread to the lymph nodes above the clavicle
- Cancer involves axillary lymph nodes and has enlarged the internal mammary lymph nodes
- Cancer involves 4 or more axillary lymph nodes, and tiny amounts of cancer are found in internal mammary lymph nodes on sentinel lymph node biopsy

Metastases (M)

MX: Presence of distant metastases cannot be assessed

M0: No distant spread

M1: Spread to distant organs is present

DCIS: Ductal carcinoma *in situ*; LCIS: Lobular carcinoma *in situ*.
Source: References 6, 12, 21.

Table 9.3: American Joint Committee on cancer staging system for breast cancer			
Stage	*T*	*N*	*M*
Stage 0	Tis	N0	M0
Stage I	T1	N0	M0
Stage IIA	T0	N1	M0
	T1	N1	M0
	T2	N0	M0
Stage IIB	T2	N1	M0
	T3	N0	M0
Stage IIIA	T0	N2	M0
	T1	N2	M0
	T2	N2	M0
	T3	N1, N2	M0
Stage IIIB	T4	N0, N1, N2	M0
Stage IIIC	Any T	N3	M0
Stage IV			

Table 9.4: Survival bound on stage	
Stage	*5-year relative survival rate*
I	94 percent
IIA	85 percent
IIB	70 percent
IIIA	70 percent
IIIB	48 percent
IV	18 percent

though definite improvement was demonstrated by the National Surgical Adjuvant Breast and Bowel Project (NSABP) in women with LCIS or atypia.[28]

SURGICAL TECHNIQUES

Excisional Biopsy with Needle Localization

The complete removal of a breast lesion with cancer-free margins is referred to as an excisional biopsy. Margins are generally examined by frozen section intraoperatively. The possibility of mastectomy should be discussed with all patients prior to the operation for the possibility of worse-than-expected findings. Subareolar and centrally located lesions should be approached via circumareolar incisions, which result in excellent scars. For lesions located outside the nipple-areolar complex, curvilinear incisions along Langer's lines should be utilized. For the inferior quadrants, radial incisions result in the best outcomes. Once excised, the lesion is marked for orientation for the pathologists using silk suture (for example, long tails for lateral margin, short tails for superior margin, air-knot for anterior margin). Hemostasis is obtained using electrocautery. While not usually necessary to approximate the subcutaneous tissue, if a large lesion was removed some approximation using absorbable suture may help prevent dimpling. A running subcuticular stitch is used to close the skin and a surgical bra is applied to prevent seroma formation. This approach is the same for stereotactic-needle biopsy lesions. A J-shaped wire is placed using mammography guidance. The surgeon then excises a core of tissue around the length of the wire. Before the skin is closed, intraoperative radiography is performed to ensure full excision of the lesion was achieved.

Sentinel Lymph Node Dissection

Sentinel lymph node dissection (SLND) is used to assess the lymph node status in women with early breast cancer and no detectable nodes on clinical exam. SLND is only useful in early breast cancer—by stages III and IV, full axillary lymph node dissection should be undertaken. It should also not be used in cases of palpable nodes, pregnancy, DCIS without mastectomy, or prior axillary surgery.

SLND can be performed using several techniques. Studies have shown that a combination of intraoperative gamma probe detection of radio-labeled colloid and methylene or lymphazurin blue for sentinel lymph node detection yields the best results. The area around the prior biopsy site (known lesion location, and/or retroareolar location) is injected with 0.5 mCi of 0.2 Technetium (Tc) 99m-labeled sulfur colloid few hours before surgery and X-ray is taken to visualize the SLN for resection. Immediately prior to the operation, 3-5 ml of methylene blue dye is injected sub-areolarly and peri-tumorally and massaged gently. Women should be notified that the methylene or lymphazurin blue may change the color of their urine to blue as well for 24-48 hours. Anaphylactic reactions are rare, though there is a slightly higher risk associated with

lymphazurin blue over methylene blue. Total radiation exposure is minimal.

Intraoperatively, a hand-held gamma probe is used to transcutaneously detect the lymph node with highest concentration of colloid. A 3 cm transverse incision along the axillary hairline should be made and dissection carefully undertaken. Attention should be paid to identifying areas of blue dye concentration. If delicate lymphatic channels can be identified and preserved, this results in cleaner dissection, less edema, and less spilling of dye onto non-nodal tissue (creating less distraction during dissection). The node with the highest gamma-probe signal (and hopefully concurrent greatest concentration of blue dye) should be removed. *Exvivo*, the node undergoes a ten-second radioactive count, which is recorded.

The remainder of the axilla is then checked for areas with a radioactive count greater than 10 percent of that of the highest count. Any node with greater than 10 percent should be excised and sent for pathology. Additionally, any node with a high concentration of blue dye should be excised. These are sent for frozen section. If found to be positive, or if greater than three nodes are suspicious, full axillary lymph node dissection should be performed.

The overall success rate in identifying the sentinel node is 97.2 percent. False-negative rate is 9.8 percent. This was found to be associated with tumors located near the axillary tail, as peri-tumor injections may have led to false results. The less lymph nodes removed, the less diagnostic the dissection. According to the NSABP B-32 trial, there was a 7.7 percent reduction in false negative rates when three lymph nodes were removed compared to two (10% versus 17.7%). Additionally, prior excisional biopsy contributes to disruption of normal lymphatics and for this reason, core biopsy is recommended when possible prior to surgery to aid in better presurgical planning and the possibility of a single, definitive surgery. Of note, peritumoral injection may help identify SNL outside of the usual expected level I and II nodes.

Complications of sentinel lymph node biopsy were as follows: wound infection 1 percent, seroma or hematoma 1.4 percent, axillary paresthesias 8.6 percent, and lymphedema in 2 percent. These numbers are greatly reduced compared to those found in patients undergoing SLND with completion of axillary lymph node dissection.[39]

Conservation Therapy

Patients may opt for breast conservation therapy, which involves resection of the primary breast lesion with assessment of regional lymph node status and radiation therapy. The surgical therapy may involve wide local excision, lumpectomy, partial mastectomy, or segmental mastectomy with a minimum of 2 mm margins. This is particularly ideal for stage I or II breast cancer because results are equivalent to those after total mastectomy with the added benefit of preservation of the breast. Six randomized trials showed equivalent disease-free survival rates with breast conserving therapy (BCT) as compared to mastectomy. BCT also is often preferred in terms of cosmesis and quality of life. It offers additional protection of sensation preservation and less psychological adjustment for women as opposed to those undergoing total mastectomy. BCT is the current standard of care for DCIS, stage 0, I and II breast cancer with postoperative radiation treatment.

SLND is the preferred staging procedure if there are no clinically-positive nodes. This should be performed prior to the excision of the primary tumor. Local recurrence in BCT is primarily determined by the adequacy of surgical margins during the primary operation. If clear margins are not able to be obtained during re-excision, the decision should be made to proceed with mastectomy.

Oncoplastic surgery may be considered at the time of segmental mastectomy. This should be considered only in situations where re-excision is not a possibility. Oncoplastic surgery should be considered when large amounts of breast tissue are removed, when there is an expected unfavorable cosmetic outcome, and when there is concern for malpositioning of the nipple.

Mastectomy

A skin-sparing mastectomy removes all breast tissue including the nipple-areolar complex and prior biopsy scars. A total mastectomy removes the aforementioned tissue with the additional removal of overlying skin. An extended simple mastectomy removes all that of a total mastectomy and level I axillary nodes. A modified radical mastectomy adds the removal of level II nodes. The Halsted, or radical mastectomy, requires removal of the pectoralis major and minor muscles, as well as all III lymph node levels. With the improvement of chemotherapy, radiation therapy and hormonal therapy, radical mastectomies are rarely required. Some women who would be good candidates for BCT may elect to proceed with mastectomy. This may be due to preferred single-stage treatment, economic reasons, or lack of access to follow-up care with chemotherapy or radiation. As always, the patient should be evaluated from a complete medical and psychosocial standpoint to yield the best personal results.

Reconstruction

There are a variety of reconstruction options once all chemotherapy and radiation have been finished. Depending on the remaining breast tissue, a pedicled flap, such as a latissimus dorsi flap or a transverse rectus abdominus flap may be utilized. Some women may elect to undergo immediate reconstruction after mastectomy with tissue expander and subsequent implants. Proper preoperative planning and discussion helps to expedite reconstruction via early involvement of all necessary specialists.

Radiation Therapy

Radiation therapy is utilized in all patients undergoing BCT to prevent local recurrence. Radiation should also be used in patients who had positive margins after undergoing mastectomy. Women with axillary involvement of 4 or more nodes or those pre-menopausal women with 1-3 positive nodes should also be considered for adjuvant radiation therapy. For stage IIIB and IV, neoadjuvant chemotherapy with segmental mastectomy should be followed by radiation of the supraclavicular lymph nodes and chest wall. Partial breast radiation via brachytherapy or external beam radiation using three-dimensional conformal radiation is increasingly being used in low-risk populations as part of prospective trials.

Adjuvant Chemotherapy

Adjuvant chemotherapy is recommended for women with blood vessel or lymphatic invasion, high nuclear grade, high histologic grade, and HER-2/neu over-expression.[40-45] A large meta-analysis that looked at the major prospective, randomized trials of chemotherapy was performed by the Early Breast Cancer Trialists Collaborative Group. It found that adjuvant chemotherapy reduced the risk of death equally in patients with node positive as well as node negative disease. Doxorubicin was found to have a slightly increased benefit over other chemotherapy. Adjuvant chemotherapy reduced the odds of death by 8 percent in women ages 60 to 69 years, and a staggering 27 percent in women under the age of 40 years.[46] The addition of a taxane to doxorubicin slightly increases the benefit to women with node-positive disease. Recently, the use of herceptin, an antibody to c-HER2-neu protein, and vinorelbine, has been the focus of new avenues of adjuvant therapy.[46] Tamoxifen acts as a selective estrogen receptor modulator (SERM). It acts against estrogen in the breast via competitive blockade of estrogen receptors. It has the added benefit of preserving bone density and lowering cholesterol as an estrogen agonist. Tamoxifen, unfortunately, also acts to increase the incidence of endometrial carcinoma. In patients who have tumors that are ER positive, PR positive, or both, tamoxifen has been found to reduce the annual odds of recurrence by 47 percent and annual odds of death by 26 percent. These results have been replicated in over 63 trials. Another avenue of interest has been aromatase inhibitors, which prevent the peripheral conversion of androgens to estrogen, such as Anastrozole. In a large randomized clinical trial, Anastrozole has shown to be slightly more effective than tamoxifen alone or when used in combination, with a more favorable side-effect profile.[47]

In meta-analysis of randomized, controlled trials, the combination of chemotherapy and tamoxifen is beneficial in all groups of women, though the side-effects in post-menopausal women must be considered. The proportional reduction in mortality must be evaluated in terms of absolute reduction to calculate the benefit for the individual patient.[48-49]

REFERENCES

1. Singletary SE. Rating the risk factors for breast cancer. Ann Surg 2003;237:474.
2. Hulka BS. Epidemiologic analysis of breast and gynecologic cancers. Prog Clin Biol Res 1997;396:17.
3. Pujol P, Galtier-Dereure F, Bringer J. Obesity and breast cancer risk. Hum Reprod 1997;1:(12 Suppl):116.
4. Goss PE, Sierra S. Current perspectives on radiation-induced breast cancer. J Clin Oncol 1998;16:338.
5. Mulholland M, et al. Greenfield's Surgery: Scientific Principles and Practice. Breast Disease, 4th edn. 2005.
6. Wynder EL, et al. Breast cancer: Weighing the evidence for a promoting role of dietary fat. J Natl Cancer Inst 1997;89:766.
7. Gail MH, et al. Projecting individualized absolute invasive breast cancer risk in African American women. J Natl Cancer Inst 2007;99:1782.
8. Edwards BK, et al. Annual report to the nation on the status of cancer, 1975-2002, featuring population-based trends in cancer treatment. J Natl Cancer Inst 2005;97:1407.
9. Kerlikowske K, et al. Efficacy of screening mammography. A meta-analysis. JAMA 1995;273:149.
10. Fisher B, et al. Tamoxifen for prevention of breast cancer: Report of the National Surgical Adjuvant Breast and Bowel Project P-1 Study. J Natl Cancer Inst 1998;90:1371.
11. Grodstein F, et al. Postmenopausal hormone therapy and mortality. N Engl J Med 1997;52(336):1769.
12. Wu K, Brown P. Is low-dose tamoxifen useful for the treatment and prevention of breast cancer? J Natl Cancer Inst 2003;95:766.
13. Martin AM, Weber BL. Genetic and hormonal risk factors in breast cancer. J Natl Cancer Inst 2000;92:1126.
14. Ford D, et al. Genetic heterogeneity and penetrance analysis of the BRCA1 and BRCA2 genes in breast cancer families. The Breast Cancer Linkage Consortium. Am J Hum Genet 1998;62:676.
15. Gowen LC, et al. BRCA1 required for transcription-coupled repair of oxidative DNA damage. Science 1998;281:1009.
16. Wooster R, Weber BL. Breast and ovarian cancer. N Engl J Med 2003;348:2339.
17. Oddoux C, et al. The carrier frequency of the BRCA2 6174delT mutation among Ashkenazi Jewish individuals is approximately 1%. Nat Genet 1996;14:188.
18. Haffty BG. Molecular and genetic markers in the local-regional management of breast cancer. Semin Radiat Oncol 2002;12:329.
19. Morabito A, et al. Prognostic and predictive indicators in operable breast cancer. Clin Breast Cancer 2003;3:381.
20. Rogers CE, et al. Molecular prognostic indicators in breast cancer. Eur J Surg Oncol 2002;28:467.
21. Esteva FJ, et al. Molecular prognostic factors for breast cancer metastasis and survival. Semin Radiat Oncol 2002;12:319.
22. Schnall MD. Breast MR imaging. Radiol Clin North Am 2003;41:43.
23. American Cancer Society: Cancer Facts and Figures 2008. Atlanta: American Cancer Society, 2008. Available at http://www.cancer.org/downloads/STT/2008CAFFfinalsecured.pdf [accessed January 29, 2009].
24. Clarke CA, et al. Recent declines in hormone therapy utilization and breast cancer incidence: Clinical and population-based evidence. J Clin Oncol 2006;24:e49.
25. Ferlay J, et al. Globocan 2002: Cancer Incidence, Mortality and Prevalence Worldwide. Lyon, France: IARC Press, 2004. IARC Cancer Base No. 5, Version 2.0.
26. Ries LAG, et al. SEER Cancer Statistics Review, 1975-2002, National Cancer Institute. Bethesda, MD, http://seer.cancer.gov/csr/1975_2002/ [accessed January 29, 2009].
27. Khan SA, Stewart AK, Morrow M. Does aggressive local therapy improve survival in metastatic breast cancer? Surgery 2002;132:620; discussion 626.
28. Townsend CM, et al. Sabiston Textbook of Surgery: Expert Consult. Breast Disease. (18th edn) Nov 2007.
29. Gallager HS, Martin JE. The study of mammary carcinoma by mammography and whole organ sectioning. Early observations. Cancer 1969;23:855.
30. Consensus conference on the classification of ductal carcinoma in situ. Hum Pathol 1997;28:1221.
31. Foote FWJ, Stewart FW. Lobular carcinoma in situ: A rare form of mammary carcinoma. Am J Pathol 1941;17:491.
32. McDivitt RW, et al. Tubular carcinoma of the breast: Clinical and pathological observations concerning 135 cases. Am J Surg Pathol 1982;6:401.
33. Bassett LW. Breast imaging. In: Bland KI, Copeland EM III (Eds): The Breast: Comprehensive Management of Benign and Malignant Diseases. Philadelphia: WB Saunders, 1998;648.
34. Birads: bestpractice.bmj.com. Accessed 7/21/10.
35. Shelty MK, Shah YP, Sharman RS. Prospective evaluation of the value of combined mammographic and sonographic assessment in patients with palpable abnormalities of the breast. J Ultrasound Med 2003;22:263-8.

36. Morrow M, Schmidt RA, Bucci C. Breast conservation for mammographically occult carcinoma. Ann Surg 1998;227:502–6.

37. Fletcher SW, Elmore JG. Clinical practice. Mammographic screening for breast cancer. N Engl J Med 2003;348:1672.

38. Holland R, Veling SH, Mravunac M, et al. Histologic multifocality of Tis, T1-2 breast carcinomas. Implications for clinical trials of breast-conserving surgery. Cancer 1985;56:979–90.

39. Hunt KK, et al. The Breast: a brief history of breast cancer therapy. Schwartz's Principles of Surgery (9th edn), 2010.

40. Tamoxifen for early breast cancer: An overview of the randomised trials. Early Breast Cancer Trialists' Collaborative Group. Lancet 1998;351:1451.

41. Polychemotherapy for early breast cancer: An overview of the randomised trials. Early Breast Cancer Trialists' Collaborative Group. Lancet 1998;352:930.

42. Fisher B, et al. Two months of doxorubicin-cyclophosphamide with and without interval reinduction therapy compared with 6 months of cyclophosphamide, methotrexate, and fluorouracil in positive-node breast cancer patients with tamoxifen-nonresponsive tumors: Results from the National Surgical Adjuvant Breast and Bowel Project B-15. J Clin Oncol 1990;8:1483.

43. Kelleher M, Miles D. The adjuvant treatment of breast cancer. Int J Clin Pract 2003;57:195.

44. Loprinzi CL, Thome SD. Understanding the utility of adjuvant systemic therapy for primary breast cancer. J Clin Oncol 2001;19:972.

45. Wood WC, et al. Dose and dose intensity of adjuvant chemotherapy for stage II, node-positive breast carcinoma. N Engl J Med 1994;330:1253.

46. Early Breast Cancer Trialists' Collaborative Group. Polychemotherapy for early breast cancer: an overview of the randomized trials. Lancet 1998;352:930–42.

47. Baum M, Buzdar A, Cuzick J, et al. Anastrozole alone or in combination with tamoxifen versus tamoxifen alone for adjuvant treatment of postmenopausal women with early-stage breast cancer: results of the ATAC (arimidex, tamoxifen alone or in combination) trial efficacy and safety update analyses. Cancer 2003;98:1802–10.

48. Schneiderman M, Axtell LM. Deaths among female patients with carcinoma of the breast treated by surgical procedure alone. Surg Gynecol Obstet 1979;148:193–6.

49. Early Breast Cancer Trialists' Collaborative Group. Tamoxifen for early breast cancer: an overview of the randomized trials. Lancet 1998;351:1451–67.

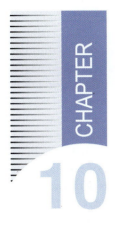

Melanoma

Richard Englehardt, Vijay Mittal

INTRODUCTION

Melanoma is currently the fastest increasing cancer. There are many possible causes for this rapid rise in cases. The factor which is felt to be the largest contributor is an increased exposure to ultraviolet radiation from sunlight. Other risk factors for melanoma include a family history, freckles, red or blonde colored hair, fair skin pigmentation, a history of at least one blistering sunburn, and the presence of multiple nevi, particularly any dysplastic nevi.

From 2003-2007, the median age at diagnosis for melanoma of the skin was 60 years of age. Approximately 0.8 percent were diagnosed under age 20; 7.5 percent between 20 and 34; 11.8 percent between 35 and 44; 18.7 percent between 45 and 54; 20.4 percent between 55 and 64; 17.8 percent between 65 and 74; 17.0 percent between 75 and 84; and 6.0 percent 85+ years of age. The age-adjusted incidence rate was 20.1 per 100,000 men and women per year (Table 10.1).[1] From 2003-2007, the median age at death for melanoma of the skin was 68 years of age. Approximately 0.1 percent died under age 20; 2.7 percent between 20 and 34; 6.3 percent between 35 and 44; 14.3 percent between 45 and 54; 19.6 percent between 55 and 64; 20.9 percent between 65 and 74; 24.1 percent between 75 and 84; and 11.9 percent 85+ years of age. The age-adjusted death rate was 2.7 per 100,000 men and women per year. These rates are based on patients who died in 2003-2007 in the US (Table 10.2).[1]

Table 10.1: Incidence of melanoma based on race and gender		
Race/Ethnicity	Male	Female
All races	25.6 per 100,000 men	16.2 per 100,000 women
White	29.7 per 100,000 men	19.1 per 100,000 women
Black	1.1 per 100,000 men	1.0 per 100,000 women
Asian/Pacific Islander	1.6 per 100,000 men	1.3 per 100,000 women
American Indian/Alaska Native	4.1 per 100,000 men	3.7 per 100,000 women
Hispanic	4.4 per 100,000 men	4.7 per 100,000 women

Table 10.2: Mortality secondary to melanoma as distributed by race and gender		
Race/Ethnicity	Male	Female
All races	4.0 per 100,000 men	1.7 per 100,000 women
White	4.5 per 100,000 men	2.0 per 100,000 women
Black	0.5 per 100,000 men	0.4 per 100,000 women
Asian/Pacific islander	0.4 per 100,000 men	0.3 per 100,000 women
American Indian/Alaska native	1.6 per 100,000 men	0.8 per 100,000 women
Hispanic	1.0 per 100,000 men	0.6 per 100,000 women

Suspicious lesions for melanoma include those that are **Asymmetric,** have an irregular **Border,** have multiple or unusual **Colors** such as gray, white, red, blue, or dark black. Lesions with a **Diameter** >5 mm or have undergone any new change should also be regarded as suspicious.[2]

Melanomas are further classified into different categories based on their patterns of growth. These classes include superficial spreading, acral lentiginous melanoma, nodular melanoma, and lentigo maligna.

Superficial spreading melanoma is the most common presentation of melanoma, comprising more than 70 percent of all melanomas. These generally arise from pre-existing nevi in sun exposed areas of the body. Growth generally occurs in a superficial pattern initially, with later development of a vertical growth phase.[3,4]

Acral lentiginous melanoma accounts for approximately 5 percent of all melanomas in the Caucasian population. In contrast it makes up between 30 and 60 percent of all cases of melanoma among black, Asian, and Hispanic races. As opposed to the superficial spreading melanomas, acral lentiginous lesions are more commonly found in non-sun exposed areas such as the nail beds, soles of the feet or palms, and the perineum. These lesions develop quickly and are often very aggressive. They tend to be very large; with an average diameter of 2.5-3 cm. Acral lentiginous melanomas are notable for their irregular borders, ulceration, and unusual color patterns.[3,4]

Nodular melanoma makes up 15 to 25 percent of the melanomas found in the Caucasian population. Nodular lesions are generally more pronounced, dome-like lesions with well-defined borders. They are more commonly found in the elderly, and are often located around the head, neck, and trunk. Nodular melanomas are notable for having an aggressive vertical growth phase, and as a result often are diagnosed as deep, invasive lesions.[3,4]

Lentigo maligna melanoma accounts for roughly 4 to 10 percent of all melanomas. While lentigo maligna lesions tend to be locally advanced with high recurrence rates following excision, they also have the lowest propensity for metastatic spread compared with the other subtypes. Lentigo maligna is generally found in sun exposed areas and is noted for having irregular borders and a more horizontal growth pattern.[3]

Genetics and Melanoma

The major familial gene associated with melanoma is *CDKN2A/p16*, cyclin-dependent kinase inhibitor 2A, which is located on chromosome 9p21. It is an upstream regulator of the retinoblastoma gene pathway, acting through the cyclin D1/cyclin-dependent kinase 4 complex. The *CDKN2A* tumor suppressor gene controls the passage of cells through the cell cycle and provides a mechanism for holding damaged cells at the G1/S checkpoint, to permit repair of DNA damage prior to cellular replication. Mutations in *CDKN2A* account for 35 to 40 percent of familial melanomas. One large case series found that *CDKN2A* mutations were present in 100 percent of families with seven to ten individuals affected with melanoma, 60 to 71 percent of families with four to six cases, and 14 percent of families with two cases. Other genetic markers associated with increased risk of melanoma include mutations to the *CDK4* and *CDK6* genes. These mutations cause disruption along a similar signaling pathway as the *CDKN2A* gene. Germline *CDK4* mutations are very rare and germline mutations in *CDK6* have not been identified in any melanoma families.[5]

Clinical testing is available to identify germline mutations in *CDKN2A*. Current practices regarding testing for germline mutations of *CDKN2A* in familial melanoma follows two different schools of thought. Arguments for genetic testing involve the benefit of identifying a possible cause of disease for the individual tested, and the reassurance of a negative test result in individuals in a mutation-carrying family. However, a negative test result in a family that does not have a known mutation is uninformative; the genetic cause of disease in these patients must still be identified. It is important to note that members of *CDKN2A* mutation–carrying families who do not carry the mutation themselves remain at increased risk of melanoma. Currently identification of a *CDKN2A* mutation does not affect the clinical management of the affected patient or family members. Close dermatologic follow-up is indicated, regardless of genetic testing result. Any genetic testing performed in this population should be accompanied with genetic counseling in order to clarify the role of the testing.[6]

Staging of Melanoma

The stage of development of the primary tumor is one of the most important prognostic factors associated with melanoma. The current microstaging method which is now the standard for classification was originally described by Breslow. In this method the primary tumor is classified according to its thickness in millimeters as measured from the top of the granular layer to the base of the tumor.[7] There are many studies which demonstrate an inverse correlation between the thickness of the tumor and the patient survival. The ulceration status and mitotic rate have also been used as independent factors which aid in the microstaging of the lesion.[6]

Prior to the use of the Breslow system for microstaging, melanomas were staged using the Clark's level classification system. The Clark's level classification stages lesions according to the level of invasion into the histologic layers of the skin. This system separates the degree of invasion into five levels with level 1 being comprised of in situ involvement only and level 5 extending to the subcutaneous tissue. Several studies have subsequently confirmed that the Breslow staging based on thickness conveys a more accurate prognostic evaluation than does the determination of the Clark's level.[8,9]

Presence of regional lymph node metastasis is associated with a worse prognosis in melanoma lesions. The degree to which the lymph node is involved (microscopic versus macroscopic disease) has demonstrated an inverse correlation with long-term survival. The use of sentinel lymph node biopsy has been instrumental in identifying a subgroup of patients with micrometastatic nodal disease who have been found to have a more favorable prognosis than those with macroscopic nodal involvement. This difference in prognosis has led to the incorporation of the type of nodal involvement into the staging system as well.[10,11]

Diagnosis of Melanoma

Examination of nodal metastases by H&E alone often leads to either overdiagnosis or underdiagnosis of metastatic disease due to hypercellularity of the lymph node and similar staining of the cells. Several antigens have been identified on melanoma cells, against which monoclonal antibodies have been generated, and used for diagnostic immunohistochemistry. Those markers which are most frequently used include S-100 protein, HMB-45, Melan-A, Mitf, and Tyrosinase.[12] Comparison of the sensitivities and specificities of the various markers is shown in (Table 10.3).

Treatment of the Melanoma

Any lesion which is felt to be suspicious for melanoma should be biopsied. The goal of any biopsy is to provide the pathologist with sufficient tissue to allow for a complete evaluation of the lesion. In order to accomplish this, the melanoma must be biopsied at its deepest portion so that the Breslow depth can be determined. Excision or punch biopsies are the preferred methods of biopsy. When possible complete excisional biopsies are preferred, however, if the lesion is large, and in an anatomic location which would make complete excision disfiguring, such as the face, scalp, or hands, a punch biopsy may be performed. Shave biopsies or curette biopsies should be avoided if melanoma is suspected.[13]

Once confirmed via biopsy, complete treatment of a primary melanoma tumor consists of complete excision with a margin of tissue determined by the depth of invasion. Previously, 5 cm margins were used for all melanomas. Multiple studies and trials have shown that narrower margins can be used without increasing the risk of local recurrence or overall survival. The narrower margins also allow for less morbidity such as the need for skin grafting. The current standard of practice determines the width of margins based on the depth of invasion of the lesion.[5,8,9]

Melanoma in situ can safely be excised with 5 mm margins. Melanoma with invasion less than 1 mm in thickness can be excised with 1 cm margins. Lesions which are between 1 to 4 mm in thickness should ideally be excised with 2 cm margins. In locations where a 2 cm margin cannot be obtained, a 1 cm margin is acceptable. Melanomas with a thickness of greater than 4 mm should undergo resection with 2 cm margins (Table 10.4). If tissue allows for a 3 cm margin around these lesions, a wider margin should be considered.[5,8,9]

In addition to obtaining adequate horizontal margins, resection should be carried down to the underlying fascia,

Table 10.3: Comparison of the sensitivity, specificity, positive and negative predictive values and likelihood ratio of S-100, HMB-45, Mitf, Melan-A, and Tyrosinase as markers for diagnosing melanomas

	Sensitivity	Specificity	Positive predictive value	Negative predictive value	Likelihood ratio
S-100	88	70	78	82	26
HMB-45	92	97	97	92	69
Mitf	100	97	97	100	90
Melan-A	95	97	97	94	75
Tyrosinase	98	84	89	96	59
S100+HMB45	80	100	100	80	59
Mitf+Melan-A	95	100	100	94	84

Table 10.4: Recommended clinical excision margins for melanoma based on thickness[5]	
Tumor thickness	*Recommended margins*
In situ	0.5 cm
<1 mm	1 cm
1-4 mm	2 cm
>4 mm	> 2 cm

although the fascia need not be excised. A number of reconstructive options exist following wide excision. A simple local advancement flap is most commonly used, often by performing the resection in an elliptical fashion. Ideally a length-to-width ratio of 3:1 should be observed in order to allow for ideal tissue closure. Rotational flaps, Z-plasty closures, or V-Y flaps, as well as pedicled or free flaps can be used in difficult situations; however they are not often necessary.

Skin grafting in general provides good closure in situations where closure by an advancement flap is not possible. Full thickness skin grafting should be used for the face, scalp, and hands. Split-thickness grafts can be used to cover larger areas, particularly in areas such as the chest, back, or proximal extremities.

SITE-SPECIFIC CONSIDERATIONS

General recommendations regarding the extent of surgical resection are applicable to most areas of the body. However, certain anatomic sites are not amenable to rigid surgical criteria. Situations which require special surgical considerations include subungual melanomas and lesions involving the digits, face, and sole of the foot.

More than 75 percent of subungual melanomas involve either the great toe or the thumb. A melanoma located on the skin of a digit or beneath the nail is usually removed by a partial digital amputation. Amputations are usually performed at the middle interphalangeal joint of the fingers or proximal to the interphalangeal joint of the thumb. More proximal amputations are not associated with improved survival and are rarely indicated. For a melanoma located on a toe, an amputation of the entire digit at the metatarsal-phalangeal joint is recomended; however, for a melanoma of the great toe, amputation can be performed proximal to the interphalangeal joint.[14]

Excision of a melanoma on the plantar surface of the foot often produces a sizable defect in a weight-bearing area. A plantar flap can provide well-vascularized local tissue for weight-bearing areas. Staged closure of some plantar

melanomas has been performed with initial use of a negative pressure wound vacuum to stimulate granulation tissue followed by skin graft application.[14]

Facial lesions usually cannot be excised with more than l cm margin because of adjacent vital structures; in these cases, the tumor diameter, tumor thickness, and tumor's exact location on the face must all be considered when margin width is planned. Mohs surgery with using repeated microscopic analysis to obtain negative margins has been used with some success for lesions involving the face. Best results have been reported for melanoma *in situ*, however, it has also been used successfully for select deeper lesions.

EVALUATION OF LYMPHATIC INVOLVEMENT

Melanomas generally metastasize through lymphatic spread using a predictable route. The most likely site of initial spread of melanoma disease is to the regional lymph nodes. Any palpable lymph node should be considered highly suspicious for metastatic disease. Presence of metastatic disease can be confirmed with fine needle aspiration biopsy. Patients with clinical evidence of nodal metastasis at the time of their initial operation should undergo lymph node dissection at the time of the initial surgery. In the majority of cases, however, the status of the regional lymph nodes is not known beforehand.[4,10,11]

The use of lymphatic mapping and sentinel lymph node biopsy allows for identification of occult lymphatic metastasis without subjecting patients to an initial morbid procedure like lymphadenectomy. Sentinel lymph node biopsy is indicated in all patients whose melanomas are 1 mm or greater in thickness. Sentinel node biopsy should be selectively used in patients with tumor thickness between 0.75 mm and 1 mm when other worrisome features such as ulceration, a high mitotic rate, young age, or a Clarks stage IV or greater. Patients who are found to be node negative on sentinel lymph node exam are more than 6 times more likely to survive than those with a positive sentinel lymph node, making the predictive value of a sentinel lymph node biopsy one of the most valuable prognostic factors. Additional evidence suggests that early removal of micrometastatic disease from the lymph node basins may improve overall survival as opposed to waiting for regional recurrence before performing a lymphadenectomy.[4,10,11]

The sentinel lymph node is defined as the first lymph node to receive lymphatic drainage from the primary tumor site. In order to identify the sentinel node either a radiocolloid such as technetium–sulfur colloid, or a blue dye such as lymphazurin or isosulfan blue dye, or both dye and radiocolloid are used. Preoperative lymphoscintigraphy is performed to identify all possible draining lymphatic basins. The site of the sentinel node can then be marked on the patient. In the operating room, before preparing the operative site, the blue dye is injected at the biopsy site as a second aid in identifying the sentinel node. The injection should be intradermal to allow for maximal passage of dye within the lymphatics. Approximately 1-2 ml of dye should be used. Sentinel lymph node dissection should be performed prior to excision of the primary melanoma.[4]

A gamma probe is used intraoperatively to confirm the location of the sentinel node prior to making incision, and intermittently following incision to localize the site of the sentinel node. The sentinel node can be identified by color or high radioactivity measured with the gamma probe. More than one sentinel node may be present, as such the nodal basin should be re-examined after removal of the first sentinel node to ensure no significant radioactivity remains. Nodes which measure within 10 percent of the highest measured lymph node should be excised.[3]

In patients with nodal metastasis a complete lymphadenectomy is the standard of care. A complete lymph node dissection is significantly more invasive that a sentinel lymph node biopsy, and carries a much higher rate of morbidity, particularly with regard to lymphedema.[3]

CHEMOTHERAPY AND RADIOTHERAPY

Traditional chemotherapeutic regimens have generally been shown to be ineffective in the treatment of melanoma. The cytokine IFN alfa-2b has been shown to improve overall survival and increase the disease free period in patients without evidence of systemic metastasis. IFN alfa-2b therapy generally requires a 12 months treatment plan, and is notable for having substantial toxic side effects. Despite this, IFN alfa-2b is currently the only approved adjuvant therapy of melanoma and all patients with high-risk melanoma should be informed of the option as well as its risks and benefits.[15]

Melanoma is traditionally thought of as a radioresistant cancer. Despite this, there is some evidence to suggest that the use of radiotherapy may decrease the risk of recurrence in lymph node dissection basins in cases where multiple lymph nodes were involved or there was gross extracapsular extension. The use of radiotherapy is not without significant risks. There is an increased risk of lymphedema following radiation therapy. In lymphatic basins such as the cervical region, where there is a higher incidence of nodal recurrence, the risks of radiotherapy may outweigh the possible complications.[13]

TREATMENT OF LOCAL RECURRENCE AND IN-TRANSIT METASTASIS

Isolated local recurrence is rare when appropriate surgical practices are followed during the initial operation. Local recurrence can be treated with a repeat wide local excision with 2 cm margins.[5]

Between 2 and 3 percent of patients who have had a primary melanoma removed will develop in-transit metastatic disease. This disease pattern is peculiar to melanoma, and results from foci of tumor cells that spread via lymphatics without reaching the lymph nodes. They present as dermal or subcutaneous lesions.[3]

Management of in-transit metastasis is dictated by the number and size of the lesions. In cases where there are a small number of lesions, the metastases may be excised with a small negative pathologic margin. More commonly however, the extent of the disease prohibits local excision and recurrences are common. Hyperthermic isolated limb perfusion is one treatment strategy for in-transit metastasis in an extremity which allows for chemotherapeutic administration to the extremity at a concentration 15-25 times higher than possible with systemic chemotherapy and without the systemic side effects. Hyperthermic isolated limb perfusion uses the drug Melphalan as the standard chemotherapeutic agent due to its efficacy and low regional toxicity. Use of isolated limb perfusion has not been shown to significantly improve survival, however, it has been shown to provide substantial palliation of local and regional symptoms when other options have been exhausted.[16]

Some centers have employed the use of local immunotherapy in patients with in-transit disease. This involves injection of bacilli Calmette-Guerin (BCG) or interferon-alpha combined with topical application of imiquimod cream. This results in local inflammation and toxicities such as erythema, ulceration, and edema. Some centers report a regression of approximately 80 percent of injected lesions, particularly among the smaller lesions.[4]

METASTATIC DISEASE

Distant metastatic disease has traditionally been seen as a contraindication for surgery. In a carefully selected subset of patients however, resection may be appropriate. Recent studies have shown that while systemic therapy has never shown an improved survival, postoperative adjuvant vaccine therapy following resection of distant metastatic disease as demonstrated a nearly 40 percent 5-year survival. Isolated small bowel metastases appear to have a particularly favorable prognosis.[14]

Preoperative staging and careful selection of appropriate patients for resection is crucial. Workup should include CT of the chest, abdomen, and pelvis, as well as PET scan and MRI of the brain. So long as all lesions can be resected, the number of metastasis does not have a major impact on the overall outcome.[8]

REFERENCES

1. Altekruse SF, Kosary CL, Krapcho M, et al (Eds). SEER Cancer Statistics Review, 1975-2007, National Cancer Institute. Bethesda, MD, http://seer.cancer.gov/csr/1975_2007/, based on November 2009 SEER data submission, posted to the SEER web site, 2010.
2. Harmful effects of ultraviolet radiation. Council on Scientific Affairs. JAMA 1989;262(3):380-4.
3. Sabel MS. Oncology. In: Doherty G (Ed). Current Diagnosis and Treatment: Surgery, (13th edn). New York: McGraw Hill 2010;1225-7.
4. Farles MB, Morton DL. Cutaneous melanoma. In: Cameron JL (Ed). Current Surgical Therapy. (9th edn). Philadelphia: Mosby 2008;1096-1100.
5. Goldsmith L, Koh HK, Bewerse B, et al. Proceedings from the national conference to develop a national skin cancer agenda. American Academy of Dermatology and Centers for Disease Control and Prevention, April 8-10, 1995. J Am Acad Dermatol 1996;34(5 Pt 1): 822-3.
6. Balch CM, Soong SJ, Gershenwald JE, et al. Prognostic factors analysis of 17, 600 melanoma patients: validation of the American Joint Committee on Cancer melanoma staging system. J Clin Oncol 2001;19:3622-34.
7. Breslow A. Tumor thickness, level of invasion and node dissection in stage I cutaneous melanoma. Ann Surg 1975;182:572-5.
8. Balch CM, Buzaid AC, Soong S, et al. Final version of the American Joint Committee on Cancer staging system for cutaneous melanoma. J Clin Oncol 2001;19:3635-48.
9. Edge SB, et al. AJCC Cancer Staging Handbook, (7th edn). Springer Publishing, 2010.
10. Morton DL, et al. Sentinel node biopsy or nodal observation in melanoma. N Engl J Med 2006; 355:1307.
11. Vaquerano J, Kraybill WG, Driscoll DL, et al. American Joint Committee on Cancer clinical stage as a selection criterion for sentinel lymph node biopsy in thin melanoma. Ann Surg Oncol 2006;13:198-204.
12. Sheffield MV, Yee H, Dorvault CC, et al. Comparison of five antibodies as markers in the diagnosis of melanoma in cytologic preparations. Am J Clin Pathol 2002;118:930-6.
13. Balch CM, et al. Cutaneous Melanoma (4th edn). Quality Medical Publishing, 2003.
14. Gershenwald JE, Hwu P. Melanoma. Holland-Frei Cancer Medicine, (8th edn). In: Hong WK, Bast RC, et al (Eds). Peoples Medical Publishing House, 2010.
15. Sabel MS, Sondak VK. Pros and cons of adjuvant interferon in the treatment of melanoma. Oncologist 2003;8:451.
16. Blazer DG, Sondak VK, Sabel MS. Surgical therapy of cutaneous melanoma. Semin Oncol 2007;34:270.

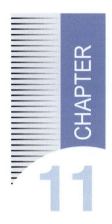
Small Bowel Neoplasms

Deepa Taggarshe, Vijay Mittal

GENERAL CONSIDERATIONS

Neoplasms of the small bowel are rare, although the small bowel itself accounts for approximately 80 percent of the total length of the gastrointestinal tract and 90 percent of its mucosal surface area. Small bowel neoplasms comprise less than five percent of all gastrointestinal cancers with an estimated incidence of 6110 cases in the United States in 2008.[1] The possible reasons for this disparity include rapid transit of the luminal contents, limiting the contact time between carcinogens and mucosa, an alkaline environment due to the presence of pancreatic enzymes, high levels of IgA in the small bowel wall and the low bacterial counts in the small bowel luminal contents. The incidence of these neoplasms, however, is increasing especially with a four-fold rise in carcinoids.[2]

Small bowel cancers are more common in men and patients are usually diagnosed in their fifth or sixth decade. Most tumors of the small bowel are benign, which are usually asymptomatic and identified at autopsy. Malignant neoplasms on the other hand, comprise a majority of symptomatic lesions leading to surgery[3] (Table 11.1 and Fig. 11.1).

Risk factors associated with adenocarcinoma of small bowel include Crohn's disease, familial adenomatosis polyposis, hereditary nonpolyposis colorectal cancer, Peutz-Jegher's syndrome, celiac sprue and biliary diversion. Consumption of red meat, smoked or cured food have also been implicated. Recent studies have shown that carcinoids are being increasingly seen in the small bowel and now constitute the most common primary malignant tumor in the small bowel.[2,4]

Table 11.1: Incidence of small bowel malignant neoplasms		
Tumor type	*Frequency*	*Predominant site*
Adenocarcinoma	30-50%	Duodenum
Carcinoid	20-30%	Ileum
Lymphoma	15%	Ileum
GIST	15%	

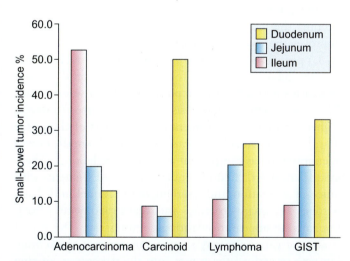

FIGURE 11.1: Incidence of small bowel tumors by histological types and anatomical locations. Adapted from Hatzaras I, Palesty A, et al. Small-bowel tumors epidemiologic and clinical characteristics of 1260 cases from the Connecticut Tumor Registry. Arch Surg 2007;142:229-35

CLINICAL PRESENTATION

The clinical presentation of small bowel tumors is non-specific and ill defined. Most benign tumors are asymptomatic. Small bowel obstruction due to luminal narrowing or intussusception; associated with intermittent abdominal pain, distention, nausea and vomiting can be seen. The second most common mode of presentation is intermittent gastrointestinal bleeding and anemia.

Patients with malignant tumors present with weight loss[3] and may already be malnourished at the time of surgery. Obstruction and bleeding can also be seen. Obstruction in case of malignant tumors is more likely to be reflective of extensive tumor infiltration and adhesions. A palpable mass may be felt in up to 25 percent of patients. Perforations from small bowel tumors are seen in 10 percent, usually due to lymphomas and sarcomas. Lesions in the periampullary duodenum can cause obstructive jaundice or pancreatitis.

DIAGNOSIS

Laboratory tests are limited for diagnosis of small bowel tumors. Complete blood counts may show anemia. Elevated 5-hydroxyindoleacetic acid (5-HIAA) is seen in carcinoids. Elevated carcinoembryonic antigen (CEA) levels are seen in small bowel adenocarcinomas with liver metastasis.

Due to the rarity of small bowel neoplasms, a high index of suspicion must be kept for these tumors to be diagnosed. Keeping the radiologist informed of a suspected diagnosis improves the chances of diagnosis by imaging studies.

Upper GI series with small bowel follow through (SBFT) studies have been used for diagnosing small bowel neoplasms and have been reported to have a sensitivity of 30 to 44 percent.[5] Enteroclysis has been reported to have a higher sensitivity at 90 percent and is the test of choice for distal small bowel tumors. Advanced small bowel adenocarcinomas can present as "apple-core lesions". These lesions are short, circumferentially narrowed segments with mucosal ulceration and overhanging proximal and distal borders. Malignant strictures are usually rigid, with a fixed, unchanging appearance during compression. The initial studies of carcinoid may show some mucosal thickening, but with growth of the tumor into the mesentery, kinking of the bowel wall, narrowing of the lumen, and angulation of the involved small bowel maybe seen. On barium studies, submucosal gastrointestinal stroma tumors (GISTs) appear as smooth, round filling defects with or without ulceration.

Plain films may show small bowel obstruction, but are ineffective at picking up tumors. Computed tomography (CT) is gaining more prominence in diagnosing small bowel neoplasms. It is particularly useful in picking up large tumors, extramural invasions of tumors and staging the cancer. The reported sensitivities vary from 57 to 63 percent. Adenocarcinomas may show as discrete small bowel mass causing intraluminal narrowing. With the improved quality of multidetector CT, even smaller carcinoids can now be diagnosed as submucosal lesions. Mesenteric extension of the carcinoid can be seen as an ill-defined calcified mesenteric mass in 70 percent.[6] The mass can also have a spiculated appearance due to desmoplastic reaction in the mesentery in response to serotonin. GIST may show up as a large smooth mass with central necrosis. Tumors of vascular origin can be diagnosed by angiography or 99 mTc radioisotope-tagged red blood cells (RBCs) scan.

Flexible gastroduodenal endoscopy and small bowel enteroscopy are useful in diagnosing tumors of the duodenum and proximal jejunum. Terminal ileum can be visualized by advancing the colonoscope into the terminal ileum. The advantages of these techniques lay in the opportunity to biopsy the lesion and obtain a tissue diagnosis. Capsule endoscopy allows for visualization of the distal jejunum and ileum; however it has its limitations mainly in the inability to re-examine the suspected area. It has a higher diagnostic yield than other tests at identifying small bowel tumors which present with GI bleeding.[7]

STAGING

The staging of malignant small bowel neoplasms is according to the American Joint Committee on cancer staging system.

Primary tumor (T)
- TX: Primary tumor cannot be assessed.
- T0: No evidence of primary tumor is present.
- Tis: Carcinoma *in situ* is present.
- T1: Tumor invades the lamina propria or submucosa.
- T2: Tumor invades the muscularis propria.
- T3: Tumor invades through the muscularis propria into subserosa or into nonperitonealized perimuscular tissue (mesentery or retroperitoneum), with extension of less than 2 cm.
- T4: Tumor penetrates the visceral peritoneum or directly invades other organs or structures.

Regional lymph nodes (N)
- NX: Regional lymph nodes cannot be assessed.
- N0: No regional lymph node metastasis is present.
- N1: Regional lymph node metastasis has occurred.

Distant metastases (M)
- MX: Presence of distant metastasis cannot be assessed.
- M0: No distant metastasis is present.
- M1: Distant metastasis has occurred.

Stage grouping
- Stage 0 — Tis, N0, M0
- Stage I — T1-2, N0, M0
- Stage II — T3-4, N0, M0
- Stage III — Any T, N1, M0
- Stage IV — Any T, Any N, M1

BENIGN NEOPLASMS

Benign neoplasms of the small bowel include adenomas, lipomas, hamartomas, and benign GISTs. Adenomas are the most common benign small bowel tumors, but GISTs are the most common symptomatic benign tumors.

Adenomas

Adenomas comprise about 15 percent of all benign small bowel tumors. They may be associated with familial adenomatous polyposis and Gardner's syndrome. There are three types of adenomas: tubular adenomas, villous adenomas and Brunner gland adenomas. Nearly half of the small bowel adenomas are found in the ileum, with 20 percent in the duodenum and 30 percent in the jejunum. Majority of the lesions are asymptomatic. Most common presenting symptoms are bleeding and obstruction. Villous adenomas have a malignant potential between 35 percent and 55 percent. The malignant potential increases with a size larger than 2 cm. Brunner's gland adenomas are hyperplastic lesions arising from the Brunner glands in the duodenum. They do not have a malignant potential.

Adenomas can be diagnosed and treated with endoscopic measures. Diagnosis can be confirmed by biopsy. Tubular adenomas and Brunner gland adenomas can be resected by simple endoscopic excision. However, with villous adenomas, especially if larger than 2 cm, endoscopic excision may be inadequate. Surgical options include segmental resection, transduodenal polypectomy and for tumors located near the ampulla of Vater, pancreaticoduodenectomy.

Lipomas

Lipomas are rarely found in the small intestine. Lipomas present as intramural lesions, located in the submucosa. They are mainly seen in the sixth and seventh decade and are more common in men. Main symptoms include obstruction and bleeding due to ulceration. Lipomas can be identified in CT scan because of their high fat content. Treatment of symptomatic lipomas is excision.

Hamartomas

Hamartomas are seen as part of the Peutz-Jegher's syndrome, which is an autosomal dominant syndrome characterized by mucocutaneous melanotic pigmentation and gastrointestinal polyps. The pigmented lesions appear as 1 - 2 mm, black or brown lesions located in the circumoral region of the face, forearms, palms, soles and the perianal region. These polyps are mainly located in the jejunum and ileum, and have the potential to cause obstruction or intermittent intussusception. Patients present with colicky intermittent abdominal pain. Bleeding is less common and patients may present with anemia.

Patients with Peutz-Jegher's syndrome have an increased risk of adenocarcinoma and should be followed closely. Extra-colonic cancers are also seen in 50 to 90 percent of these patients, mainly cancers of the small intestine, stomach, pancreas, lung, breast, ovary and uterus. If patients are symptomatic, resection may be necessary, but should be limited to the segment of bowel involved in active disease. Due to the widespread nature of the disease, extensive resection is not curative and unnecessary.

Benign GISTs

Gastrointestinal stroma tumors are defined by their expression of the transmembrane tyrosine kinase receptor KIT (CD117). These tumors arise from the interstitial cell of Cajal, an intestinal pacemaker cell and are identified by staining with the monoclonal antibody for KIT.

Benign GISTs are three to four times more common than malignant GISTs. They are usually seen in the fifth decade with an equal incidence in men and women. The tumors can cause obstruction due to intramural growth, or bleeding. Patients may present with abdominal pain or symptoms of obstruction or GI bleeding. Due to the slow growth of these tumors, patients may remain asymptomatic for a long time. These tumors are submucosal and have a smooth appearance on barium studies. On CT scan, the tumor may appear smooth and if large, may show areas of central necrosis. Treatment is by surgical resection. Increased risk of local recurrence has been reported with tumors with mitotic counts higher than 2 per 50 high-powered fields.[8,9]

MALIGNANT NEOPLASMS

Carcinoid Tumors

Carcinoid tumors arise from the enterochromaffin cells (Kulchitsky cells) found in the crypts of Lieberkühn. These cells can be stained by silver compounds and hence are called *Argentaffin cells*. Carcinoid tumors may be derived from the foregut (respiratory tract, thymus), midgut (stomach, proximal duodenum, jejunum, ileum, and right colon), and hindgut (distal colon and rectum). The most common sites for gastrointestinal carcinoids are appendix, followed by the ileum. In the small bowel, nearly 80 percent of the carcinoids occur within the last two feet of the ileum. Carcinoids secrete various products, including 5-hydroxytryptamine (serotonin), 5-hydroxytryptophan, dopamine and somatostatin.

Carcinoids are small, submucosal tumors that are yellow in color. They can be multicentric in 20 to 30 percent of patients. As the tumors are slow-growing, most are found incidentally during surgery. Desmoplastic reaction is seen with the invasion of the tumor into the mesentery, secondary to the local effects of serotonin and other growth factors, leading to mesenteric fibrosis and obstruction.

Patients present with vague abdominal pain. Obstructive symptoms are more common than bleeding or perforation. Obstruction can be either due to intussusception of the tumor or the desmoplastic reaction mentioned earlier. **Carcinoid syndrome** is seen in 10 percent of patients with carcinoid tumors, and is caused by high levels of serotonin, 5-hydroxytryptophan, histamine, dopamine and other amines. Carcinoid syndrome is more commonly associated with small bowel carcinoids; these patients usually have widespread hepatic metastases at the time of presentation. Symptoms include diarrhea, flushing, sweating, wheezing and abdominal pain. The cutaneous flushing in patients may vary from short lived flushing of the face, neck and chest to prolonged flushes lasting 2-3 days, involving the entire body and associated with hypotension and edema. Cardiac lesions include tricuspid and pulmonary stenosis. Carcinoid tumors utilize the majority of body's tryptophan for serotonin production and patients may manifest symptoms of pellagra—dermatitis, dementia and diarrhea.

Carcinoids can be diagnosed by elevated urinary levels of 5-hydroxyindoleacetic acid. The measurement of 24-hour urinary 5-HIAA is useful because it provides a summation of tumor secretory activity that may occasionally be missed by random plasma peptide sampling if secretion is paroxysmal.[10] However, this test is time consuming and can be altered by various medications. Plasma levels of substance P and serotonin may be elevated. If these tests are equivocal, provocative tests, using calcium, epinephrine or pentagastrin may be employed, but with the advancement of current diagnostic tests, these are rarely used nowadays. On barium studies, carcinoid tumors present as smooth, solitary, intraluminal defects but may also exhibit narrowing, and obstruction. CT scan can show the extent of bowel and mesenteric involvement, hepatic metastases and retroperitoneal extension. A spiculated mesenteric mass with radiating strands of fibrosis is pathognomic for carcinoids.[11] An Octreotide scan, using In-111 Octreotide (6 mCi administered intravenously) can identify carcinoids, which express serotonin receptors. This has a sensitivity of >90 percent and can also be used to detect metastases. Elevated Chromogranin A levels correlates well with metastatic disease and has also been shown to be indicative of a poor prognostic outcome in patients with liver metastases.[12]

Treatment of carcinoids (Fig. 11.2) is based on tumor size and the presence of any metastases. Primary tumors less than 1 cm in diameter can be resected if there is no evidence of spread to lymph nodes. Wide excision of bowel and mesentery is employed for multiple tumors or lymph node involvement. Small duodenal tumors can be removed by enucleation; however larger tumors may require a pancreaticoduodenectomy. In ileal and jejunal carcinoids, enbloc resection is required, with lymph node metastases. Debulking surgery has been shown to provide symptomatic relief.[13] Hepatic metastases are treated by surgical resection or ablation. In case of widespread hepatic metastases, embolization has shown good results. Carcinoid crisis may be precipitated by anesthesia, and hence Octreotide should be readily available in the operating room.

Medical therapy for carcinoids is directed towards symptomatic relief, by using somatostatin analogues like Octreotide. Adjuvant chemotherapy with streptozocin and 5-fluorouracil is used in patients with metastatic disease who are unresponsive to other treatments. The response rate to chemotherapy varies from 20-30 percent.

The overall 5 years survival rate is 60 percent. Patients with small, nonmetastatic disease, have 5 years survival rates of 100 percent after resection. Even with distant metastases, survival rates approach 25-35 percent and with resection of liver metastases, survival rates improve to 50 percent.

Lymphomas

Lymphomas are the third most common malignant type of small bowel neoplasm, accounting for about 15 percent of small bowel tumors. However, in children younger than 10 years, they are the most common intestinal neoplasms. They may be primarily from the GI tract or involve the small bowel as part of systemic involvement.

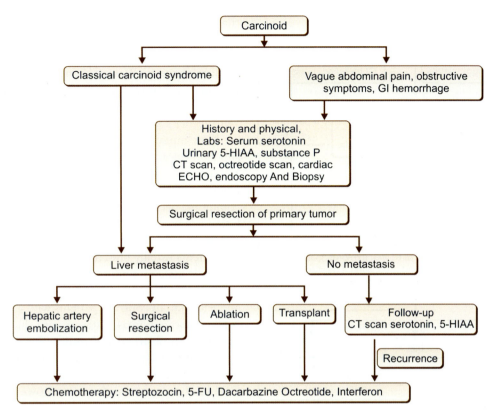

FIGURE 11.2: An overview of diagnosis and management of small bowel carcinoids

Most patients present in the fifth or sixth decade and it is slightly more common in men. Lymphomas are usually associated with immunosuppressive states like transplant recipients, AIDS, Crohn's disease and systemic lupus erythematosus. These neoplasms are usually non-Hodgkin's B-cell lymphomas with intermediate or high-grade,[14] and are more commonly found in the ileum.

Patients usually present with abdominal pain, fatigue, malaise and weight loss. With systemic involvement, patients may have fever. Patients may also present with features of obstruction or GI bleeding. About a quarter may have perforation. Generalized lymphadenopathy is suggestive of systemic involvement. Patients may have a palpable abdominal mass.

Diagnosis can be made using CT, where the lymphoma can be seen as a homogenous mass causing mural thickening and may have enlarged nodes. Submucosal lymphomatous proliferation may show multiple filling defects on barium studies.

Staging of Lymphoma (Ann Arbor Classification)

IE: Limited to the intestine with focal/multifocal spread.
IIE: Involvement of organ and regional nodes on the same side of the diaphragm
      IIE$_1$: Involvement of local nodes
      IIE$_2$: Involvement of non-continuous nodes.
IIIE: Involvement of organ and regional nodes on both sides of the diaphragm.
IVE: Involvement of distant organs and extra lymphatic organs.

Initial management of small bowel lymphomas involves surgical resection of the affected small bowel with its mesentery.[15,16] This can immediately palliate the symptoms, and prevent a potential perforation. A good exploratory laparotomy is essential at the time of surgery for staging the disease (Fig. 11.3). Debulking is considered to be of benefit. Chemotherapy with CHOP (cyclophosphamide,

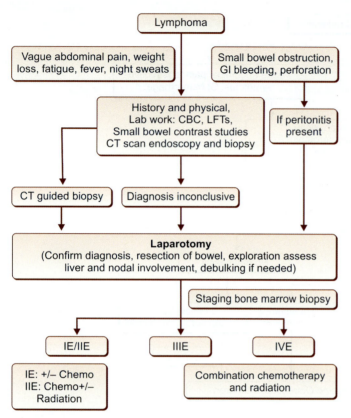

FIGURE 11.3: An overview of the diagnosis and management of small bowel lymphomas. Chemotherapy usually involves CHOP (cyclophosphamide, doxorubicin, vincristine and prednisolone)

doxorubicin, vincristine, and prednisolone) is used in patients with advanced staged tumors, and has been shown to be of benefit in Stage IE and IIE.[17] Patients with stage IIE (regional nodal or extranodal involvement confined to one side of the diaphragm) chemotherapy with combined radiation is recommended. Combination chemotherapy is primarily used in patients with stage IIIE or IVE (involvement of nodes on both sides of the diaphragm or extra nodal involvement, i.e. of bone marrow or liver). Radiation therapy is used for bulky tumors and treatment of residual disease after chemotherapy.[18]

The overall prognosis is poor and dependant on the stage. Twenty to forty percent of patients with localized disease survive five years, whereas the survival for disseminated disease is less than a year.

Adenocarcinoma

Adenocarcinomas constitute about 30 to 50 percent of small bowel malignant neoplasms, although recent reports suggest that carcinoid may now outnumber adenocarcinoma in frequency. Epidemiologically, adenocarcinomas of the small bowel are similar to colorectal adenocarcinomas, with predominance in Western countries, and in patients with certain conditions like familial adenomatosis polyposis, Crohn's disease, hereditary nonpolyposis colorectal cancer, Peutz-Jegher's syndrome and celiac sprue.

K-ras mutation and *p53* overexpression is common in small-bowel adenocarcinoma as in colorectal carcinoma. Mutation of the *APC* tumor suppressor gene, which is characteristic of colorectal carcinoma, however, does not commonly occur in small bowel adenocarcinoma.[19,20] Small bowel adenocarcinomas also show mutation of the *SMAD/DPC4* gene.[21]

Patients usually present in the seventh decade and there is a slight male preponderance. The most common location is the proximal small bowel, with a majority in the duodenum and jejunum. In contrast, patients with Crohn's disease have ileal adenocarcinomas. Patients with duodenal tumors may present with obstructive jaundice. Symptoms are otherwise nonspecific, with vague abdominal pain, weight loss and feeling of fullness. Features of intestinal obstruction and GI bleeding may be present, however perforation is uncommon. On physical examination, patients may have abdominal distension due to obstruction. Peritonitis if present is suggestive of perforation.

Laboratory investigations may show anemia due to blood loss, and in periampullary tumors, liver function tests may be deranged. Elevated carcinoembryonic antigen maybe seen with small bowel adenocarcinomas. Duodenal tumors can be diagnosed by endoscopy and biopsy. In case of distal tumors, small bowel contrast studies show an "apple-core" or annular lesion with adenocarcinomas. Plain abdominal radiographs may show small bowel obstruction, but otherwise is unhelpful. On computed tomography (CT), small bowel adenocarcinomas may appear as a discrete tumor mass, with possible overhanging edges or as an ulcerative lesion. Sometimes annular narrowing of the lumen is present. The proximal tumors tend to be more polypoid, whereas distal tumors are more annular in nature. Gradual narrowing of the lumen leads to partial or complete small bowel obstruction. The mass itself usually shows moderate enhancement after the intravenous administration of contrast material.[22]

Treatment of small bowel adenocarcinomas, primarily involves wide resection of the small bowel including the involved lymph nodes[23] (Figs 11.4A and B). Due to the higher local nodal involvement, a wide resection of the mesentery

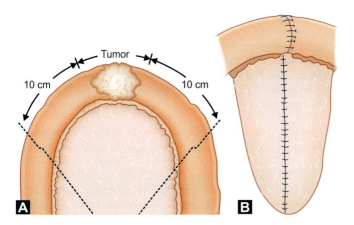

FIGURES 11.4A and B: Small bowel resection for adenocarcinoma of the bowel with wide resection (A) and primary anastomosis (B)

is essential. Removal of involved nodes has been shown to decrease the rate of local recurrence. Periampullary tumors need a pancreaticoduodenectomy (Whipple's procedure).

Presence of liver or widespread peritoneal metastases is a contraindication to curative resection. However, patients can also present late, due to the indolent nature of the symptoms and surgical curative resection is not possible. In such cases, a palliative resection should be performed to prevent future episodes of obstruction and hemorrhage. If resection is not possible, a bypass procedure can provide symptomatic relief. Some studies involving small number of patients have shown minor response of small bowel adenocarcinomas to chemotherapy agents commonly used in colorectal cancers, i.e. 5-Fluorouracil, oxaliplatin, etc.[24] The role of adjuvant chemotherapy and radiation remains yet undefined.

Only 50 percent of patients have lesions amenable to a curative resection. About a quarter of the patients present with metastatic disease. In a National Cancer Database based Review, by Howe et al the prognosis was dependant on age, site of tumor (worse in duodenal), stage and nature of surgical resection.[25] In their review, patients who did not have a curative resection had a more than twofold increased risk of death related to the cancer, compared with patients who underwent curative surgery. A negative margin after curative surgery has been shown to be associated with longer survival.[26] The overall 5-year survival remains poor at 25 to 30 percent.[25,27]

Malignant GIST

Gastrointestinal stromal tumors constitute the majority of gastrointestinal sarcomas and are thought to arise from the interstitial cell of Cajal. These tumors occur as a result of mutation of the c-KIT oncogene, found on chromosome 4q, leading to increased expression of the tyrosine kinase receptor KIT (CD117). Expression of KIT is considered the most specific criterion for diagnosis.[28] Activation of KIT, leads to activation of other enzyme cascades which leads to cellular proliferation. This is a common feature to both benign and malignant GISTs. Malignant GISTs can be identified by the presence of metastases or local invasion. However, the aggressiveness of GISTs can be difficult to predict by pathology. The GIST workshop, convened by the NIH in 2000 proposed a criterion[29] to grade the malignant risk of GISTs based on their size and mitotic rate as follows:

Most patients present with nonspecific abdominal symptoms such as abdominal discomfort, GI bleeding, and with or without a palpable mass.[30] GISTs are typically fast growing neoplasms and hence develop a necrotic centre due to outgrowing their blood supply. When this encroaches onto the lumen, profuse bleeding can occur. Small bowel GISTs may also cause obstruction, or jaundice if present in the duodenum.

On barium studies, GISTs are seen as smooth masses causing extrinsic compression. CT scan offers the best imaging modality for GISTs which appear as smooth masses with the presence of central ulceration. It provides information on the exact location, size and extent of the tumor, and presence of any metastases.

Surgery remains the primary treatment modality for localized and locally advanced GISTs. Complete resection of the tumor with 2-3 cm margins, even in case of locally

	Size	Mitotic count
Very low risk	<2 cm	<5 per 50 High power field (HPF)
Low risk	2-5 cm	<5 per 50 HPF
Intermediate risk	<5 cm	6-10 per 50 HPF
	5-10 cm	<5 per 50 HPF
High risk	>5 cm	>5 per 50 HPF
	>10 cm	any mitotic rate
	Any size	>10 per 50 HPF

advanced tumors is associated with better survival.[31] For small bowel GISTs, this entails a segmental resection of the small bowel with primary anastomosis. As these tumors do not spread by lymphatic dissemination, lymphadenectomy is not essential. Periampullary lesions may require a pancreaticoduodenectomy.

Imatinib (Gleevec) is the first effective systemic therapy for patients with metastatic or locally advanced GIST. Imatinib which is a selective C-KIT inhibitor has been shown to decrease GIST cell proliferation and increase induction of apoptosis.[32] It holds the progression of the tumor, and occasionally causes shrinkage, but complete response is rare. Dose is usually 400 mg per day, given orally and in the current setting lifetime therapy is indicated. Side effects include diarrhea, nausea, rash, abdominal cramps and periorbital edema.

Recurrence rate of GIST is 20 to 50 percent, usually within the first two years after surgery. NCCN guidelines recommend abdominal and pelvic CT every 3 to 6 months for the first 5 years post-surgery. PET scan is also useful in identifying recurrences. Prior to the use of Imatinib, the overall 5 years survival rate was estimated to be 44 percent, and up to 64 percent with completely excised localized tumors.

Metastatic Neoplasms in Small Bowel

Metastatic neoplasms of the small bowel are more common than primary neoplasms of the small bowel. The primary sites for these metastases are usually other intraabdominal organs, including the ovaries, colon, stomach, kidney, cervix and pancreas. The small bowel involvement is due to direct extension of the tumor or implantation of tumor cells. Extra-abdominal tumors involving the breast, lung and skin (melanoma) also metastasize to small bowel. The most common extra-abdominal source for small bowel metastases is melanoma of the skin, with small bowel involvement seen in more than half of the patients dying of metastatic melanoma. Patients may present with symptoms of small bowel obstruction, weight loss and bleeding. Diagnosis is usually made at surgery for obstruction or bleeding. Treatment involves small bowel resection. If the tumor is extensive or there are widespread metastases, either a palliative resection or bypass can relieve symptoms. Adjuvant therapy is dependant on the type of primary tumor.

REFERENCES

1. Jemal A, Siegel R, Ward E, Hao Y, Xu J, Murray T, et al. Cancer Statistics 2008. CA Cancer J Clin 2008;58:71-96.
2. Bilimoria KY, Bentrem DJ, Wayne JD, Ko CY, Bennett CL, Talamonti MS. Small Bowel Cancer in the United States: changes in epidemiology; treatment, and survival over the last 20 years. Ann Surg 2009;249(1):63-71.
3. Mittal VK, Bodzin JH. Primary malignant tumors of the small bowel. Am J Surg 1980;140(3):396-9.
4. Maggard MA, O'Connell JB, Ko CY. Updated population-based review of carcinoid tumors. Ann Surg 2004;240(1):117-22.
5. Coit DG. Cancer of the small intestine. In: DeVita VT, Hellman S, Rosenberg SA (Eds): Cancer: Principles and Practice of Oncology, 6th edn. Philadelphia: Lippincott Williams and Wilkins, 2001, p.1204.
6. Gore RM, Mehta UK, Berlin JW, Rao V, Newmark GM. Diagnosis and staging of small bowel tumors. Cancer Imaging 2006;6:209-12.
7. Cobrin GM, Pittman RH, Lewis BS. Increased diagnostic yield of small bowel tumors with capsule endoscopy. Cancer2006;107(1): 22-7.
8. Kim CJ, Day S, Yeh KA. Gastrointestinal stromal tumors: analysis of clinical and pathological factors. Am Surg 2001;67(2):135-7.
9. Yao KA, Talamonti MS, Langella RL, Schindler NM, Rao S, Small W Jr, et al. Primary gastrointestinal sarcomas: analysis of prognostic factors and results of surgical management. Surgery 2000; 128(4):604-12.
10. Modlin IM, Tang LH. Approaches to the diagnosis of gut neuroendocrine tumors: the last word (today). Gastroenterology 1997;112(2):583-90.
11. Pantongrag-Brown L, Buetow PC, Carr NJ, Lichtenstein JE, Buck JL. Calcification and fibrosis in mesenteric carcinoid tumor: CT findings and pathologic correlation. AJR Am J Roentgenol 1995;164(2):387-91.
12. Ahmed A, Turner G, King B, Jones L, Culliford D, McCance D, et al. Midgut neuroendocrine tumors with liver metastases. Results of the UKI NETS study. Endocr Relat Cancer 2009: May 20 epub ahead of print.
13. Kulke MH, Mayer RJ. Carcinoid tumors. N Engl J Med. 1999;340(11):858-68.
14. Ha CS, Cho MJ, Allen PK, Fuller LM, Cabanillas F, Cox JD. Primary non-Hodgkin lymphoma of the small bowel. Radiology 1999;211(1):183-7.
15. Romaguera JE, Velasquez WS, Silvermintz KB, Fuller LB, Hagemeister FB, McLaughlin P, et al. Surgical debulking is associated with improved survival in stage I-II diffuse large cell lymphoma. Cancer 1990;66(2):267-72.
16. Turowski GA, Basson MD. Primary malignant lymphoma of the intestine. Am J Surg 1995;169(4):433-41.
17. Daum S, Ullrich R, Heise W, Dederke B, Foss HD, Stein H, et al. Intestinal non-Hodgkin's lymphoma: a multicenter prospective clinical study from the German study group on Intestinal Non-Hodgkin's Lymphoma. J Clin Oncol 2003;21(14):2740-6.
18. Rawls RA, Vega KJ, Trotman BW. Small bowel lymphoma. Current Treat Options Gastroenterol 2003;6(1):27-34.
19. Arai M, Shimizu S, Imai Y, Nakatsuru Y, Oda H, Oohara T, Ishikawa T. Mutations of the Ki-ras, p53 and APC genes in adenocarcinomas of the human small intestine. Int J Cancer 1997;70(5):390-5.
20. Wheeler JM, Warren BF, Mortensen NJ, Kim HC, Biddolph SC, Elia G, et al. An insight into the genetic pathway of adenocarcinoma of the small intestine. Gut 2002;50(2):218-23.

21. Blaker H, von Herbay A, Penzel R, Gross S, Otto HF. Genetics of adenocarcinomas of the small intestine: frequent deletions at chromosome 18q and mutations of the SMAD4 gene. Oncogene 2002;21(1):158-64.

22. Buckley JA, Fishman EK. CT evaluation of small bowel neoplasms: spectrum of disease. Radiographics 1998;18(2):379-92.

23. Ouriel K, Adams JT. Adenocarcinoma of the small intestine. Am J Surg 1984;147(1):66-71.

24. Bettini AC, Beretta GD, Sironi P, Mosconi S, Labianca R. Chemotherapy in small bowel adenocarcinoma associated with celiac disease: a report of three cases. Tumori 2003;89(2):193-5.

25. Howe JR, Karnell LH, Menck HR, Scott-Conner C. The American College of Surgeons Commission on Cancer and the American Cancer Society. Adenocarcinoma of the small bowel: review of the National Cancer Database 1985-1995. Cancer 1999;86(12): 2693-706.

26. Bakaeen FG, Murr MM, Sarr MG, Thompson GB, Farnell MB, Nagorney DM, et al. What prognostic factors are important in duodenal adenocarcinoma? Arch Surg 2000;135(6):635-41.

27. Agrawal S, McCarron EC, Gibbs JF, Nava HR, Wilding GE, Rajput A. Surgical management and outcome in primary adenocarcinoma of the small bowel. Ann Surg Oncol 2007;14(8):2263-9.

28. Logrono R, Jones DV, Faruqi S, Bhutani MS. Recent advances in cell biology, diagnosis and therapy of gastrointestinal stromal tumor (GIST). Cancer Biol Ther 2004;3(3):251-8.

29. Fletcher CD, Berman JJ, Corless C, Gorstein F, Lasota J, Longley BJ. Diagnosis of gastrointestinal stromal tumors: a consensus approach. Int J Surg Pathol 2002;10(2):81-9.

30. Machado-Aranda D, Malamet M, Chang YJ, Jacobs MJ, Ferguson L, Silapaswan S, et al. Prevalence and management of gastro—intestinal stromal tumors. Am Surg 2009;75(1):55-60.

31. Conlon KC, Casper ES, Brennan MF. Primary gastrointestinal sarcomas: analysis of prognostic variables. Ann Surg Oncol 1995;2(1):26-31.

32. Demetri GD. Targeting c-kit mutations in solid tumors: scientific rationale and novel therapeutic options. Semin Oncol 2001;28 (5 Suppl 17):19-26.

Diseases of Pancreas

Vijay Mittal, Sumeet Virmani

SURGICAL EMBRYOLOGY AND ANATOMY

The pancreas develops during the fourth week of fetal life from dorsal and ventral outgrowths of endoderm that arise from the caudal portion of the foregut. In the seventh week, the ventral bud fuses with the dorsal bud as the duodenum rotates to the right. The dorsal pancreatic duct joins with the duct of ventral pancreas to form the main pancreatic duct (duct of Wirsung) that merges with common bile duct (CBD); however, a small part remains as accessory duct (duct of Santorini) that drains directly into the duodenum. In 5–10 percent of people, the ventral and dorsal pancreatic ducts do not fuse, and most regions of the pancreas drain through the duct of Santorini through the orifice of the minor papilla. Failed fusion of pancreatic ducts (pancreatic divisum: Fig. 12.1) may result in pancreatitis arising from the stenosis of the duct of Santorini. Another embryonic anomaly may occur if the second part of duodenum gets trapped in the pancreatic band leading to annular pancreas.

The pancreas is a retroperitoneal organ located in the upper part of abdomen and weighs 70-100 gm in an adult. The pancreas can be divided into following regions: head (including uncinate process), neck, body and tail. The head is located between L1 and L2 vertebra in the C-loop of duodenum. Blood supply is derived from branches of the celiac and superior mesenteric arteries (SMA). The pancreatic head is supplied from superior and inferior pancreaticoduodenal arteries. The body is supplied by great, inferior and caudal pancreatic arteries (all branches from splenic artery) and the tail is supplied from branches of splenic, gastroepiploic and dorsal pancreatic arteries. Venous drainage is via the portal system. Lymphatic drains into the celiac and SMA nodes.

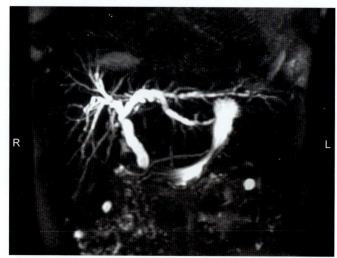

FIGURE 12.1: MRI (3D reconstruction) of abdomen showing moderate intra- and extrabiliary ductal dilatation. Pancreatic duct draining the tail, body and anterior aspect of pancreas drains directly into the duodenum. Posterior aspect of pancreatic head mass drains through a second orifice consistent with pancreatic divisum

PHYSIOLOGY

The exocrine pancreas secretes about 1-2 liters/day of clear, alkaline (pH 7-8.5) solution rich in digestive enzymes. Secretin, cholecystokinin (CCK) and parasympathetic vagal discharge stimulate the pancreatic exocrine secretion, whereas somatostatin and pancreatic polypeptide inhibit their release. Ductal cells contain carbonic anhydrase and secrete HCO_3^-, while acinar cells secrete Cl^- and digestive enzymes. Digestive enzymes include amylase, lipase, trypsinogen, chymotrypsinogen, carboxypeptidase and

HCO3-. Amylase is the only pancreatic enzyme secreted in its active form.

Endocrine pancreas secretes glucagon (alpha cells), insulin (beta cells), somatostatin (delta cells), pancreatic polypeptide (F cells), vasoactive intestinal polypeptide (VIP), serotonin and neuropeptide Y (islet cells).

ACUTE PANCREATITIS

Introduction

Acute pancreatitis is an acute inflammatory process of the pancreas with severity ranging from mild self-limiting disease to one with high morbidity and mortality. It is important to differentiate "acute" from "chronic" pancreatitis which is based on the functional and structural integrity of the gland before and after the attack rather than duration of the disease. Mild cases of acute pancreatitis are often successfully treated conservatively while severe cases may require urgent ICU admission. The incidence is higher in male population as compared to female. Overall mortality from the disease is approximately 5 percent, but may reach 20 to 30 percent in the presence of multiorgan failure.[1] Acute pancreatitis is a challenging disease to manage, with a significant morbidity, mortality and financial costs.

Etiology

The leading cause of acute pancreatitis in developed countries is gallstones including microlithiasis, with alcohol abuse as a close second. Together they account for 80 percent of the cases. Endoscopic retrograde cholangio-pancreatography (ERCP) induced pancreatitis is responsible for

another 5 percent. Major and less common causes of acute pancreatitis have been summarized in Table 12.1. In children, this disorder may be associated with abdominal trauma, hemolytic uremic syndrome, Kawasaki disease, mumps, Reye's syndrome and viral illnesses.

The exact mechanism causing pancreatitis is not known. However, the disease process is said to start with pancreatic acinar cell injury. The enzymes normally secreted by the pancreas in an inactive form become activated inside the pancreas and start to digest the pancreatic tissue. Subsequently trypsin activates the complement, kallikrein-kinin, coagulation, and fibrinolysis cascades leading to acinar cell injury. This process termed "auto digestion" activates the inflammatory response and in severe cases ultimately leads to necrosis of pancreatic parenchyma. Lipase activation produces the necrosis of fat tissue in pancreatic interstitium and peripancreatic spaces. With further progression of the disease a systemic inflammatory response syndrome (SIRS) is triggered leading to acute respiratory distress syndrome (ARDS), shock, metabolic disturbances and renal failure. Phospholipase A_2 causes injury to alveolar membranes of the lungs. Enzyme rich peri-pancreatic fluid collection often occurs in about 40 percent of the patients. Fifty percent of these resolve spontaneously while others become infected or form pseudocysts.

Fifty percent of deaths occur within the first 2 weeks after the onset of symptoms; these deaths are primarily the result of SIRS-induced multisystem organ failure. Most of the remaining deaths occur 2 to 3 weeks after presentation and result from complications of pancreatic necrosis, especially infection.

Table 12.1: Major and less common causes of acute pancreatitis	
Major causes	*Less common causes*
Gallstones including microlithiasis	Autoimmune pancreatitis
Alcohol abuse	Abnormalities of bile and pancreatic ducts
ERCP	(e.g. long common duct)
Infection: Mumps, Epstein-Barr virus; cytomegalovirus; rubella; hepatitis A, B, non-A, non-B; coxsackie B, mycoplasma pneumonia, campylobacter	Genetic factors (hereditary pancreatitis) Pancreatic divisum
Drug induced: Estrogens, corticosteroids, thiazide diuretics, isoniazid, tetracycline and azathioprine	Fatty necrosis
Hypercalcemia	Pregnancy
Traumatic injury	Cystic fibrosis
Pancreatic surgical procedures	Pancreatic cancer
Ascaris species	Sphincter of Oddi dysfunction
Vasculitis	
Idiopathic	

Clinical Findings

The signs and symptoms vary depending upon the severity of an attack. Acute pancreatitis usually begins after a large meal or alcohol consumption and is associated with abdominal pain radiating to the back, nausea, vomiting and anorexia. Pain often reduces by sitting upright and leaning forward or lying on the side with knees flexed. Some patients complain of pale, foul-smelling and oily stools (steatorrhea). Dehydration, tachycardia and hypotension, resulting from intravascular hypovolemia, are often seen in patients requiring hospitalization. Abdominal examination may reveal epigastric tenderness with guarding or rigidity depending upon the severity of attack. Bowel sounds are usually decreased or absent. An abdominal mass on palpation may indicate a phlegmon, pseudocyst or an abscess. Low-grade fever is secondary to pancreatic inflammation while high-grade fevers are indicative of intra- or extrapancreatic infection. Diaphragmatic irritation may cause shallow respirations and dyspnea may occur in patients with associated pleural effusion. Jaundice may be evident in the presence of cholangitis. Bluish discoloration in the flank (Grey Turner's sign) or periumbilical area (Cullen's sign) or inguinal region (Fox's sign), indicate retroperitoneal hemorrhage. Other less common findings include subcutaneous nodular fat necrosis known as panniculitis (due to circulating lipases), thrombophlebitis in the legs, and polyarthritis.

Differential Diagnosis

Biliary colic, cholecystitis, small bowel obstruction, severe gastritis, acute mesenteric ischemia, perforation, and ruptured aortic aneurysm need to be considered while evaluating a patient presenting with acute upper abdominal pain. However, blood investigations and imaging tests are often very useful in excluding other causes of acute abdomen.

Laboratory Findings

Complete blood count (CBC) with differential count, liver function test (LFT), blood urea nitrogen (BUN), serum creatinine, serum amylase and lipase are often the initial tests ordered. Acute pancreatitis results in significant third space losses, and may result in hemoconcentration and a high hematocrit. WBC count is increased because of pancreatic inflammation. Serum amylase level increases within 6 to 12 hours of attack and then return to normal (half-life: 10 hours) over next 3 to 5 days in an uncomplicated attack. However, hyperamylasemia is nonspecific and occurs in a number of other conditions (e.g. acute cholecystitis, parotitis, trauma, radiation, acidosis or ketoacidosis, macroamylasemia, anorexia nervosa/bulimia, renal failure, and malignancy with ectopic amylase production). Measurement of P-isoamylase (amylase of pancreatic origin) improves diagnostic accuracy.

The sensitivity of serum lipase for the diagnosis of acute pancreatitis ranges from 85 to 100 percent. However, like amylase, lipase is not specific to pancreas and can be elevated in diseases of salivary glands, perforated viscous and ischemic bowel disease. Other enzymes like phospholipase A, trypsin, carboxylester lipase, carboxypeptidase A, and co-lipase may also be elevated. Levels of pancreatitis-associated protein (PAP), a heat shock protein, are markedly increased in acute pancreatitis, however, its sensitivity for the detection of acute pancreatitis appears to be no better than conventional tests.

Patients with recurrent idiopathic pancreatitis are now screened for mutations in the genes for cationic trypsinogen (PRSS1), pancreatic secretory trypsin inhibitor (PSTI or SPINK1), and cystic fibrosis transmembrane conductance regulator (CFTR) gene.

Imaging

An abdominal X-ray may show localized ileus of a segment of small intestine (sentinel loop) or the "colon cutoff sign". Chest X-ray (CXR) may reveal pleural effusions, basal atelectasis and pulmonary infiltrates especially on left side. Abdominal ultrasound may reveal gall stones. A diffusely enlarged, hypoechoic pancreas is the classic ultrasonographic image of acute pancreatitis. However, about 1/4th of patients have bowel gas thus, making the study inconclusive.

A CT scan is often not required on the first day of hospital admission, unless there are other possible diagnoses. However, it is always the first radiological investigation and is indicated in patients with severe acute pancreatitis. Dynamic spiral CT scanning is used to determine the presence and extent of pancreatic necrosis. The patients are given oral and intravenous contrast (if normal renal function), to identify any areas of pancreatic necrosis which are seen as unenhanced areas (Fig. 12.2). Diffuse glandular enlargement is the most common finding. Abdominal CT scans also provide prognostic information based on the following grading scale developed by Balthazar (Table 12.2).

MRI and MRCP are being increasingly used in the diagnosis of suspected biliary or pancreatic duct obstruction in the setting of pancreatitis. The advantages include: (a) ability of MRI to better categorize fluid collection as acute fluid collections, necrosis, abscess, hemorrhage and pseudocyst, and (b) greater sensitivity of MRI to detect mild acute pancreatitis compared to CT. ERCP is usually contraindicated during the acute attack, except when pancreatitis is caused by an impacted common bile duct stone. Under those conditions, sphincterotomy and stone retrieval result in significant reduction in morbidity and mortality.

Endoscopic ultrasonography (EUS) is an endoscopic procedure that allows a high-frequency ultrasound transducer to be inserted into the gastrointestinal tract to visualize the pancreas and the biliary tract. EUS is often helpful in evaluating the cause of severe pancreatitis, particularly microlithiasis and biliary sludge. It can help to identify periampullary lesions better than any other imaging

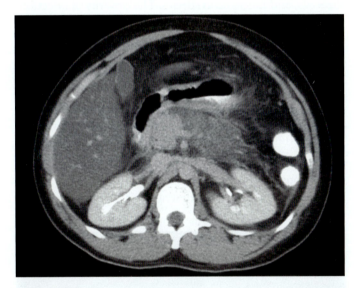

FIGURE 12.2: CT scan of the abdomen with contrast showing fluid around the pancreas consistent with pancreatitis. Some hypo-enhancement of the body of the pancreas is also seen suggestive of pancreatic necrosis or impending necrosis

modalities. Secretin-stimulated EUS study may reveal resistance to ductal outflow at the level of the papilla.

PREDICTORS OF SEVERITY OF ACUTE PANCREATITIS

Clinical, laboratory, and radiologic risk factors can not be used to predict severity of acute pancreatitis. The Atlanta classification divided acute pancreatitis into two broad categories: Mild (edematous and interstitial) acute pancreatitis and severe (usually synonymous with necrotizing) acute pancreatitis. The criteria for severe acute pancreatitis included any of the following: a Ranson's score (Table 12.3) of 3 or more and/or an Acute Physiology and Chronic Health Evaluation-II (APACHE II) score of 8 or more within the first 48 hours, organ failure (respiratory, circulatory, renal, and/or gastrointestinal bleeding), and/or local complications (pancreatic necrosis, abscess, or pseudocyst). Those with actual or predicted severe disease and those with other severe comorbid conditions should be considered for triage to an intensive care or intermediate medical care unit.

Serum markers of immune activation IL-6, IL-8, IL-10, TNF, PMN elastase, and C-reactive protein, predict an unfavorable outcome of acute pancreatitis. Levels of C-reactive protein above 150 mg/dl at 48 hours discriminate severe from mild disease. C-reactive protein at 48 hours have a sensitivity and specificity of 80 and 76 percent respectively, using a cut-off of 150 mg/L. Early and persistent organ failure is a reliable indicator of a prolonged hospital stay and increased mortality.

TREATMENT OF ACUTE PANCREATITIS

Treatment of acute pancreatitis is aimed at alleviating the symptoms of nausea, vomiting and pain; hemodynamic stabilization; adequate nutrition; limiting the severity of

Table 12.2: CT scan based Balthazar grading system for acute pancreatitis. CT scan severity index (points for grade of acute pancreatitis) + (points for degree of pancreatic necrosis); Interpretation: Minimum score 0, maximum score 10.

Criteria	CT finding	Points
Grade of acute pancreatitis	Normal	0
	Gland enlargement,	1
	peripancreatic inflammation	2
	Single extrapancreatic fluid collection	3
	extensive extrapancreatic fluid collection, pancreatic abscess	4
Degree of pancreatic necrosis	No necrosis	0
	Necrosis of one-third of pancreas	2
	Necrosis of one half of the pancreas 4	4
	Necrosis of more than one half of the pancreas	6

Table 12.3: Ranson criteria for predicting the severity of acute pancreatitis	
At admission	*At 48 hours*
Age in years > 55 years	Serum calcium < 2.0 mmol/L (< 8.0 mg/dl)
WBC count > 16000 cells/mm^3	PO2 < 60 mm Hg
Blood glucose > 200 mg/dl (> 11 mmol/L)	Hematocrit fall > 10%
Serum SGOT (AST) > 250 IU/L	BUN increased by 5 or more mg/dl (1.8 or more mmol/L) after IV fluid hydration
Serum LDH > 350 IU/L	Base deficit (negative base excess) > 4 mEq/L (> 4 mmol/L)
	Fluids sequestration > 6 L

attack; and management of acute organ failure. Attempts should be made to correct any underlying predisposing factors which may include: (a) reversal of hypercalcemia, (b) cessation of possible causative drugs, (c) administration of insulin to the poorly controlled diabetic usually associated with marked hypertriglyceridemia and (d) an early ERCP in patients with gallstone pancreatitis (Fig. 12.3) who have obstructive jaundice or biliary sepsis.[2] Mild pancreatitis is treated for several days with supportive care including pain control, aggressive fluid repletion, and nothing by mouth. The algorithm for managing the patients with acute pancreatitis has been outlined in Figure 12.4.

Supportive Treatment

A multidisciplinary approach holds the key to successful management of this disease.[3] In severe pancreatitis, intensive care unit monitoring and support of pulmonary, renal, circulatory, and hepatobiliary function may minimize systemic sequelae. Fluid resuscitation is particularly important, as patients with necrotizing pancreatitis accumulate vast amounts of fluid in the injured pancreatic bed. At least 250 to 300 cc of intravenous fluids per hour are required for initial 48 hours (guided by CVP). On the other hand, in some patients, a low urine output may already reflect the development of acute tubular necrosis rather than persistent volume depletion. Arterial oxygen saturation should be maintained ≥ 95 percent.

Pain Management

Abdominal pain is often the dominant symptom. Intravenous opiates, usually in the form of a patient controlled analgesia (PCA) pump are preferred. Morphine causes an increase in sphincter of Oddi pressure, and hence should be avoided; instead meperidine can be used.

Antibiotics

About one-third of patients with pancreatic necrosis develop infected necrosis. Antibiotics should be restricted to patients

with proven infection, exception being a decompensating patient in whom infection is strongly suspected but not yet proved. The important organisms causing infection in necrotizing pancreatitis are usually from the intestine including but not limited to *Escherichia coli*, *Pseudomonas*, *Klebsiella*, and *Enterococcus* species. The majority of infections (75%) are monomicrobial. Imipenem, third generation cephalosporins, piperacillin, mezlocillin, fluoroquinolones, and metronidazole are the antibiotics of choice because of higher penetration in pancreatic tissue. Gut decontamination also helps to reduce the incidence of pancreatic associated infection.

Nutrition

Patients with mild pancreatitis can often be managed with intravenous fluids, however, nutritional support is required in patients with severe pancreatitis.[4] Acute pancreatitis

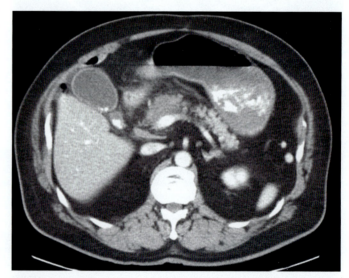

FIGURE 12.3: CT scan of the abdomen with contrast showing significant peri-pancreatic fat stranding and ascites. There is hypoattenuation of the proximal pancreatic body suspicious for pancreatic necrosis. Also seen are innumerable tiny gallstones highly suspicious for causing the gallstone pancreatitis

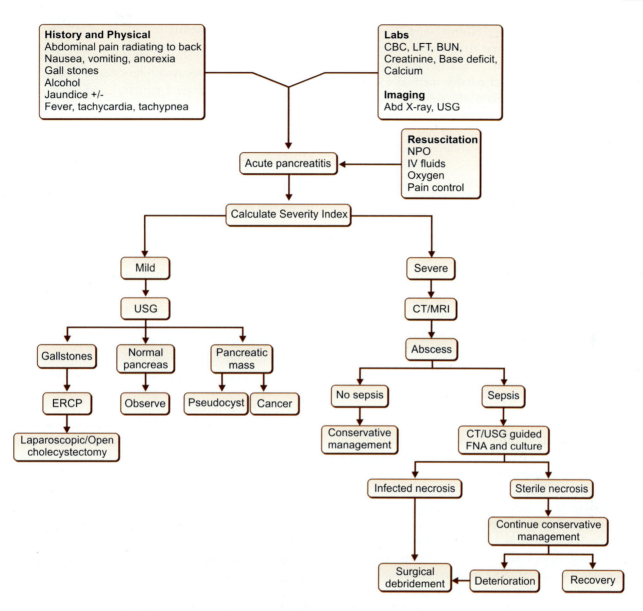

FIGURE 12.4: Algorithm summarizing the management of acute pancreatitis

creates a state of catabolic stress, promoting a systemic inflammatory response and nutritional deterioration. Oral alimentation is the preferred route and it can be resumed once the pain and abdominal tenderness subside. Enteral feeding has been shown to be safe, less expensive, well tolerated and as effective as total parenteral nutrition (TPN). It helps to maintain mucosal function, and limits the absorption of endotoxins and cytokines from the gut. Pancreatic stimulation can be avoided by placement of them enteral feeding tube distal to the Treitz ligament. If enteral feeding is not tolerated after five days, TPN should be used to meet caloric and protein requirements.

INDICATIONS FOR SURGERY

There are several clear indications for operative intervention in acute pancreatitis. Patients with an acute abdomen in whom the diagnosis is unclear or those who develop a complication (e.g. hemorrhage, bowel infarction, or perforation) will need surgical intervention. However, focus should be directed first to identify patients with infected pancreatic necrosis.[5,6] CT guided fine needle aspiration (FNA) is a safe and reliable method to look for areas of necrosis/pus and remains the gold standard. Gram stain and culture of the aspirate is accurate for the diagnosis of infection, with both a positive and negative predictive value of around 90 percent. The ability to safely delay any interventions to allow better demarcation and liquefaction of pancreatic necrosis offers a higher success rate for any pancreatic intervention.

CHRONIC PANCREATITIS

Introduction

"Chronic pancreatitis" as the name suggests refers to "progressive inflammation" of the pancreas. It results in permanent structural damage eventually leading to impairment or loss of exocrine and endocrine function. Clinically it presents as a syndrome of persistent/recurrent abdominal pain, steatorrhea, diabetes and/or pancreatic calcification.[7]

Etiology

Chronic pancreatitis is often caused by chronic alcohol abuse (>150 gm/day for 6 to 12 years). Other frequent causes include gallstone-associated pancreatitis, chronic steroid or anti-inflammatory drug use, hereditary, and autoimmune pancreatitis (Table 12.4). Tropical pancreatitis is a form of idiopathic pancreatitis occurring in young non-alcoholic individuals. This entity is seen in countries like India, Indonesia and Africa and has been linked to genetic mutations such as the SPINK1 gene mutation and various environmental factors.[8] In children cystic fibrosis and severe protein-energy malnutrition are the most common causes of chronic pancreatitis.

Table 12.4: Causes of chronic pancreatitis
Causes of chronic pancreatitis
• Chronic alcohol abuse
• Gallstone-associated pancreatitis
• Chronic steroid or anti-inflammatory drug use
• Tropical pancreatitis
• Auto immune chronic pancreatitis
• Recurrent or severe acute pancreatitis
• Cystic fibrosis

Clinical Presentation

The two primary clinical manifestations of chronic pancreatitis are: (a) recurrent episodes of acute pancreatitis in a chronically damaged pancreas and/or; (b) persistent pain with or without malabsorption. Initially the pain may occur in discrete attacks located deep in the epigastric region often radiating to the back. However, as the condition progresses, the pain becomes more continuous and often increases in severity. The pain in chronic pancreatitis is thought to be caused by inflammation in the pancreatic tissue and perineural sheath. Another hypothesis relates to the increased pressure within the pancreatic duct and parenchyma.

Many patients with chronic pancreatitis do not show any clinically significant protein or fat deficiencies until over 90 percent of pancreatic function is lost. Pancreatic insufficiency leads to maldigestion and malabsorption of nutrients. Diabetes is a common complication due to the chronic pancreatic damage and may require treatment with insulin. Considerable weight loss, due to malabsorption, is evident in a high percentage of patients. The patient may also complain of abdominal pain related to their food intake, especially those meals containing a high percentage of fats and protein. Pancreatic insufficiency affects fat absorption more as compared to protein or carbohydrate digestion. Protein digestion is aided by gastric pepsin while carbohydrate digestion is aided by salivary and intestinal amylase. Fat-soluble vitamin deficiency (vitamins A, D, E and K) in addition to magnesium, calcium and essential fatty acids deficiencies may occur late in the disease and are directly related to fat malabsorption. Apart from chronic pancreatitis other causes of exocrine pancreatic insufficiency include cystic fibrosis and Shwachman-Diamond syndrome.

Diagnosis

Diagnosis of chronic pancreatitis is usually based on tests on pancreatic structure and function. Direct biopsy of the pancreas is not done routinely due to the increased risks. Serum amylase and lipase levels are rarely elevated except in cases of acute or chronic episodes. Serum bilirubin and alkaline phosphatase if elevated, indicate stricturing of the common bile duct due to edema, fibrosis or cancer. Elevations in ESR, IgG4, rheumatoid factor, ANA and antismooth muscle antibody may suggest an auto immune process.

A secretin-cholecystokinin stimulation test is considered the gold standard functional test for diagnosis of chronic pancreatitis with a 95 percent sensitivity rate in early stages of disease. Pancreatic enzyme activity as well as bicarbonate levels are measured in duodenal juice after stimulation with secretin and cholecystokinin. Pancreatic fluid with bicarbonate concentration of < 80 mEq/L and bicarbonate output below 15 mEq/30 min indicates pancreatic insufficiency. Pancreolauryl test, PABA excretion test and fecal fat balance test are also used to evaluate pancreatic exocrine function. The most sensitive and specific test is the measurement of fecal elastase (ELISA test). A value less than 200 ug/g indicates pancreatic insufficiency.

Imaging

Radiological investigations are now commonly used to make a diagnosis of chronic pancreatitis and include abdominal X-rays, ultrasound, EUS, CT scan, MRI, ERCP and MRCP. Pancreatic calcification can often be seen on plain abdominal X-rays. CT scan may show pancreatic atrophy, calcifications (Fig. 12.5), ductal dilatation, pseudocysts, splenic artery pseudoaneurysm, and/or biliary obstruction. ERCP is a highly sensitive radiographic test to detect chronic pancreatitis with a sensitivity and specificity of more than 90 percent. With the availability of more safer and less invasive techniques the role of ERCP in the diagnosis of pancreatic cancer has decreased. However, it can be both

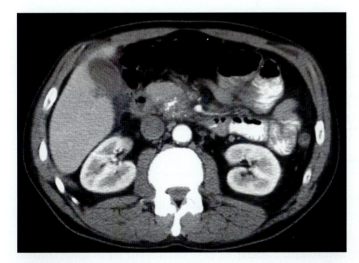

FIGURE 12.5: CT scan of the abdomen with contrast showing pancreatic calcification in the head of pancreas suggestive of chronic pancreatitis. Also seen is the fluid located on the medial and superior to the pancreas with peripancreatic inflammatory change

diagnostic as well as therapeutic. Sensitivity of MRCP varies between 70 and 92 percent with ERCP considered as the gold standard. Heavy T2 weighted images allow better visualization of fluid-filled structures, and hence, pancreatic duct.

Treatment

Treatment modalities for management of chronic pancreatitis include medical measures, therapeutic endoscopy and surgery (summarized in Fig. 12.6). Treatment is directed to the underlying cause, relief of pain and malabsorption, correction of glucose levels and management of complications. Patients with chronic alcohol use are counselled against taking any alcohol. Although, the damage to pancreas is irreversible, abstinence from alcohol often results in reduction of both chronic and acute abdominal pain in more than half of cases. Diabetes may occur and need long term insulin therapy. The abdominal pain often times is very severe and may require high doses of analgesics. Analgesics should be given prior to meals, as the pain is maximal postprandially. Disability and mood problems are common, although early diagnosis and support can make these problems manageable.

Pancreatic Enzyme Supplementation

Replacing pancreatic enzymes are helpful in treating the malabsorption and steatorrhea. It is indicated if patient looses > 10 percent body weight or excretes > 15 gm/day of fat in stools. Treatment with these enzymes is usually lifelong. Pancreatic enzyme supplements may also relieve pain in some patients. Patients with idiopathic pancreatitis and those without involvement of large ducts benefit from enzyme supplementation while patients with alcoholic pancreatitis are less likely to respond. Pancreatic enzyme products (PEPs) such as pancrelipase are supplemented with diet.[9] They help in the breakdown of fats (lipases), proteins (proteases) and carbohydrates (amylases) into units that can be digested by patients with exocrine pancreatic insufficiency.

Pain Management

Abdominal pain remains the most important symptom in patients with chronic pancreatitis and is the one that is difficult to control. For best results a stepwise approach starting with some general measures is recommended. Abstinence from alcohol, small frequent meals (low in fat), and pancreatic enzymatic supplementation along with judicious use of analgesics improves the pain in vast majority

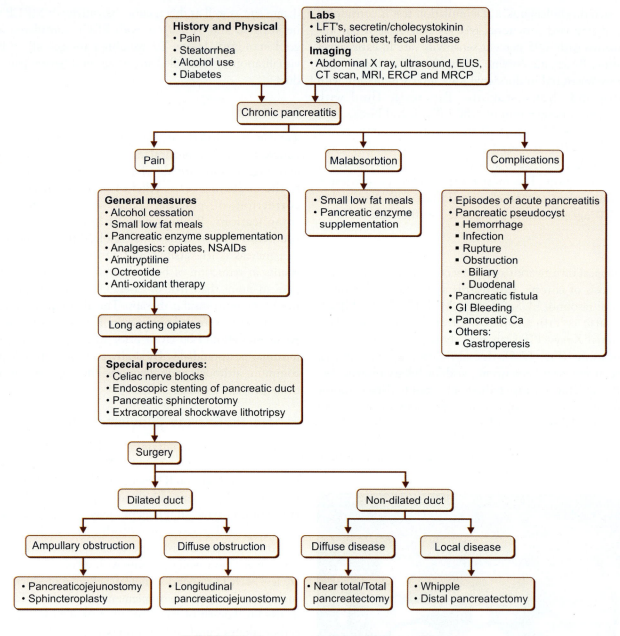

FIGURE 12.6: Management of chronic pancreatitis

of patients. Pancreatic enzyme supplementation reduces pain in some patients.

Short course of opiates along with a low dose of amitryptiline and NSAIDs will break the pain cycle. Admission to the hospital and keeping the patient nil orally on IV fluid supplementation decreases the pancreatic stimulation and hence, the abdominal pain. Chronic opioid use is only recommended in patients with severe chronic pain. Use of long acting agents such as morphine sulphate and fentanyl patch is usually advised later in the course of disease progression. Benefits from octreotide, and antioxidant[10] therapies have been reported in some studies.

Patients with severe pain refractory to medical management benefit from celiac nerve block, endoscopic stenting of pancreatic duct/pancreatic sphincterotomy, extracorporeal shock wave lithotripsy.[11]

Surgery

Surgery for chronic pancreatitis tends to be divided into two areas-resectional and drainage procedures depending on the extent of pancreatic disease (diffuse vs localized) and/or dilated on nondilated duct (Fig. 12.7). Timing of surgery is controversial. Early surgery may prevent progression of disease and its complications but at the same time complications of major surgery cannot be ignored.[7,12,13] Many patients choose surgery as the last option. Surgical procedures that have been described are: (a) Decompression/drainage procedures; (b) Pancreatic resections; (c) Denervation procedures.[14]

PANCREATIC PSEUDOCYST

A pancreatic pseudocyst is a collection of fluid in the lesser sac. The fluid collection is usually the pancreatic fluid that has leaked out of a damaged pancreatic duct as a result of acute or chronic pancreatitis but may occur after trauma. Unlike, true cysts, which are lined by epithelium; pseudocysts are lined with granulation tissue. In acute pancreatitis, the ductal disruption is secondary to necrosis of part of the pancreas with subsequent duct leakage. However, patients with chronic pancreatitis may have elevated pancreatic duct pressures resulting from strictures, ductal calculi, or other causes. This results in a small ductal disruption, frequently leading to a pseudocyst formation.

Patient usually presents with abdominal pain, fever, weight loss or even with features of bowel obstruction from compression. Abdominal USG, CT or MRI helps in the diagnosis of pancreatic pseudocyst. Treatment (Fig. 12.8) depends on the size of the pseudocyst and whether or not the cyst is causing the symptoms. Many pseudocysts resolve on their own. Those that remain longer than 6 weeks and are larger than 5 cm in diameter and/or are symptomatic and continuously increasing in size may require surgery. Patients with symptomatic or growing pseudocyst need MRCP or ERCP to check for duct involvement.[15] CT guided percutaneous drainage of cyst may be done if duct is not involved. In case, a duct involvement is suspected, endoscopic drainage through the gastric or duodenal wall with placements of stents or surgical drainage into an adjacent hollow viscous, e.g. cystojejunostomy or cystogastrostomy, is preferred. Resection of the pseudocyst along with some pancreatic parenchyma may be done if the pseudocyst is located in tail of pancreas.

PANCREATIC FISTULAS

Disruption of the pancreatic duct or rupture of a pseudocyst usually leads to a leakage of pancreatic secretions and may result in either an external or internal pancreatic fistula. Pancreatic fistulas can be caused by pancreatic disease, trauma, or surgery. Pancreaticocutaneous fistula results in the loss of bicarbonate-rich pancreatic fluid leading to hyperchloremic or normal anion gap metabolic acidosis. An internal pancreatic fistula develops in patients with chronic pancreatitis with the development of pancreatic ascites. Patients usually complain of abdominal distension or dyspnea. Amylase level in fluid is usually elevated (> 18,000 IU/L). Most pancreatic fistulas respond to medical management (Fig. 12.7) which includes, nil orally, use of TPN, repeated fluid drainage and octreotide to decrease pancreatic secretions. Patients with failed medical management may benefit from ERCP, sphincterotomy and pancreatic stent placement.[16] Surgery is reserved for patients who fail medical and endoscopic therapy and may include connecting the fistulous tract with a Roux-en-Y loop or rarely pancreatectomy.

PANCREATIC CANCER

Incidence and Epidemiology

Pancreatic cancer is the fifth leading cause of cancer-related deaths in US. It is more common in men and 80 percent of cases are above 60 years in age. Risk factors include: (a) High-protein and high-fat diet; (b) Cigarette smoking (doubles the risk); (c) Exposure to industrial carcinogens; (d) Family history of pancreatic cancer; (e) Hereditary or chronic pancreatitis; and (f) Alcohol abuse.

Molecular Biology

Ninety percent of patients with pancreatic cancers demonstrate codon 12 mutations of the K-ras oncogene. Mutations of the $p53$ tumor suppressor gene (75% of pancreatic cancers) along with other tumor suppressor genes, like $p16$, SMAD-4/DPC, and DCC have also been reported. Growth factors like epidermal growth factor (EGF) receptor, insulin-like growth factor receptor (IGFR), platelet derived growth factor receptor (PDGFR) and transforming growth factor beta receptor are also up-regulated. K-ras mutations and HER2/neu over expression are the earliest changes to occur. Alterations in $p16$ are found primarily in PanIN-2 and PanIN-3.

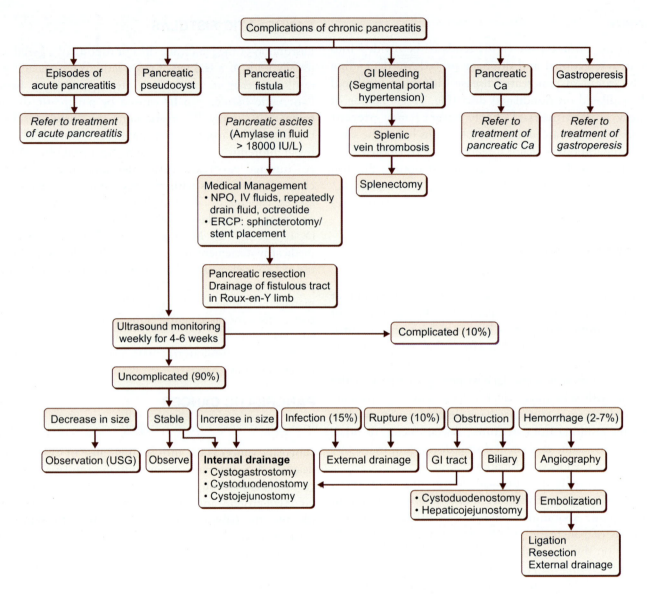

FIGURE 12.7: Algorithm summarizing the management for the complications of chronic pancreatitis

The incidence of pancreatic cancer is increased in families with hereditary nonpolyposis colon cancer (HNPCC), familial breast cancer (*BRCA2* mutation), Peutz-Jeghers syndrome, ataxia-telangiectasia, and familial atypical multiple mole melanoma (FAMMM) syndrome.[17] Patients with hereditary pancreatitis are also at increased risk for developing pancreatic cancer.

Pathology

Solid Epithelial Tumors

Ductal adenocarcinoma and its variants account for 80 to 90 percent of all pancreatic neoplasms and for an even greater fraction of the malignant tumors. Approximately 70 percent of ductal cancers arise in the pancreatic head or uncinate process. In more than 80 percent of the patients at the time of diagnosis, tumor ≤12 is > 3 cm in diameter, with both nodal involvement and distant metastases. Perineural growth of the tumor is highly characteristic of this cancer ultimately invading the neighboring neural plexuses resulting in severe upper abdominal and back pain.

Much like colon cancers pancreatic tumors also demonstrate progression to malignant from benign precursor lesions. The precursor lesions are referred to as pancreatic intraepithelial neoplasia (PanIN). PanIN-1A and PanIN-1B are proliferative lesions without remarkable nuclear abnormality that have a flat and papillary architecture, respectively. PanIN-3 is associated with severe architectural and cytonuclear abnormalities (loss of nuclear polarity, dystrophic goblet cells, mitoses, nuclear irregularities and prominent nucleoli), but invasion through the basement membrane is absent. True cribriforming, budding off of small clusters of epithelial cells into the lumen and luminal necrosis also suggests the diagnosis of PanIN-3. PanIN-2 is an intermediate category and is associated with a moderate degree of architectural (mucinous epithelial lesions—flat or papillary) and cytonuclear abnormality (some loss of polarity, nuclear crowding, enlarged nuclei, pseudo-stratification and hyperchromatism).[18]

Adenosquamous carcinomas are a rare variant of ductal adenocarcinoma with both glandular and squamous differentiation and occurs in patients with previous history of chemoradiation. *Acinar cell carcinomas* account for only 1 percent of pancreatic exocrine tumors. These tumors are more common in males and tend to be larger than ductal adenocarcinomas, often being larger than 10 cm. *Giant cell carcinomas* account for less than 5 percent of nonendocrine pancreatic tumors, often with average diameters more than 15 cm. Histologically they show pleomorphic cells and have a poor prognosis. *Pancreatoblastoma* is a rare form of pancreatic cancer that usually presents in young children and contain both epithelial and mesenchymal elements. Nonepithelial cancers of all types, including leiomyosarcomas, liposarcomas, plasmacytomas, and lymphomas, can also develop within the pancreas, however are quite rare.

Cystic Epithelial Tumors

Cystic neoplasms of the exocrine pancreas are less frequent than ductal adenocarcinomas and occur more commonly in females. Almost 70 percent of the cystic lesions in pancreas are pseudocyst. However, it is important to differentiate these from cystic neoplasms (Fig. 12.5) because of their malignant potential.[19,20]

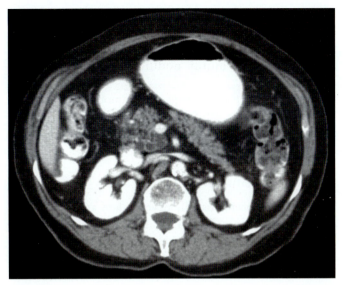

FIGURE 12.8: CT scan of the abdomen with contrast showing 2 cm multi-loculated cystic mass located in the uncinate process of pancreatic head with mildly prominent duct

Also known as serous cystadenomas, *serous cystic neoplasm (SCN)* are lined by simple, glycogen-rich cuboidal epithelium and occur more commonly in females. SCN can exhibit macroscopic variations and subdivided into serous microcystic and serous oligocystic adenomas. On CT scan SCN show a honeycomb pattern of microlacunae, with thin septa separating different segments. These tumors can have a sunburst pattern of central calcification. Although benign, with very low malignant potential, symptomatic lesions or those > 4 cm in size, or those that cannot be differentiated from other potentially malignant cysts should be considered for surgical resection.

Mucinous cystic neoplasms (MCN) are formed by mucus-producing cells and are associated with ovarian-like stroma. All MCN are considered potentially malignant and should undergo surgical resection.

Intraductal papillary-mucinous neoplasms (IPMNs) are intra-ductal mucin producing neoplasms with tall, columnar, mucin-containing epithelium with or without papillary projections. IPMNs are divided into: (a) main-duct; and (b) branch-duct type according to the involvement of the pancreatic ducts. IPMNs are usually found in elderly patients 60 to 80 years in age and appear to be more common in head, neck and uncinate process of pancreas but can occur through out the gland. CT scan often reveals a cystic mass located in the head of pancreas with a pancreatic duct communication. ERCP confirms the communication with the pancreatic duct along with mucin oozing out from ampulla of Vater. All main-duct type IPMN should be resected because of the high malignancy rate whereas branch-duct type IPMN demonstrating favorable features (<3 cm size and absence of mural nodules) may be managed conservatively.[21]

Solid and cystic papillary neoplasms (Hamoudi tumors) occur in females in their 4th-5th decade of life. These tumors show solid, cystic and papillary components and range from 5 to 15 cm in diameter.

Signs and Symptoms

Signs and symptoms usually develop late and depend on the site of the tumor (Table 12.5). Eighty percent of patients have metastasis before clinical symptoms arise. Tumors located in pancreatic head may cause biliary, pancreatic or duodenal obstruction. Symptoms include unexplained episodes of pancreatitis, painless jaundice, nausea, vomiting, steatorrhea, and unexplained weight loss (>10% of original body weight or 1-2 kg/month). Unlike the pancreatic head tumors, tumors in the pancreatic neck, body, or tail usually do not develop jaundice or gastric outlet obstruction. Their symptoms may be limited to unexplained weight loss and vague upper abdominal pain until the tumor has grown extensively and spread beyond the pancreas. These patients may later develop epigastric pain/back pain when peripancreatic nerve plexuses are involved. Initial metastasis is to the regional lymph nodes followed by hematogenous metastasis to liver (80%) and lungs (50%). Cancers in body or tail may cause splenic vein obstruction, splenomegaly, gastric/esophageal varices and GI hemorrhage. New-onset diabetes mellitus is occasionally the first symptom of an otherwise occult pancreatic cancer.[22]

Table 12.5: Clinical features of pancreatic cancer depending upon location	
Pancreatic head cancers	*Pancreatic body or tail cancers*
Loss of weight	Weight loss
Abdominal pain	Anorexia
Jaundice	Weakness
Dark urine	Nausea/Vomiting
Light stool	Abdominal pain
Anorexia	
Nausea/Vomiting	
Weakness	
Pruritus	
Palpable gallbladder	

Unexplained migratory thrombophlebitis (Trousseau's syndrome), Metastatic subumbilical (Sister Mary Joseph node) and pelvic peritoneal (Blumer's shelf) deposits, as well as left supraclavicular lymphadenopathy (Virchow's node) indicate the presence of distant metastases. Malignant ascites, caused by peritoneal carcinomatosis, may also be present.

Periampullary tumors originate from head of the pancreas, ampulla of Vater, distal common bile duct and the duodenum. They constitute 30 percent of malignant tumors arising from pancreatic head region. Distal common bile duct obstruction caused by the tumor often leads to bile duct and gallbladder distention. Thus, a palpable gallbladder in a patient with painless jaundice (i.e. Courvoisier's sign) suggests the presence of a periampullary neoplasm.

Blood Tests

Patients with pancreatic head lesions or with liver metastasis frequently have increased serum total bilirubin, alkaline phosphatase and gamma-glutamyl transferase levels. Transaminases may be elevated but usually not to the same extent as alkaline phosphatase. In patients with localized cancer of the body and tail of the pancreas, laboratory values are frequently normal. Normochromic anemia and hypoalbuminemia are seen secondary to the nutritional consequences of the disease. In patients with jaundice, the prothrombin time can be abnormally prolonged. This usually is an indication of biliary obstruction, which prevents bile from entering the gastrointestinal tract and leads to malabsorption of fat-soluble vitamins and decreased hepatic production of vitamin K-dependent clotting factors. Serum amylase and lipase levels are usually normal in patients with pancreatic cancer. More than 25 percent of patients with pancreatic cancer may present with increased glucose levels or worsening of pre-existing diabetes. This has been related to secretion of an anti-insulin hormone "islet amyloid polypeptide" (IAPP).

CEA and the Lewis blood group carbohydrate antigen CA 19-9 (both tumor markers for pancreatic cancer) are frequently elevated and are often used to monitor the disease. With normal upper limit of 37 U/ml, the accuracy of the CA 19-9 level in identifying patients with pancreatic adenocarcinoma is only about 80 percent. Increasing the cutoff value to 200 U/mL increases the accuracy to 95 percent. Levels of CA 19-9 have been correlated with prognosis and tumor recurrence. Higher CA 19-9 values before surgery indicate an increased size of the primary tumor and often correlates well with unresectability. They are also used to monitor the results of neoadjuvant and adjuvant chemoradiation therapy. Postoperative increase in CA 19-9 indicates recurrence or progression of disease, whereas decreasing levels indicate a better prognosis.

Imaging Studies

Radiological imaging plays a key role in diagnosis and staging of pancreatic cancer. Abdominal ultrasound due to its wide availability, low cost and non-invasiveness is considered as the screening test for most abdominal conditions. It is considered to be operator-dependent but can demonstrate pancreatic masses (solid or cystic) (Fig. 12.9); dilated intrahepatic and extrahepatic bile ducts, liver metastases, ascites, and enlarged peripancreatic lymph nodes. Its sensitivity ranges from 60 to 100 percent and specificity from 44 to 99 percent. Contrast-enhanced CT scan with a dual-phase intravenous contrast study is currently the preferred noninvasive imaging test. Recent advances in this imaging modality have contributed to early tumor detection and thus higher resectability rate. It usually demonstrates hypodense mass (Figs 12.10 and 12.11) with poorly demarcated edges with invasion into local structures or metastatic disease if present. Sensitivity depends on the size of the tumor, exceeding 95 percent for tumors larger than 2 cm in diameter. Positron emission tomography (PET) may

be of value in diagnosing small pancreatic tumors that escape CT or MRI detection. It uses the increased glucose metabolism of cancer cells and effectively differentiates benign from malignant lesions.

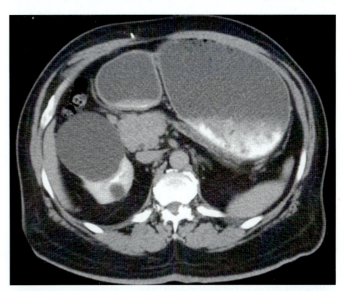

FIGURE 12.10: CT scan of the abdomen with contrast showing a 3 cm hypodense pancreatic head mass resulting in bowel obstruction at the level of second part of duodenum with marked gastric distension

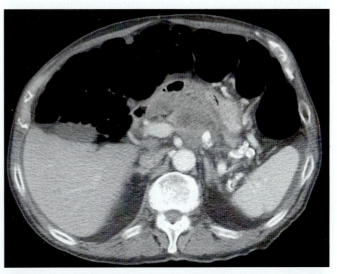

FIGURE 12.11: CT scan of the abdomen with contrast showing a 7.4 cm × 6.5 cm mass in the body of pancreas with subtle enhancement and encasement of left renal vein and splenic artery with splenic vein thrombosis and gastric varices

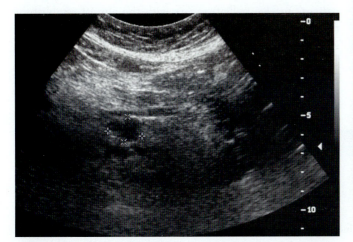

FIGURE 12.9: Abdominal ultrasound showing a 1.5 cm hypo-echoic cystic lesion in the head of pancreas

ERCP may be particularly helpful in evaluating patients with obstructive jaundice without a detectable mass on CT or MRI. The finding of a long, irregular stricture in an otherwise normal pancreatic duct is highly suggestive of a pancreatic cancer. It helps in: (a) identifying stones or other nonmalignant causes of obstructive jaundice, (b) define the location of the bile duct obstruction, (c) identify ampullary and periampullary lesions, and (d) to establish the diagnosis of IPMN if mucus is seen extruding through a fish-mouth papillary opening. Diagnostic ERCP should be reserved for patients with high index of suspicion for pancreatic cancer with or without jaundice with negative imaging studies. Role of EUS is very limited and was developed to eliminate interface with bowel gas. EUS is operator dependent and its applicability to preoperative staging is dependent on the locally available expertise.[23] Its role is justified in patients with uncertain diagnosis. EUS helps to detect and localize the smaller lesions (<3 cm) better (high resolution) and at the same time gives an opportunity to obtain tissue samples for histological confirmation.

Staging of Pancreatic Cancer

The goal of preoperative staging (Table 12.6) is to identify unresectable or metastatic disease and to select the patients who qualify for and will benefit from surgical resection. The TNM staging of pancreatic cancer takes into account the size of the tumor (T), lymph node involvement (N), and the distant metastasis (M). American Joint Committee for Cancer (AJCC) system is the most commonly used classification system. Absence of extrapancreatic disease, a patent superior mesenteric vein (SMV)-portal vein confluence, no evidence of encasement to the celiac axis or superior mesenteric artery and no extrapancreatic disease suggest a resectable pancreatic tumor. The role of staging laparoscopy is controversial. Twenty to fourty percent of

patients with stage I or II disease have unrecognized small metastases to peritoneal surfaces and can be detected laparoscopically, thus precluding a laparotomy.[24] In contrast it is argued that these patients can still benefit by performing prophylactic bilioenteric, and possibly gastroenteric, bypass. However with the advent of laparoscopic ultrasound, biopsy and peritoneal cytology it is now possible to detect the locally advanced disease.

Surgery

For resectable tumors of the head, neck, and uncinate process of the pancreas, pancreaticoduodenectomy, with or without preservation of the pylorus and proximal duodenum, is the surgical treatment of choice. Mortality rate for pancreaticoduodenectomy is 2 to 4 percent. Anastomotic leaks, intra-abdominal abscesses, gastrointestinal bleeding and delayed gastric emptying account for most of the perioperative complications after pancreaticoduodenectomy. Five-year survival rates of 15 to 20 percent have been reported.

For resectable tumors located in the body or tail of pancreas distal pancreatectomy with splenectomy is preferred. Complications include subphrenic abscess (5-10%) and pancreatic duct leak (up to 20%). Management of pancreatic carcinoma has been summarized in Figure 12.12.

Palliative Treatment of Pancreatic Cancers

Eighty percent of all pancreatic cancer patients present with unresectable disease at the time of diagnosis. Thus, most patients receive palliative care with the aim of establishing the diagnosis and to relieve symptoms of pain, jaundice, gastric outlet obstruction, depression and weight loss. Tissue diagnosis is usually achieved by CT or ultrasound-guided percutaneous fine-needle aspiration of either the tumor/metastatic lesion. Transduodenal fine-needle aspiration of

Stage	Tumor size	Nodal status	Metastasis
	Table 12.6: American Joint Committee on cancer: TNM system for staging of pancreatic cancer		
Stage 0	Tis	N0	M0
Stage IA	T1 (<2 cm)	N0	M0
Stage IB	T2 (>2 cm)	N0	M0
Stage IIA	T3 (direct extension of tumor to duodenum, bile duct, peripancreatic tissues)	N0	M0
Stage IIB	T1	N1	M0
	T2	N1	M0
	T3	N1	M0
Stage III	T4 (direct extension of tumor to stomach, spleen, colon, adjacent large vessels)	Any N	M0
Stage IV	Any T	Any N	M1

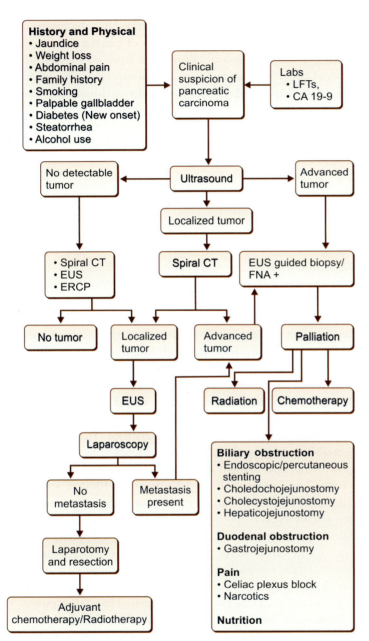

FIGURE 12.12: Algorithm summarizing the management of pancreatic carcinoma

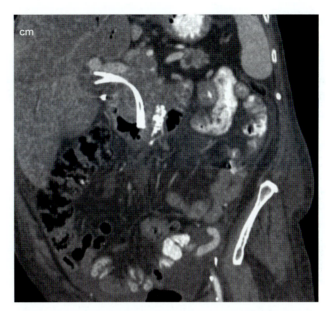

FIGURE 12.13: CT scan of the abdomen with 3D reconstruction showing a stent in the common bile duct

stents (Fig. 12.13) is the preferred method. Endoscopic approach has a higher success rate and a low complication rate as compared to percutaneous transhepatic stenting. Alternative to endoscopic stenting include cholecysto-jejunostomy or a choledochojejunostomy. The former is most appropriate for patients with nondilated ducts in whom the cystic duct—common bile duct confluence is distant from the tumor. Choledochojejunostomy, is considered when bile duct is > 1 cm in diameter[25] and the tumor is close to or at the cystic duct—common bile duct confluence. These drainage procedures often decrease the serum bilirubin levels in majority of patients.

To relieve duodenal obstruction expandable endoluminal metal stents are placed into the duodenum. For lesions that are not amenable to stents, surgical gastrojejunostomy may be required. Role of prophylactic gastric bypass is debatable as only 20 percent of patients with pancreatic head tumors will ultimately develop gastric outlet obstruction (Fig. 12.10).

Pain control is the most important aspect of palliative management and is often times most difficult to control. NSAIDs, COX-2 inhibitors or opiates may be used. Percutaneous CT or EUS guided celiac plexus block eliminates/reduces pain in majority of patients. This can also be done intraoperatively or via laparoscopically. Use of chemotherapy (especially gemcitabine) and radiation have also decreased pain in pancreatic cancer patients.

the tumor with endoscopic ultrasound guidance and duct cytology obtained by brushings is an alternative method of establishing the diagnosis.

For most patients with unresectable pancreatic cancer presenting with biliary tract obstruction, decompression can be achieved endoscopically or percutaneously. Endoscopic biliary decompression with plastic or expandable metal

Radiation and Chemotherapy

Patients with locally advanced pancreatic cancer receive chemotherapy and/or radiation therapy, however, the response rate is only 10-15 percent with a marginal improvement in survival. **Chemoradiation therapy comprises of** radiation therapy combined with either 5-fluorouracil or gemcitabine. Intraoperative radiation therapy, as adjuvant treatment, has been evaluated, but has not shown to improve the survival rates.

PANCREATIC NEUROENDOCRINE TUMORS

Introduction

Pancreatic neuroendocrine tumors (PET) are rare neoplasms of the pancreas accounting for less than 5 percent of all primary pancreatic malignancies. They include insulinomas, gastrinomas, glucagonoma and somatostatinomas. Collectively these neoplasms are classified as functional PETs. When a PET is not associated with a clinical syndrome due to hormone over secretion it is referred to as a non-functioning PET.[26]

Nonfunctional Endocrine Tumors

They represent one-third of all PETs but almost 90 percent of them are malignant. Unlike patient with functional PETs who clinically present due to hormone overproduction, non-functional PETs usually present with features of mass effect or metastatic lesions. Nonfunctioning PETs are pancreatic tumors with endocrine differentiation but lack a clinical syndrome of hormone hypersecretion. Although these tumors are hormonally "silent" they may produce a precursor hormone that is functionally inert, or at an amount that is too small to cause symptoms. Nonfunctioning tumors are slow growing and occur most commonly in the head of the pancreas.

Functional Endocrine Tumors

Insulinoma

Insulinomas are PETs arising from the insulin producing islet beta cells, and are the commonest type of PET. Ninety percent of them are benign. Insulinomas present with symptoms of hypoglycemia due to uncontrolled insulin production and can vary from confusion, behavioral changes, blurred vision, fatigue, seizures, and coma to even death. The classic Whipples' triad of: (a) fasting hypoglycemia; (b) low serum glucose (< 50 when symptomatic); and (c) relief of symptoms with IV administration of glucose. The

diagnosis can be made by the demonstration of high serum insulin and low blood sugar. A ratio of plasma insulin to glucose > 0.3 is diagnostic. Proinsulin levels more than 40 percent suggest malignant islet cell tumor. High resolution CT scan, MRI and EUS often help in localizing the insulinomas. Intraoperative ultrasound combined with surgeon palpation and full mobilization of the pancreas, results in localization of >95 percent of insulinomas. Enucleation is recommended for lesions < 2 cm in size while a formal resection is advocated if lesion is > 2 cm in size. For metastatic disease streptozocine, octreotide and 5-FU are recommended.

Gastrinoma (Zollinger-Ellison Syndrome)

Gastrinomas are the second commonest PET and arise from non-beta islet cells of the pancreas. They are most frequently diagnosed in the 5th and 6th decades of life. Fifty percent of gastrinomas are malignant and 50 percent are multiple. Seventy five percent of these tumors occur spontaneously while 25 percent are associated with MEN I syndrome. Ninty percent of gastrinomas are located in gastrinoma triangle—CBD, neck of pancreas and third portion of the duodenum. Ten percent of the tumors may be found in ectopic sites including duodenum. Patients present with abdominal pain (refractory peptic ulcer disease) and diarrhea. The diagnosis is established by the demonstration of marked fasting hyper-gastrinemia and marked gastric acid hypersecretion. Serum gastrin levels are usually > 200. Value > 1000 is almost diagnostic of gastrinoma. Secretin stimulation test increases the gastrin levels > 200 in patients with suspected Zollinger-Ellison syndrome (ZES). High resolution CT scan, MRI and EUS often help in localizing the gastrinomas. Somatostatin receptor scintigraphy is the single best study for localizing the tumors. The symptoms of acid hypersecretion can be effectively controlled by proton pump inhibitors in majority of patients with ZES. Enucleation is recommended for lesions < 2 cm in size while a formal resection is advocated if lesion is > 2 cm in size. High levels of gastrin may be present in G-cell hyperplasia. This can be distinguished from gastrinoma by the sharp rise of gastrin levels (> 200%) in response to meals as compared to minimal or no increase in patients with gastrinoma.

Glucagonoma

Glucagonoma is one of the most malignant functional PET with majority of tumors located in distal pancreas. They arise from alpha cells of the pancreas. The patients usually present with diabetes, dermatitis, deep vein thrombosis and depression. The pathognomic rash (necrolytic migratory erythema) is present in 70 percent of patients. Following treatment and normalization of glucagon levels, supplemented with zinc, amino acids and fatty acids this rash generally resolves. The diagnosis is established by the demonstration of elevated plasma glucagon levels which increase, paradoxically, when challenged with intravenous tolbutamide. Treatment with somatostatin analogues may benefit symptoms.

VIPoma (Verner Morrison Syndrome)

VIPoma is also one of the most malignant functional PET with majority of tumors located in distal pancreas. Ten percent of the VIPomas may be extrapancreatic. VIPomas produce pancreatic cholera syndrome. Patients usually present with watery diarrhea, hypokalemia and hypochlorhydria or achlorhydria. The treatment is aimed at the correction of dehydration and electrolyte abnormalities. As with other PETs, complete resection is the only chance for complete cure. Even in the presence of metastatic disease, debulking may assist in the postoperative management of VIP hypersecretion.

Somatostatinoma

Somatostatinoma is also one of the rare but most malignant functional PET with majority of tumors located in head of the pancreas. Fasting somatostatin level >14 mol/L is diagnostic. Patients present with diabetes, gall stones with a dilated gallbladder, steatorrhea, anemia and hypochlorohydria. Most of the patients have metastasis at the time of presentation. The diagnosis is established by demonstration of high serum levels of somatostatin. Surgery offers the only curative treatment by excising the primary tumor and all lymph node metastases. Cholecystectomy may be performed at the time of resection.

REFERENCES

1. Pannala R, Kidd M, Modlin IM. Acute pancreatitis: a historical perspective. Pancreas 2009;38(4): 355-66.
2. Petrov MS. Early management of severe acute biliary pancreatitis: wind of change. Gut 2008;57(9):1337-8; author reply 1338.
3. Hasibeder WR, et al. Critical care of the patient with acute pancreatitis. Anaesth Intensive Care 2009;37(2):190-206.
4. Petrov MS, Pylypchuk RD, Uchugina AF. A systematic review on the timing of artificial nutrition in acute pancreatitis. Br J Nutr 2009;101(6):787-93.
5. Bakker OJ, et al. Prevention, detection, and management of infected necrosis in severe acute pancreatitis. Curr Gastroenterol Rep 2009;11(2):104-10.
6. Werner J, et al. Management of acute pancreatitis: from surgery to interventional intensive care. Gut 2005;54(3):426-36.
7. Church NI, et al. Chronic pancreatitis: diagnosis and management of complications. Gut 2007;56(9):1189-90.
8. Tandon RK, Garg PK. Tropical pancreatitis. Dig Dis 2004;22(3):258-66.
9. Waljee AK, et al. Systematic review: pancreatic enzyme treatment of malabsorption associated with chronic pancreatitis. Aliment Pharmacol Ther 2009;29(3):235-46.
10. Forsmark CE. Antioxidants for chronic pancreatitis. Curr Gastroenterol Rep 2009;11(2):91-2.
11. Gachago C, Draganov PV. Pain management in chronic pancreatitis. World J Gastroenterol 2008;14(20):3137-48.
12. Buchler MW, Klar E. Introduction. Complications of pancreatic surgery and pancreatitis. Dig Surg 2002;19(2):123-4.
13. Johnson CD, Fitzsimmons D. Quality of life after surgery for chronic pancreatitis. Pancreatology 2006;6(5):497-8; author reply 498.
14. Gourgiotis S, Germanos S, Ridolfini MP. Surgical management of chronic pancreatitis. Hepatobiliary Pancreat Dis Int 2007;6(2):121-33.
15. Singh S. Surgical management of complications associated with percutaneous and/or endoscopic management of pseudocyst of the pancreas. Ann Surg 2006;244(4):630.
16. Mahvi D. Defining, Controlling, and Treating a Pancreatic Fistula. J Gastrointest Surg 2009.
17. Greenhalf W, et al. Screening of High-Risk Families for Pancreatic Cancer. Pancreatology 2009;9(3):215-22.
18. Sipos B, et al. Pancreatic intraepithelial neoplasia revisited and updated. Pancreatology 2009;9(1-2):45-54.
19. Gonzalez Obeso E, et al. Pseudocyst of the pancreas: the role of cytology and special stains for mucin. Cancer Cytopathol 2009;117(2):101-7.
20. Ng DZ, et al. Cystic neoplasms of the pancreas: current diagnostic modalities and management. Ann Acad Med Singapore 2009;38(3):251-9.
21. Freeman HJ. Intraductal papillary mucinous neoplasms and other pancreatic cystic lesions. World J Gastroenterol 2008;14(19):2977-9.
22. Pannala R, et al. New-onset diabetes: a potential clue to the early diagnosis of pancreatic cancer. Lancet Oncol 2009;10(1):88-95.
23. Saftoiu A, Vilmann P. Role of endoscopic ultrasound in the diagnosis and staging of pancreatic cancer. J Clin Ultrasound 2009;37(1):1-17.
24. Pisters PW, et al. Laparoscopy in the staging of pancreatic cancer. Br J Surg 2001;88(3):325-37.
25. Hwang SI, et al. Surgical palliation of unresectable pancreatic head cancer in elderly patients. World J Gastroenterol 2009;15(8):978-82.
26. O'Grady HL, Conlon KC. Pancreatic neuroendocrine tumours. Eur J Surg Oncol 2008;34(3):324-32.

Large Bowel Tumors

Deepa Taggarshe, Vijay Mittal

GENERAL CONSIDERATIONS

Cancer of the colon and rectum is the third most common cancer in the United States in both men (after prostate and lung cancer) and women (after breast and lung cancer). The estimated new cases of colon cancer in 2008 in the US were 108,070 (53,760 men and 54,310 women). The predicted deaths in 2008 due to colon cancer were 49,960 with 24,260 men and 25,700 women predicted to die due to this condition in the US.[1] According to the World Health Organization, 639,000 deaths occur every year across the world due to colorectal cancer. The incidence of colorectal cancer has decreased at an annual rate of 2.3 percent from 1998 to 2004 and similarly the mortality due to colorectal cancer decreased at an annual rate of 4.7 percent from 2002 to 2004.[2]

Tumors of the left side include those of the descending colon, sigmoid colon, rectosigmoid junction, and the rectum and these account for more than half of all colorectal cancers as shown in Figure 13.1.

EPIDEMIOLOGY

Some of the risk factors involved with colorectal cancer are as follows:

1. **Hereditary risk factors:** Colorectal cancer occurs in hereditary or familial forms. Hereditary syndromes of susceptibility to colorectal cancer are characterized by strong family history, early onset, and the presence of specific genetic defects. Hereditary non-polyposis colorectal cancer (HNPCC) syndrome and familial adenomatosis polyposis (FAP) are the two most common and widely researched forms of hereditary colorectal cancer.

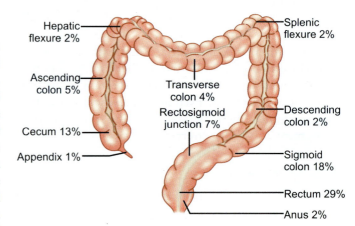

FIGURE 13.1: Percentage distributions of colorectal cancer cases at different sites in the large bowel. Cases in England from 1997 to 2002[2]

The familial form of colorectal cancer increases in lifetime risk for a person if one or more first-degree relatives have colorectal cancer, especially if diagnosed at a young age. The risk increases as the number of family members with colorectal cancer increases. An individual who is a first-degree relative of a patient diagnosed with colorectal cancer at an age younger than 50 is twice as likely as the general population to develop the cancer.[3]

2. **Age:** The incidence of colorectal cancer increases with age, with more than 90 percent of the patients diagnosed with colorectal cancer being over 50 years at the age of diagnosis. Colorectal screening programs in the United States are therefore geared towards asymptomatic people over 50 years.

3. **Diet:** Dietary fiber has been considered to be protective against colorectal cancer, by decreasing intestinal transit time, and acting as a diluent thus decreasing the exposure of intestinal mucosa to potential carcinogens.[4] Studies have shown strong associations between dietary fiber intake and decreased incidence of colorectal adenomas and carcinomas.[5] A diet high in animal fat and saturated fat increases the risk of colorectal cancer whereas vegetable fiber is protective.

4. **Inflammatory bowel disease:** Patients with long standing colitis are at increased risk of colorectal cancer, presumably due to the chronic inflammation of the mucosa predisposing a malignant change. In ulcerative colitis, the risk of cancer is approximately 2 percent after 10 years, 8 percent after 20 years, and 18 percent after 30 years. Patients with colitis due to Crohn's also have an increased risk of cancer. Patients with inflammatory bowel disease are therefore screened with annual colonoscopy after 8-10 years of the disease.

5. **Other factors:** Lack of physical exercise, smoking and alcohol, have all been associated with a higher risk of colorectal cancer. Altered bile metabolism after previous gastrectomy or vagotomy has also been implicated to increase the risk.[6] Patients with ureterosigmoidostomy also have an increased risk of colorectal cancer.[7]

COLORECTAL CARCINOGENESIS

Colorectal carcinogenesis constitutes the transition from normal epithelium to adenoma to invasive carcinoma, and is associated with a number of characteristic genetic changes.

The human colon and rectum consists of millions of crypts (Fig. 13.2) and stem cells, which reside at the bottom of the crypts, divide slowly and asymmetrically, so regenerating themselves at the same time as producing the epithelial cells that will populate the rest of the crypts and the mucosal surface. The risk of mutational events increases with each cell division of the stem cells due to errors during DNA replication and chromosomal segregation and this can in turn increase the risk of colorectal carcinogenesis.

The genetic changes involved in the multistep process of colorectal carcinogenesis (adenoma-carcinoma sequence) were first described by Fearon and Vogelstein (Fig. 13.3).[8] The accumulated genetic and epigenetic changes drive the progression to carcinoma and most of these tumors display some form of genomic instability.

The earliest event is the mutation of the *adenomatosis polyposis coli* (APC) gene, which is a tumor suppressor gene located on *5q21*. Mutations of the APC gene in colonic epithelial cells, very often resulting in truncated APC proteins very similar to those observed in **Familial adenomatous polyposis** patients, or deletions are also seen in about 80-85 percent of sporadic colorectal cancers.[9] APC acts as a "gatekeeper" of epithelial cell proliferation. Abnormal cells with mutations or deletions of both copies of APC accumulate in the crypt leading to formation of a dysplastic polyp.

Accumulation of further mutations as in *K-ras, p53* and genes on *18q* leads to progression towards cancer. *K-ras* is a proto-oncogene involved in intracellular signal transduction via the G-protein pathway. Ras proteins exist in two states: the active guanine triphosphate (GTP)-bound state and the inactive state bound to guanine diphosphate (GDP). GTPase-activating protein enhances the intrinsic capacity of Ras proteins to hydrolyse GTP into GDP, thereby returning Ras into the inactive form. Mutant Ras proteins have impaired GTPase activity, which makes them resistant to inactivation, thus leading to increased cellular division.

Other genes involved in colorectal cancer include *SMAD4, SMAD2,* and possibly *DCC* located on chromosome *18q*. The most frequently deleted gene is *SMAD4*, located on *18q21*, encoding a protein, which is involved as a downstream regulator in the transforming growth factor α

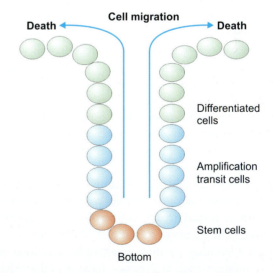

FIGURE 13.2: A colorectal mucosal crypt. The crypt is maintained by the stem cells at the base (shown in black). The amplification-transit cells divide rapidly (cells shown in brown) and migrate to the top, where they undergo differentiation (cells shown in green); and eventually die by apoptosis. Adapted from Kim K, Shibata D (Methylation reveals a niche: stem cell succession in human colon crypts. Oncogene 2002:21; 5441-549)

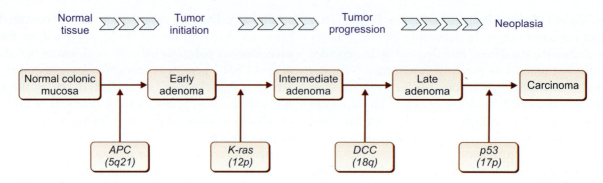

FIGURE 13.3: Genetic changes associated with the adenoma-carcinoma sequence in sporadic and hereditary colorectal cancers

(TGF-α) signalling pathway that regulates epithelial cell growth and apoptosis and is a critical factor in sustaining the peripheral immunological tolerance that characterizes the microenvironment of many tumors.

Mutations in *p53* are present in ~60 percent of colorectal cancers. This occurs late in the adenoma-carcinoma sequence. *p53* is a tumor suppressor gene, which under normal conditions acts in response to cellular stress or damage such as DNA damage or hypoxia by either inducing apoptosis or cell cycle arrest.

This remains one of the best-known models for the multistep process of colorectal carcinogenesis. The supporting evidence for the adenoma-carcinoma sequence is as follows:

1. The prevalence of adenomas correlates well with that of carcinomas. The average age of patients diagnosed with adenomas is five to ten years younger than patients diagnosed with carcinoma.[10] A polyp larger than 1 cm has an estimated cancer risk of 8 percent in 10 years.

2. Benign adenomatous tissue is often found accompanying cancers, suggesting progression of the cancer from the adenomatous cells.

3. Patients with familial adenomatous polyposis (FAP) have a 100 percent risk of developing colorectal cancers. The adenomas found in sporadic colorectal cancers are histologically identical to those in FAP patients.

4. Larger adenomas are more likely to have cellular atypia than smaller ones and hence have a higher risk for cancer.[8] The risk also increases with the type of polyp; villous adenomas having a higher risk than tubular adenomas. The risk for cancer in a tubular adenoma smaller than 1 cm in diameter is less than 5 percent, whereas the risk for cancer in a tubular adenoma larger than 2 cm is 35 percent. A villous adenoma larger than 2 cm in size carries a 50 percent chance of containing a cancer.

5. The incidence of colorectal cancer has been decreasing with increased colorectal screening and polypectomy.[11]

There is a second pathway, the "mutator phenotype" pathway, which is due to early mutations in DNA repair genes responsible for maintenance of genomic stability, i.e. the DNA mismatch repair genes *hMLH1* and *hMSH2*. This leads to accelerated accumulations of mutations in critical target genes and progression to neoplasia. The phenotype is recognisable by the presence of high frequency variation in microsatellites (regions of short repetitive DNA sequences) or microsatellite instability.[12] This is seen in patients with **hereditary non-polyposis colorectal cancer (HNPCC)** syndrome and in 15 percent of sporadic colorectal cancers.

Genomic instability is a common feature of human cancer and is an important contributor to carcinogenesis. Two types of genomic instability have been described in colorectal cancer: chromosomal instability (CIN) and microsatellite instability (MSI). CIN is characterized by significant losses and gains of chromosomes or parts thereof and is detected as aneuploidy (Figs 13.4A and B).

Chromosomal instability (CIN) is seen in 60-80 percent of all colorectal cancers, and has been claimed to be associated with a poor outcome.[13] Microsatellite instability (MSI) is the second major type of genomic instability, which can be detected as alterations in the length of short tandem repeat DNA sequences secondary to defects in the mismatch repair (MMR) system.[12] This is characteristic of tumors from patients with HNPCC syndrome, who have germline mutations in one of the mismatch repair genes, mainly in *hMLH1* and *hMSH2*.[14] It is also seen in approximately 15 percent of sporadic colorectal cancers, where *hMLH1* inactivation by promoter hypermethylation is often found.

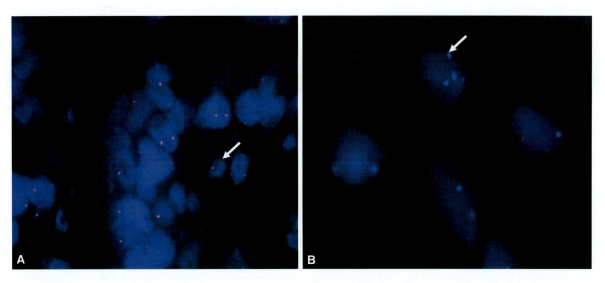

FIGURES 13.4A and B: Image of fluorescence *in situ* hybridization (FISH) of chromosome unstable colorectal cancer cells which show losses or gains of entire or part of chromosomes. (A) Cell with a single chromosome 6 (white arrow) due to loss of chromosome and (B) Cell with four copies of chromosome 7 (white arrow) due to gain of parts of chromosomes

Sporadic MSI tumors are more often found in the right colon and have been suggested to have a better prognosis in some studies.[15]

COLORECTAL POLYPS

A polyp is any mass projecting into the lumen from the surface of the mucosa of the colon. Polyps can be classified into:

1. **Hamartomatous polyps:** These are polyps usually seen in childhood and associated with *Peutz-Jegher's syndrome, Cronkite-Canada syndrome or Cowden's syndrome.* These polyps are not usually premalignant and can sometimes present only in adulthood. Symptoms associated with these include, bleeding and obstruction due to intussusception and the treatment is polypectomy. *Peutz-Jegher's syndrome* is characterized by polyps of the small intestine and to a smaller extent of the colon and rectum. Patients also have pigmented lesions in the mucosa of the cheeks and lips. They have an increased risk of cancer and are therefore screened with a baseline colonoscopy and upper endoscopy at age 20 years, followed by annual flexible sigmoidoscopy thereafter. *Cronkite-Canada syndrome* is characterized by gastrointestinal polyposis, alopecia, cutaneous pigmentation, and atrophy of nails. Patients present with diarrhea, vomiting and may develop malabsorption. Surgery is usually reserved for obstruction.

Cowden's syndrome is characterized by gastrointestinal polyposis, facial trichilemmomas, breast cancer and thyroid disease.

2. **Hyperplastic polyps:** Hyperplastic polyps are the most common polyps in the colon. They are usually small and not premalignant and characterized by hyperplasia on histology. Treatment is polypectomy.

3. **Inflammatory polyps:** These are usually pseudopolyps seen in colitis due to inflammatory bowel disease, amebic or schistosomal colitis. These are removed as they sometimes cannot be distinguished from neoplastic polyps.

4. **Neoplastic polyps:** Neoplastic polyps or adenomas are premalignant as these polyps have dysplasia. They can be either sessile (flat or without stalk) or pedunculated (with a stalk). They are classified into three types: tubular (with branched tubular glands), villous (with long finger-like projections) and tubulovillous adenomas (with both patterns). Tubular adenomas are the most common and seen in 65 to 80 percent of patients with polyps, whereas villous adenomas are seen in only 5 to 10 percent. Tubular adenomas are more likely to be pedunculated and have fewer dysplastic changes, whereas villous adenomas are more likely to be sessile and have severe dysplastic changes. The risk of malignancy depends on the size and type of adenoma. Cancer is likely to be present in about 5 percent of tubular adenomas, whereas upto 40 percent of villous adenomas that may harbor cancer.

This risk increases to 50 percent when the villous adenoma is larger than 2 cm.

Treatment of polyps is with polypectomy. In case of pedunculated polyps, this can be performed by snaring with colonoscopy. Sessile polyps can be challenging, and are elevated from the deeper layers using saline injection to enable polypectomy by endoscopic measure. If this is not feasible or there is a concern for perforation, a segmental colectomy is usually performed.

As mentioned before, adenomas are premalignant and may sometimes contain cancer. **Carcinoma *in situ*** is the condition when the malignant cells are confined to the mucosa. This cancer does not metastasize and complete polypectomy is adequate.

Invasive cancer on the other hand is the condition in which the malignant cells have extended beyond the mucosa and through the muscularis mucosae of the polyp (Fig. 13.5). These have a higher risk of lymph node involvement and local recurrence and may need more extensive surgery.

Haggitt's criterion classifies polyps with invasive cancer, depending on the level of invasion as shown in Figure 13.5.
• *Level 0:* Carcinoma *in situ* cancer limited to the mucosa.
• *Level 1:* Carcinoma invades through the muscularis mucosae into the submucosa but is limited to the head of the polyp.
• *Level 2:* Carcinoma invades the level of the neck of the polyp (junction between the head and the stalk).
• *Level 3:* Carcinoma invades any part of the stalk.
• *Level 4:* Carcinoma invades into the submucosa of the bowel wall below the stalk of the polyp but above the muscularis.

Sessile polyps with invasive cancer are Level 4 by Haggitt's criteria, as by definition, they do not have a stalk. A polyp with poorly differentiated adenocarcinoma or with lymphovascular invasion has a risk of metastases of greater than 10 percent. Sessile polyps with invasive cancer have a 10 percent risk of involvement of lymph nodes. Complete polypectomy (margins clear - 2 mm) is adequate in case of well-differentiated adenomas without lymphovascular invasion, especially in case of pedunculated adenomas with invasion upto level 3 (Fig. 13.6). For well or moderately differentiated sessile polyps in the colon with invasive cancer, with no lymphovascular invasion, prognosis after complete polypectomy depends on the level of invasion. All adenomas with the poor prognostic features and all sessile adenomas with invasive cancer in the rectum must be treated aggressively.

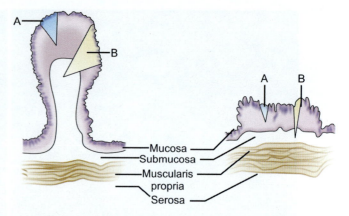

FIGURE 13.5: Diagrammatic representation of cancer in polyps. On the left is a pedunculated polyp whereas the polyp on the right is a sessile polyp. A—Carcinoma in situ in which the malignant cells are confined to the mucosa. B—Invasive cancer in which the malignant cells have extended through the muscularis mucosa into the submucosa

INHERITED COLORECTAL CANCERS

Although most of the colorectal cancers are sporadic in nature, some are inherited. Two well known familial syndromes are familial adenomatosis polyposis (FAP) and hereditary non-polyposis colorectal cancer (HNPCC).

Familial Adenomatosis Polyposis

Familial adenomatosis polyposis (FAP) is a rare autosomal dominant syndrome which has been well studied. The genetic abnormality in FAP is a mutation of the *APC* gene located on *5q21*. The gene is expressed in 100 percent of the patients with the mutation. About 20 percent of the patients may have a negative family history, and in these cases the abnormality is due to a spontaneously acquired mutation.

Patients have multiple colonic polyps, gastric and duodenal polyps and may also have extra intestinal features such as osteomas (Gardner's syndrome), desmoid tumors, epidermoid cysts and brain tumors (Turcot's syndrome). Patients will have hundreds to thousands of colonic polyps by puberty. The lifetime risk of colorectal cancer in these patients is 100 percent. APC gene testing is used to identify family members with the inherited mutation.

Family members with the mutation are then screened for colorectal and other cancers as follows:

Colorectal cancer: Colonoscopy every year, starting at age 10-12 years.

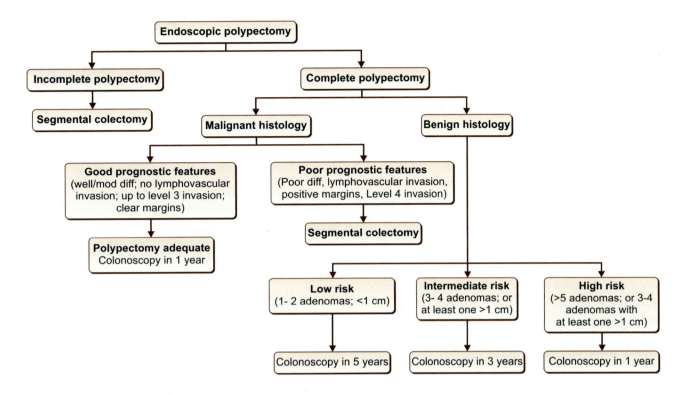

FIGURE 13.6: An algorithm showing the management of patients after polypectomy

Duodenal cancer: Upper GI endoscopy every 1-3 years, starting at age 20-25 years.

Pancreatic cancer: Abdominal ultrasound periodically.

Thyroid cancer: Annual physical examination.

CNS tumors: Annual physical examination.

Treatment once polyps are identified involves surgical excision of the affected colorectal mucosa. The most common recommended surgery is restorative proctocolectomy with ileal pouch-anal anastomosis (IPAA), with the anastomosis fashioned between the ileal pouch and the dentate line of the anal canal. A distal rectal mucosectomy is usually performed to decrease the risk of cancer by removing all the premalignant colonic mucosa. This procedure is usually satisfactory for patients and has a smaller incidence of pouchitis, but is technically difficult due to the necessary pelvic dissection, with the accompanying risk of injury to the autonomic nerves. Alternative procedure is a total abdominal colectomy with ileorectal anastomosis. This procedure removes the risk of impotence due to autonomic nerve injury, but patients must be advised about the risk of developing new cancerous polyps in the rectum.

This risk has been shown to be 4 percent, 5.6 percent, 7.9 percent, and 25 percent at 5, 10, 15, and 20 years after the operation, respectively.[16] These patients should therefore have proper surveillance with proctoscopic examination every six months. COX-2 inhibitors (Sulindac, celecoxib) have been suggested to cause slowing or prevent the development of polyps.[17]

Attenuated FAP is a variant of FAP characterized by fewer colonic adenomas (typically less than 100), a high variability of polyp number, later age of onset of colorectal polyposis (15 years later than patients with classic FAP), later age of onset of colorectal cancer and a more limited expression of the extracolonic features.[18] APC mutation may be positive in 60 percent, and then family members must be screened. Treatment involves total abdominal colectomy and ileorectal anastomosis.

Hereditary Nonpolyposis Colorectal Cancer

Hereditary nonpolyposis colorectal cancer (HNPCC) or Lynch syndrome is the most frequent occurring hereditary colorectal cancer and is seen in three percent of all colorectal cancers. It is characterized by replication errors or unstable microsatellites; due to defects in the mismatch repair systems. Mutations in *hMLH1* and *hMSH2* account for more than 90 percent of the mutations seen in patients with HNPCC. Defective mismatch repair presumably facilitates malignant transformation by the accumulation of mutations in genes with key functions in the cell. Patients usually present at a younger age, with right sided tumors, mucinous or poorly differentiated adenocarcinomas, and have increased numbers of synchronous or metachronous lesions. Nevertheless the prognosis is good after surgery. Extra colonic cancers are also common including gastric, endometrial, ovarian and renal cancers. **Lynch I syndrome** has patients with proximal colonic cancers at a young age; whereas **Lynch II syndrome** is the presence of colorectal cancer and extra colonic cancers, including cancers of endometrial, ovarian, gastric, small intestinal, pancreatic, and ureteral and renal pelvic origin.

Modified Amsterdam Criteria

This is used as clinical criteria to identify patients with HNPCC syndrome.

At least three relatives with colon cancer or any HNPCC associated cancer (endometrial, ovarian, gastric, small intestinal, ureteric, renal pelvis) and all of the following:
- One affected person is a first-degree relative of the other two affected persons
- Two successive generations affected
- At least one case of cancer diagnosed before age 50 years
- Familial adenomatous polyposis excluded.
  Screening for HNPCC is as follows:
  Colon cancer: Colonoscopy every year, starting at either age 20 to 25 years or 10 years younger than the youngest age at diagnosis in the family, whichever comes first.
  Endometrial carcinoma: Transvaginal ultrasound or endometrial aspiration biopsy every year, starting at age 25 to 35 years.

Total colectomy with ileorectal anastomosis is recommended once adenomas or a colon carcinoma is diagnosed as there is a 40 percent risk of developing a second colon cancer. Annual proctoscopy is necessary because the risk of developing rectal cancer remains high. Similarly, prophylactic hysterectomy and bilateral salpingo-oophorectomy should be considered in women who have completed childbearing.

SCREENING FOR COLON CANCER

Colon cancer screening programs rely on early diagnosis and treatment of premalignant adenomas, as it is known that most cancers of the colon arise from adenoma. In addition, screening may diagnose asymptomatic cancers at an early stage, when they can be curable. Screening measures are for the asymptomatic population at-risk for cancer.

Fecal Occult Blood Test—Guaiac Test

This test detects the presence of blood in the stool by the pseudoperoxidase activity of heme or hemoglobin. Individuals are advised to avoid non-steroidal anti-inflammatory agents, aspirin, Vitamin C, red meat, poultry, fish and some vegetables prior to testing as these can interact and cause high false-positive and false-negative results. Studies have shown that fecal occult blood test (FOBT) has reduced cancer related mortality by upto 33 percent.[19] Sensitivity of the test varies from 37 to 79 percent; based on the brand and variant of test used.[20] Only upto 50 percent of the cancers are diagnosed in most series. Specificity is also variable. However, annual screening with FOBT, especially with the high sensitive variants, have been shown to detect a majority of colon cancers and is recommended by national guidelines for screening in average-risk adults aged 50 years or above. Individuals who test positive should undergo a follow-up colonoscopy.

Flexible Sigmoidoscopy

This is an endoscopic examination of the distal colon (standard sigmoidoscope length is 60 cm). It has been associated with a 60 to 80 percent reduction in colorectal cancer mortality.[21,22] Flexible sigmoidoscopy is 60-70 percent as sensitive as colonoscopy,[23,24] but is less sensitive in African-Americans compared to Whites. Current recommendations state that flexible sigmoidoscopy performed for screening should be performed every five years by an endoscopist skilled at performing polyp biopsies; and the scope be inserted to 40 cm or beyond.[25] The main limitation of sigmoidoscopy is the inability to examine the proximal colon; hence all patients with polyps or cancers detected by sigmoidoscopy should undergo a colonoscopy.

Colonoscopy

Colonoscopy is the most complete examination of the mucosa of the colon from the appendiceal orifice to the dentate line. It allows biopsy and even treatment by polypectomy. Nevertheless, bowel preparation is critical for accuracy of colonoscopy and patients need sedation as the procedure can be very uncomfortable. Colonoscopy miss rate for large adenomas (≥ 1 cm) has been reported to be 6 to 12 percent[26,27] and the miss rate for cancer is about 5 percent.[26] Current recommendations for screening state that a colonoscopy should be performed every 10 years, starting at age 50.

Virtual Colonoscopy

Virtual colonoscopy is minimally invasive and uses computed tomography with image acquisitions of 1-2 mm thin slices and 3D reconstructions. Patients need a bowel preparation and air is then insufflated into the colon via a rectal catheter and both 2D and 3D images generated. Pickhardt et al reported 94 percent sensitivity for large adenomas.[28]

Double Contrast Barium Enema

This test evaluates the entire colon by coating the mucosal surface with high-density barium and distending the colon with air introduced through a rectal catheter. It has high sensitivity (90%) for detecting large polyps (>1 cm). No randomized trials have been performed evaluating this test for screening for colon cancers. It requires bowel preparation, is uncomfortable for patients and does not provide for biopsy. Double contrast barium enema (DCBE) every 5 years is acceptable for patients older than 50 years with an average risk for colon cancer.

In summary, the current national guidelines[25] recommend the following screening options for asymptomatic average risk individuals above 50 years.

1. **Tests that detect adenomatous polyps and cancer**
   Flexible sigmoidoscopy every 5 years, or
   Colonoscopy every 10 years, or
   Double-contrast barium enema every 5 years, or
   Computed tomographic colonography every 5 years.
2. **Tests that primarily detect cancer**
   Annual guaiac-based fecal occult blood test with high test sensitivity for cancer, or
   Annual fecal immunochemical test with high test sensitivity for cancer, or
   Stool DNA test with high sensitivity for cancer, interval uncertain.

SPORADIC COLON CANCER

Sporadic colorectal cancer generally occurs in the absence of a significant family history, mostly affects older people (60-80 years), and is usually seen as isolated colonic or rectal tumors.

PRESENTATION

The symptoms of colon cancer can be non-specific and varied. Symptoms depend on the location of the tumor, and the degree of obstruction caused by it. Right sided tumors typically present with anemia, as the liquid stools and the wider diameter preclude obstructive symptoms. With left sided tumors, the most common symptoms are change in bowel habit and rectal bleeding. Although left sided tumors are more likely to cause obstruction, any advanced tumor will cause the same. Tumors of the sigmoid colon can cause colovesical or colovaginal fistulas. With advanced tumors, patients may have an abdominal mass.

ROUTES OF SPREAD

Direct Spread

This can occur longitudinally, transversely and radially spreading to organs close by. If located in the retroperitoneal colon, the spread may involve the ureter, duodenum and posterior abdominal wall. It may also spread to the small intestine and the pelvic organs.

Lymphatic Spread

The cancer spreads initially to the paracolic nodes along the main blood vessels supplying the colon and then onto the para-aortic nodes. The risk of nodal metastases increases with poor differentiation, lymphovascular invasion and depth of invasion. Cancers limited to the bowel wall may have 5 to 20 percent associated lymph node metastases, whereas tumors that have invaded through the bowel wall or extended to adjacent organs, have >50 percent risk of associated nodal metastases.

Hematologic Spread

The most common site for distant metastases is the liver, due to spread via the portal system. Up to 37 percent of patients may have liver metastases at the time of surgery, and 50 percent are at risk of developing overt disease at some time.[29] Lung metastases are the next most common and seen in 10 percent.

STAGING

TNM staging is now widely used for staging colon cancers and is based on the tumor depth, presence or absence of nodal or distant metastases.

Tumor Stage (T)

Tx Primary tumor cannot be assessed.
T0 No evidence of primary tumor.
Tis Carcinoma *in situ*; tumor limited to mucosa.
T1 Tumor invades the submucosa.
T2 Tumor invades the muscularis propria.
T3 Tumor invades through the muscularis propria into the subserosa or into non-peritonealized pericolic or perirectal tissues.
T4 Tumor invades other organs or structures and/or perforates the visceral peritoneum.

Nodal Stage (N)

Nx Regional lymph nodes cannot be assessed.
N0 No regional lymph node metastasis.
N1 Metastasis in 1 to 3 regional lymph nodes.
N2 Metastasis in 4 or more regional lymph nodes.

Distant Metastasis (M)

Mx Distant metastasis cannot be assessed.
M0 No distant metastasis.
M1 Distant metastasis.

Stage Grouping

0	Tis, N0, M0
I	T1-2, N0, M0
IIA	T3, N0, M0
IIB	T4, N0, M0
IIIA	T1-2, N1, M0
IIIB	T3-4, N1, M0
IIIC	Any T, N2, M0
IV	Any T, Any N, M1

PREOPERATIVE EVALUATION

Colonoscopy is the gold-standard test, since it allows for biopsying the lesion. Even if a cancer is detected by other measures, a colonoscopy should be performed to evaluate the colon for synchronous tumors which may be present in 5 percent of patients. A CT scan of the abdomen and pelvis and a chest radiograph should be performed to detect any metastases. If a chest radiograph is positive, this can be further evaluated with a chest CT. Preoperative CEA is obtained and is more useful for postoperative follow-up. When patients present with obstruction, a water-soluble contrast enema is useful to understand the anatomic location of obstruction.

TREATMENT

Colon Resection

A curative resection entails complete removal of the primary cancer with anatomically complete lymphadenectomy of the regional nodes and en-bloc resection of any involved adjacent organs. About 80 to 90 percent of the patients are fit for a curative resection. The length of bowel resected depends on the vascular supply, as the lymphatics accompany the arterial supply. In order to achieve resection of the pericolic and paracolic nodes, the main vascular pedicles need to be ligated and divided. If this cannot be achieved, a palliative procedure may be considered, including colonic stenting for obstructive left sided tumors.

Tumors of the cecum and ascending colon are managed by a *right hemicolectomy*, which entails division of the ileocolic, right colic and right branch of the middle colic arteries. An *extended right hemicolectomy* may be used for hepatic flexure or proximal transverse colon tumors, and involves extension of the standard right hemicolectomy to include division of the main middle colic vessel at its base. *Transverse colectomy* involves division of the middle colic vessel and resection of transverse colon with a colo-colonic anastomosis, but an extended right hemicolectomy with an ileo-colonic anastomosis is safer and preferred. For splenic flexure and descending colon tumors, a *left hemicolectomy* is performed, dividing the left branches of the middle colic, the left colic and the first branches of the sigmoid arteries. *Sigmoid colectomy* is used for sigmoid colon tumors, and requires division of the sigmoid branches of inferior mesenteric artery. *Total abdominal colectomy* which entails removal of the entire colon from the ileum to the rectum, with an ileorectal anastomosis is performed in patients with multiple tumors, HNPCC or rarely with obstructive sigmoid colon cancer.

In case of obstruction, the patients must be resuscitated and taken for an emergent laparotomy. If the tumor is in the right side, a right hemicolectomy with primary anastomosis can be performed in most cases, even with an unprepared bowel. Management of left sided tumors can be challenging. Traditionally, due to the higher risk of

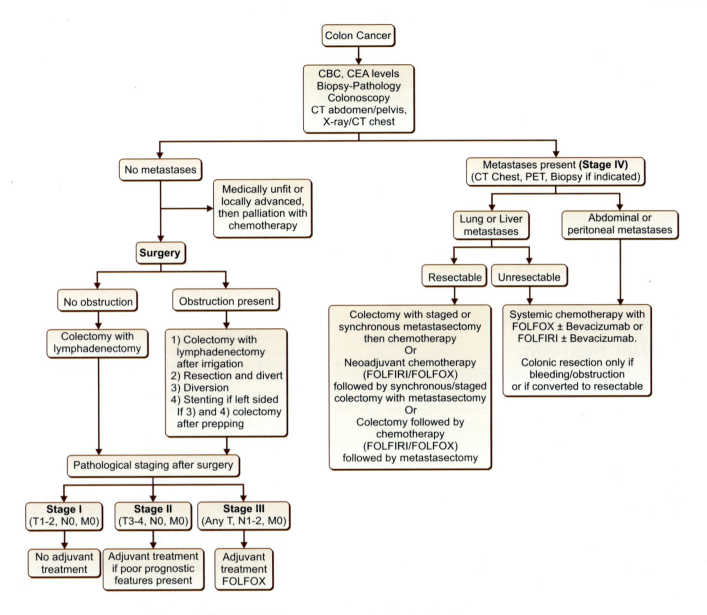

FIGURE 13.7: The management of patients with colon cancer

anastomotic leak with a primary anastomosis, these patients were managed by resection of the colon with the cancer, suture closure of the distal colon (sigmoid or rectum) and the creation of an end colostomy from the proximal colon (Hartmann's procedure). Recently, however the trend is towards a sub-total colectomy (removal of tumor and the entire colon proximal to it, with an ileosigmoid anastomosis) or a left hemicolectomy (performed after resection of the colon with cancer, and irrigation of the proximal colon with warm saline inserted through a catheter in the appendix or ileum).

Surgical Management of Metastases

About 20 percent of the patients with liver metastases can have a potentially curative resection. Survival in these patients is improved (20-40% at 5 years). Segmental resection of pulmonary metastases is also associated with 5-year survival rates of 20-40 percent.

Laparoscopic Colectomy

The results from three large randomized multi-center trials (COST, CLASICC and COLOR) show that the overall and disease free survival rates of laparoscopic colectomy are similar to those achieved by open colectomy.[30-32] Furthermore, laparoscopic colectomy resulted in shorter hospital stays, earlier return of bowel function and better pain management. The national guidelines do suggest that laparoscopic colectomy for cancer is acceptable in the hands of experienced surgeons who adhere to the surgical principles of colon resection for cancer.

LYMPH NODE ASSESSMENT

Lymph node assessment is not only important for accurate staging but plays an important role in further management as patients with nodal metastases from colon cancer need further adjuvant chemotherapy. The National Comprehensive Cancer Network (NCCN) recommends that a minimum of 12 nodes must be examined microscopically to determine the nodal status accurately. If fewer nodes are examined, this may lead to understaging of the patients.

ADJUVANT TREATMENT

Stage I and II: Majority of these patients are cured with a surgical resection. Few patients with stage I disease develop local or distant recurrence and hence adjuvant chemotherapy does not improve survival. More than 40 percent of Stage II patients, who have had a curative resection die from the disease. Adjuvant chemotherapy has, therefore, been recommended for few Stage II patients with poor prognostic features—poorly differentiated tumors, lymphovascular invasion, bowel obstruction, < 12 lymph nodes examined or T4 lesions.

Stage III: Current recommendations are that all medically fit Stage III patients should receive 5 FU based adjuvant chemotherapy. Treatment options include 5FU + leucovorin alone or FOLFOX- 5FU + Leucovorin + Oxaliplatin. FOLFOX regime was shown to have improved disease free survival over 5FU and Leucovorin by the MOSAIC trial.[33]

Stage IV: Chemotherapy regimens include FOLFOX with Bevacizumab, or FOLFIRI (5FU, leucovorin, irinotecan) with Bevacizumab (Fig. 13.7).

PROGNOSIS

TNM staging and 5-year survival rates:[34]

Stage I	70-95%
Stage II	54-65%
Stage III	39-60%
Stage IV	0-16%

SURVEILLANCE

History and physical: Every 3-6 months for 2 years; then every 6 months for a total of 5 years.

CEA: Every 3-6 months for 2 years, then every 6 months for a total of 5 years.

CT chest/abd/pelvis: Every year for 3 years in patients with high risk of recurrence.

Colonoscopy: In 1 year.

PET scan: Not routinely recommended.

REFERENCES

1. Jemal A, Siegel R, Ward E, Hao Y, Xu J, Murray T, et al. Cancer Statistics, 2008. CA Cancer J Clin 2008;58(2):71-96.
2. Toms JR (Ed). Cancer Stats Monograph 2004. Cancer Research UK: London 2004.
3. St John DJ, McDermott FT, Hopper JL, Debney EA, Johnson WR, Hughes ES. Cancer risk in relatives of patients with common colorectal cancer. Ann Intern Med 1993;118(10):785-90.
4. Burkitt DP. Epidemiology of cancer of the colon and rectum. Cancer 1971;28(1):3-13.
5. Bingham SA, Day NE, Luben R, Ferrari P, Slimani N, Norat T, et al. European Prospective Investigation into Cancer and Nutrition. Dietary fibre in food and protection against colorectal cancer. The European Prospective Investigation into Cancer and Nutrition (EPIC): an observational study. Lancet 2003;361(9368): 1496-501.
6. Bundred NJ, Whitfield BC, Stanton E, Prescott RJ, Davies GC, Kingsnorth AN. Gastric surgery and the risk of subsequent colorectal cancer. Br J Surg 1985;72(8):618-9.
7. Woodhouse C. British Society for Gastroenterology; Association of Coloproctology for Great Britain and Ireland. Guidelines for monitoring of patients with ureterosigmoidostomy. Gut 2002;51(Suppl V):v15-6.
8. Vogelstein B, Fearon ER, Hamilton SR, Kern SE, Preisinger AC, Leppert M, et al. Genetic alterations during colorectal -tumor development. N Eng J Med 1988;319:525-32.
9. Smith KJ, Johnson KA, Bryan TM, Hill DE, Markowitz S, Willson JK, et al. The APC gene product in normal and tumor cells. Proc Natl Acad Sci USA 1993;90(7):2846-50.
10. Muto T, Bussey HJ, Morson BC. The evolution of the cancer of the colon and rectum. Cancer 1975;36(6):2251-70.
11. Mandel JS, Church TR, Bond HJ, Ederer F, Geisser MS, Mongin SJ, et al. The effect of fecal occult-blood screening on the incidence of colorectal cancer. N Eng J Med 2000;343(22):1603-7.
12. Toft NJ, Arends MJ. DNA mismatch repair and colorectal cancer. J Pathol 1998;185(2):123-9.
13. Garrity MM, Burgart LJ, Mahoney MR, Windschitl HE, Salim M, Wiesenfeld M, et al. North Central Cancer Treatment Group. Prognostic value of proliferation, apoptosis, defective DNA mismatch repair, and p53 overexpression in patients with resected Dukes' B2 or C cancer: A North Central Cancer Treatment Group Study. J Clin Oncol 2004;22(9):1572-82.

14. Lynch HT, Smyrk T. Hereditary nonpolyposis colorectal cancer (Lynch Syndrome). An updated review. Cancer 1996;78(6):1149-67.

15. Parc Y, Gueroult S, Mourra N, Serfaty L, Flejou J-F, Tiret E, et al. Prognostic significance of microsatellite instability determined by immunohistochemical staining of MSH2 and MLH1 in sporadic T3N0M0 colon cancer. Gut 2004;53(3):371-5.

16. Heiskanen I, Jarvinen HJ. Fate of the rectal stump after colectomy and ileorectal anastomosis for familial adenomatous polyposis. Int J Colorectal Dis 1997;12(1):9-13.

17. Steinbach G, Lynch PM, Phillips RK, Wallace MH, Hawk E, Gordon GB, et al. The effect of celecoxib, a cyclooxygenase-2 inhibitor, in familial adenomatous polyposis. N Engl J Med 2000;342(26): 1946-52.

18. Knudsen AL, Bisgaard ML, Bulow S. Attenuated familial adenomatous polyposis (AFAP). A review of the literature. Fam Cancer 2003;2(1):43-55

19. Mandel JS, Bond JH, Church TR, Snover DC, Bradley GM, Schuman LM, et al. Reducing mortality from colorectal cancer by screening for fecal occult blood. Minnesota Colon Cancer Control Study. N Engl J Med 1993;328(19):1365-71.

20. Allison JE, Tekawa IS, Ransom LJ, Adrain AL. A comparison of fecal occult-blood tests for colorectal-cancer screening. N Engl J Med 1996;334(3):155-9.

21. Selby JV, Friedman GD, Quesenberry CP Jr, Weiss NS. A case-control study of screening sigmoidoscopy and mortality from colorectal cancer. N Engl J Med 1992;326(10):653-7.

22. Newcomb PA, Norfleet RG, Storer BE, Surawicz TS, Marcus PM. Screening sigmoidoscopy and colorectal cancer mortality. J Natl Cancer Inst 1992;84(20):1572-5.

23. Imperiale TF, Wagner DR, Lin CY, Larkin GN, Rogge JD, Ransohoff DF. Risk of advanced proximal neoplasms in asymptomatic adults according to the distal colorectal findings. N Engl J Med 2000;343(3):169-74.

24. Lieberman DA, Weiss DG, Bond JH, Ahnen DJ, Garewal H, Chejfec G. Use of colonoscopy to screen asymptomatic adults for colorectal cancer. Veteran Affairs Cooperative Study Group 380. N Engl J Med 2000;343(3):162-8.

25. Levin B, Lieberman DA, McFarland B, Smith RA, Brooks D, Andrews KS, et al. American Cancer Society Colorectal Cancer Advisory Group; US Multi-Society Task Force; American College of Radiology Colon Cancer Committee. Screening and Surveillance for the Early Detection of colorectal cancer and adenomatous polyps, 2008: a joint guideline from the American Cancer Society, The US Multi-Society Task Force on Colorectal cancer and the American college of Radiology. CA Cancer J Clin 2008;58(3):130-60.

26. Rex DK, Cutler CS, Lemmel GT, Rahmani EY, Clark DW, Helper DJ, et al. Colonoscopic miss rates of adenomas determined by back-to-back colonoscopies. Gastroenterology 1997;112(1):24-8.

27. Pickhardt PJ, Nugent PA, Mysliwiec PA, Choir JR, Schindler WR. Location of adenomas missed by optical colonoscopy. Ann Intern Med 2004;141(5):352-9.

28. Pickhardt PJ, Choi JR, Hwang I, Butler JA, Puckett ML, Hildebrandt HA, et al. Computed tomographic virtual colonoscopy to screen for colorectal neoplasia in asymptomatic adults. N Engl J Med 2003;349(23):2191-200.

29. Cedermark BJ, Shultz SS, Bakshi S, Parthasarathy KL, Mittelman A, Evans JT. The value of liver scan in the follow-up study of patients with adenocarcinoma of the colon and rectum. Surg Gynecol Obstet 1977;144(5):745-8.

30. Jayne DG, Guillou PJ, Thorpe H, Quirke P, Copeland J, Smith AM, et al. UK MRC CLASICC Trial Group. Randomized trial of laparoscopic- assisted resection of colorectal carcinoma: 3 years results of the UK MRC CLASICC Trial Group. J Clin Oncol 2007;25(21):3061-8.

31. The Clinical Outcomes of Surgical Therapy Study Group. A Comparison of laparoscopically assisted and open colectomy for colon cancer. N Engl J Med 2004;350(20):2050-9.

32. The Colon Cancer Laparoscopic or Open Resection Study Group. Survival after laparoscopic surgery versus open surgery for colon cancer: long term outcome of a randomised clinical trial. Lancet Oncol 2009;10(1):44-52.

33. Andre T, Boni C, Mounedji-Boudiaf L, Navarro M, Tabernero J, Hickish T, et al. Multicenter International Study of Oxaliplatin/ 5-Fluorouracil/Leucovorin in the Adjuvant treatment of Colon Cancer (MOSAIC) Investigators. Oxaliplatin, Fluorouracil, and Leucovorin as Adjuvant Treatment for Colon Cancer. N Engl J Med 2004;350(23):2343-51.

34. Greene FL, Page DL, Fleming, et al. AJCC Cancer Staging Manual (6th edn). New York: Springer-Verlag, 2002.

Carotid Artery Atheromatous Disease

S Rai, MP McMonagle, RK Vohra

INTRODUCTION

The extracranial carotid arteries are vulnerable to a number of atheromatous and non-atheromatous disorders. In the western world stroke is the third most common cause of death only preceded by cardiac diseases and cancer. In UK about 125,000 patients suffer their first stroke each year. It is the most common cause of disability in USA and Europe. The resulting disability has a crippling effect and leads to socioeconomic burden to the patient, his/her family and the society. American Heart Association estimated the financial impact of stroke in USA to be $57.9 billion in year 2006.[1] Though the overall mortality from stroke has decreased due to improved survival-rate, the overall incidence of stroke could increase significantly in the next 20 years due to an increasing elderly population.

Stroke is defined as an acute loss of focal cerebral function with symptoms exceeding 24 hours with no apparent cause other than that of a vascular origin. Stroke also includes acute loss of global cerebral function due to vascular origin, e.g. in cases of coma and subarachnoid hemorrhage. Transient ischemic attack (TIA) is defined as an acute loss of focal cerebral function or monocular visual loss (amaurosis fugax) due to vascular origin, with symptoms lasting less than 24 hours. The risk of recurrent event after a TIA is highest in the first month (8-10% risk at seven days, 11-15% at 30 days). Crescendo TIAs involve repeated TIAs within a short period of time in which the neurological deficit should have fully recovered before the onset of next event. 'Stroke in evolution' means repeated episodes of stroke in which the subsequent stroke occurs prior to the complete recovery of the previous stroke. Both these clinical situations often imply that there is an acutely unstable intra-arterial plaque with overlying thrombus. Reversible ischemic neurologic deficit (RIND) describes a focal neurological deficit that lasts longer than 24 hours but resolves completely within 1 week.

About 36,000 patients suffer TIA in UK each year. The incidence of stroke and TIA increases with age. In a typical western population of 200,000, approximately 168 TIAs or non-disabling strokes occur every year. Of these, 18 cases will have a carotid stenosis of >70 percent. 1500 people in the same community will have an asymptomatic carotid stenosis.[2]

ANATOMY OF CAROTID ARTERIES

There is one common carotid artery (CCA) on each side of neck. The right CCA originates from the brachiocephalic trunk while the left CCA originates directly from the arch of aorta. After arising in thorax it runs through the neck towards the cranial cavity. At the upper border of the thyroid cartilage, which generally corresponds to the level of fourth cervical vertebra, CCA bifurcates into external carotid artery (ECA) and internal carotid artery (ICA). ECA usually arises medial and anterior to ICA. There is a dilated segment at the level of CCA bifurcation which is called carotid sinus. Carotid sinus has extensive nerve endings which act as baroreceptors controlling the blood pressure. Carotid body lies within the adventitia of the posterior aspect of the CCA bifurcation and works as a chemoreceptor. It is responsible for the monitoring of blood gases and pH. ECA normally supplies extra-cranial muscles and parotid gland through various branches. ICA runs vertically upwards from the origin to the carotid foramen at the base of skull. During its course in the neck it is accompanied by internal jugular vein (IJV) which lies posterolateral to ICA with vagus nerve running in between. This segment of ICA may have loops, kinks or tortousity. After entering the carotid foramen ICA runs in the petrous part of temporal bone vertically for about 1 cm and then turns anteriorly and medially becoming horizontal and emerging at the apex of petrous bone. The intracranial segment of ICA has a precavernous, cavernous and supraclinoid segment. The ICA bifurcates into anterior and middle cerebral artery.

The vertebral artery (VA) arises from the proximal part of subclavian artery in the neck. It ascends to enter the transverse process foramen of fifth or sixth cervical vertebra. The paired VAs unite to form the basilar artery bifurcating into terminal posterior cerebral arteries. Most of the brain is supplied by the central anastomotic network formed by the anastomosis between two internal carotids and vertebrobasilar arteries, called the circle of Willis, shown in Figure 14.1.

In about 90 percent of cases some form of complete circular arterial channel between the ICA, posterior cerebral

and anterior cerebral arteries exists. The greatest variation in length is found in the anterior communicating artery; and in diameter, in the posterior communicating artery.

The nature and severity of the initial neurological deficit is unpredictable and depends upon the chronicity and degree of ICA stenosis and the extent of collateral vessel development.

ETIOLOGY AND RISK FACTORS

Eighty percent of all strokes are ischemic, 20 percent are hemorrhagic. Up to 80 percent of all ischemic strokes occur in the carotid territory. For every 100 patients who present with ischemic infarction in carotid territory, 50 are due to thromboembolism of either the ICA or middle cerebral artery (MCA), 25 are secondary to small vessel disease affecting lenticulostriate arteries, 15 are due to embolism from the heart whereas in remaining 5-10 have a hematological or non-atheromatous condition accounting for stroke. The risk factors for stroke are mentioned in Table 14.1.

PATHOPHYSIOLOGY

Carotid atherosclerotic disease covers a wide spectrum of atherosclerosis from intima-medial thickness to complete occlusion. Various factors determine the evolution from one stage to the next. With increasing age the incidence and degree of ICA stenosis due to atherosclerosis increases. Though the evolution of atherosclerosis is well-known, the triggers behind the transformation of carotid atherosclerotic plaque (Fig. 14.2A) from 'asymptomatic' to 'symptomatic' remain elusive. Similar to the concept of "vulnerable" coronary artery plaque leading to acute coronary event, a mechanism for cerebral manifestation due to carotid artery disease is evolving. Unstable (vulnerable) plaque carries a greater risk of stroke or recurrent TIAs due to embolization from the plaque. These plaques have a thin fibrous cap and a necrotic but biologically active lipid core (Fig. 14.2B). There is a significant amount of inflammation with infiltration of T-lymphocyte and activated macrophages. Upon activation these inflammatory cells secrete proteolytic enzymes such as matrix metallo-proteinases (MMPs) which degrade the collagenous extra-cellular matrix and weaken the plaque leading to an increase in the risk of plaque rupture. Direct interaction with the vascular smooth muscle cells (VSMC) also leads to the promotion of VSMC apoptosis which increases the vulnerability of the plaque by weakening the fibrinous cap. There have been attempts to utilize cellular and molecular biological events as a marker of plaque

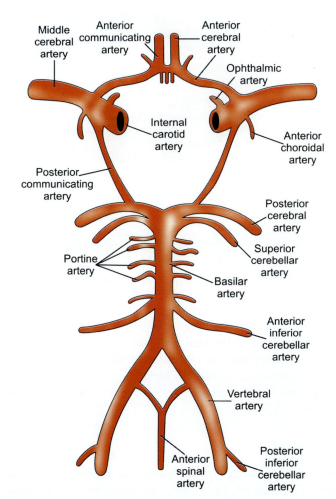

FIGURE 14.1: Circle of Willis

Table 14.1: Risk factors for stroke	
Modifiable	*Nonmodifiable*
Hypertension	Age >55 years (double every 10 years)
Cardiac diseases	Race: Afro-Americans, Hispanics > Caucasians
More common: AF, recent MI, mural thrombus,	Family history
valvular heart disease	
Lesser common: Patent foramen ovale, aortic arch	
atheroma	
Hyperlipidemia	
Smoking	
Diabetes mellitus	
Physical inactivity	
Carotid artery stenosis	
Transient ischemic attack	
Oral contraceptive pills	
Substance abuse: Crack cocaine, heroin	

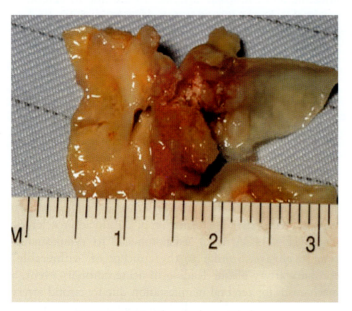

FIGURE 14.2A: Ulcerated carotid plaque

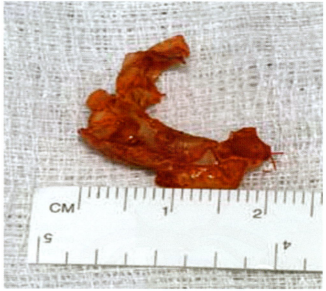

FIGURE 14.2B: Thin vulnerable carotid plaque

instability. These markers are associated with various processes of atherosclerosis and plaque instability, e.g. inflammation, proteolysis, lipid accumulation, infection and thrombosis. Important amongst these markers are MMP-2, MMP-9, soluble intercellular adhesion molecule–1 (sICAM-1), osteoprotegerin, fibrinogen, homocysteine and anti-chlamydial pneumoniae antibodies.

It is debatable whether the elevated level of these biomarkers is an effect or a cause of TIA/stroke. The fact is that most of these findings have not been tested on asymptomatic patients. Therefore, they cannot predict safely the occurrence of future stroke/TIA. These biomarkers also lack the specificity for atherosclerosis affecting ICA. There is a concern that the degree of stenosis alone may not be able to predict the risk of cerebral embolization especially in asymptomatic patients and for these patients cellular and molecular biomarkers may become particularly useful in future.

Presentation

Extracranial carotid artery disease can present in various ways (Flow chart 14.1). The spectrum of presentation includes asymptomatic disease, TIAs, RIND and stroke.

Flow Chart 14.1: Clinical features of atheromatous carotid and large cerebral arteries disease

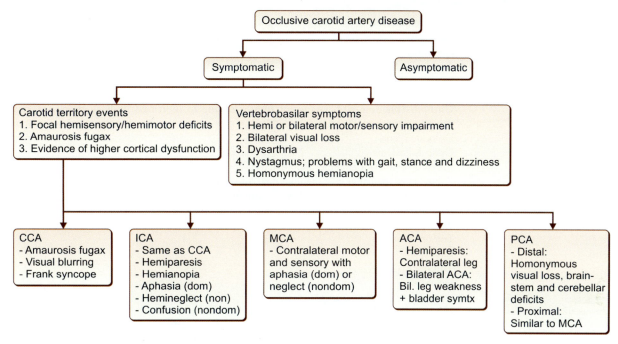

Carotid territory TIAs involve only eyes causing amaurosis fugax (transient monocular blindness) which refers to sudden loss of vision that is unilateral, transient in nature and is due to ischemia or vascular insufficiency of the retina or optic nerve head. There is a loss of vision in the top or bottom half of the visual field described by patients as a curtain coming down over their eyes. This episodic loss may be partial or complete with a typical duration of several minutes but may vary from few seconds to hours. The "curtain" may be perceived as black, gray, or white. The recovery of vision is as rapid as occurrence and is in reverse fashion. There are no positive visual phenomena such as flashes of light, bright shapes, fortification spectra, etc. These positive phenomena are more characteristic of migranious visual loss which are typically bilateral, usually followed by other features, e.g. headache, nausea, photophobia. The risk of stroke after an episode of amaurosis fugax is 2 percent per year compared to 8 percent per year after cerebral TIA. The causes of amaurosis fugax are listed in Table 14.2.

The diagnosis of TIA is based entirely on history and it may not be straight forward in many situations. TIAs are sudden in onset with maximal symptoms at the onset. There is focal neurological deficit. Most TIAs last 5-15 minutes and symptoms lasting less than 30 seconds are unlikely to be due to a TIA. TIA symptoms correspond to recognized neurological territory. Other information which helps in differentiating TIA is summarized in Table 14.3.

Management

The management algorithm for a TIA patient is outlined in Table 14.4. The carotid bruit is auscultated with the diaphragm of the stethoscope as it is a high pitched bruit. It should be emphasized that presence or absence of carotid bruit is not of any diagnostic significance. The tightest stenosis may not have any audible bruit as the flow may be insufficient whereas carotid bruit may be present in various other conditions apart from ICA stenosis, e.g. external carotid artery stenosis, common carotid artery stenosis, subclavian artery stenosis, referred murmurs from heart and hyperdynamic circulation due to contralateral carotid artery stenosis/occlusion, anemia, hyperthyroidism and pregnancy.

After the initial management it is important to stratify the patients according to their risk of future events. ABCD2 scoring system is a reasonable one. These recommendations are in line with guidelines issued by the National Institute for Health and Clinical Excellence (NICE), UK and the Royal College of Physicians Intercollegiate Stroke Working

Table 14.2: Causes of amaurosis fugax	
Ocular	Giant cell arteritis
	Congenital optic nerve abnormalities (e.g nerve drusen)
	Glaucoma
	Anterior ischemic optic neuropathy
	Retinal vein or artery obstruction
	Tear-film abnormalities
	Uhthoff's phenomenon (transient blindness due to increased body temperature, indicates demyelinating disease)
	Dislocated lens
	Optic disk edema
	Vitreous or anterior chamber hemorrhage
Orbital	Orbital mass (hemangioma, meningioma, osteoma)
	Compressive optic neuropathy (thyroid/tumor related)
Intracranial	Increased intracranial pressure
	Aneurysm
	Tumor
Carotid	Embolism
	Thrombosis
	Dissection
	Stenosis or occlusion
Cardiovascular	Hypotension/bradycardia
	Malignant hypertension
	Arrhythmia
Hematological	Anemia
	Polycythemia
	Thrombocytosis
	Sickle cell disease
	Plasma cell disorders (macroglobulinemias)
Miscellaneous	Seizure
	Migraine
	Functional

Table 14.3: Exclusion and differential diagnosis of transient ischemic attacks[3]	
Symptoms that do not suggest TIA	*Conditions mimicking TIA*
Loss of consciousness	Migraine
Acute confusion	Partial seizure
Seizure	Syncope
Loss of memory	Vestibular disorder
Isolated dizziness, light-headedness, or vertigo	Neuropathy and radiculopathy
Gradual progression of symptoms	Ocular disorders
Multiple recurrent symptoms	Hypoglycemia
Severe headache	Tumors of central nervous system

Party (RCP ICSWP) and are confirmed by various studies in different population-group. On the basis of this evidence, the NICE Guideline Development Group defined a risk of greater than 4 percent over 7 days as high risk requiring urgent referral to be seen within 24 hours.[4] This risk is equivalent to an ABCD2 score of 4 or greater.

Investigations

The goals of the investigation for patients with suspected carotid atherosclerosis are:
1. To ascertain whether or not carotid stenosis is present.
2. To determine whether or not the patient's symptoms are due to carotid lesion.

Table 14.4: Algorithm for the management of a TIA patient

A. General supportive measures (if applicable)

1. ABC (airway, breathing, circulation)
2. Pulse oximetry and O_2 supplements
3. IV access
4. Obtain blood samples for: Full blood count, blood urea, serum creatinine, serum electrolytes, fasting blood sugar, lipid profile
5. Measure blood pressure
6. Cardiac monitoring

B. Examination

1. Check pulse rate and rhythm
2. Listen to heart sounds
3. Brief neurological examination including: Speech, cranial nerves, motor, sensory, co-ordination, gait

C. Investigations

1. Non-contrast head CT scan (differentiate between ischemic and hemorrhagic infarct
2. Carotid duplex Doppler (for ischemic infarct)
3. Echocardiogram (to detect embolic source)
4. MRI brain (to define infarct) and MRA of head and neck (to look at carotid artery and cerebral circulation)

D. Referral for further management

Use of the ABCD2 scoring system to assess the risk of stroke early after a transient ischemic attack (TIA) so that high-risk people are immediately identified, urgently assessed and secondary prevention initiated.

ABCD2 scoring system:

- A — Age: 60 years of age or older, 1 point.
- B — Blood pressure at presentation: 140/90 mm Hg or greater, 1 point.
- C — Clinical features: Unilateral weakness, 2 points; speech disturbance without weakness, 1 point.
- D — Duration of symptoms: 60 minutes or longer, 2 points; 10–59 minutes, 1 point.
- D — Presence of diabetes: 1 point.

Points from the individual items are added to give the ABCD2 score.

People with a score of 4 or more are regarded as being at high risk of an early stroke.

The ABCD2 scoring system excludes certain populations who may be at particularly high risk, such as:
- People who have had two or more transient ischemic attacks (TIAs) within 1 week—they are at higher risk for early stroke.
- People on anticoagulation treatment—brain imaging is required to exclude intracranial bleeding.
- They also may not be relevant to people who present days after a TIA.

3. To assess the severity of carotid stenosis, any unusual features and its operability.

Duplex ultrasound is the current standard for non-invasive assessment of the carotid artery stenosis. "Duplex" refers to the combination of pulsed Doppler and B-mode ultrasound in the same device, where the "B" stands for "brightness". The transducer in the scanhead of the ultrasound machine converts electrical energy into vibration energy and conversely converts vibration energy of returning echoes into electrical signals. A pulsed Doppler uses the same transducer to generate and receive echoes. For carotid examination 5 to 7.5 MHz provides optimal tissue penetration. When sound waves encounter moving reflectors, such as red blood cells (RBCs) within the lumen of the carotid artery, the frequency of the reflected waves change from that of the original generated by the transducer. The magnitude of this frequency shift depends upon the velocity of the moving reflector and its angle with the sound wave. Traditionally the examination is conducted as close as possible to a Doppler angle of 60 degrees. At this angle, errors in velocity calculations secondary to misreading of the Doppler angle are small as a percentage of the true

Stenosis (%)	PSV (cm/s)	EDV (cm/s)	Spectral analysis
		Table 14.5: University of Washington criteria for categorizing carotid artery stenosis	
0	<125		Normal
1-15	<125		No flow reversal in bulb
16-49	<125		Spectral broadening during entire systole
50-79	>125	<140	Marked spectral broadening
80-99	>125	>140	Marked spectral broadening
Occlusion	–	–	No flow

PSV = Peak systolic velocity; EDV = End diastolic velocity

velocity. A color flow image is produced by assigning color to Doppler shifts. Though the technologist can adjust the color settings usually 'red' indicates flow towards the probe whereas 'blue' indicates away from the probe. The addition of color flow scanning has made it easier to recognize ICA occlusion and differentiation between an ICA occlusion from very high-grade stenosis (string sign). Color-flow Duplex imaging also helps in seeing tortuous ICA, carotid aneurysm and carotid body tumor.

There are various spectral criteria for classifying stenosis in the ICA. The criteria developed at the University of Washington are, however, the most commonly used. These are mentioned in Table 14.5. The peak systolic velocity ratio between ICA to CCA of 4.0 detected a 70-99 percent stenosis by NASCET criteria. A peak systolic velocity of > 290 cm/s and end-diastolic velocity of > 80 cm/s represents 60 percent

stenosis of ICA which is the criterion used for offering CEA in ACAS trial for asymptomatic patients.[5]

Duplex ultrasound also evaluates plaque density and surface morphology. There are two limitations of Duplex imaging: 1. It is operator dependent. 2. It does not show arch, great vessel origins and intracranial vasculature. Intracranial vasculature can be seen noninvasively using transcranial Doppler (TCD).

Catheter angiography has been the gold standard for the evaluation of atherosclerotic disease and the degree of stenosis in patients for possible CEA (Figs 14.3A to E). Intra-arterial digital subtraction angiography (DSA) has allowed use of smaller contrast doses, catheter, and exposure time. DSA has largely replaced the cut-film angiography. Carotid angiography has evolved from direct percutaneous cervical arterial puncture to transfemoral catheterization. A variety

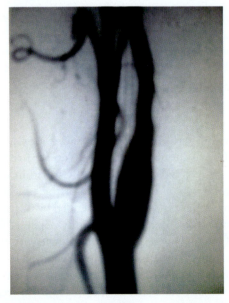

FIGURE 14.3A: Normal carotid digital subtraction angiogram

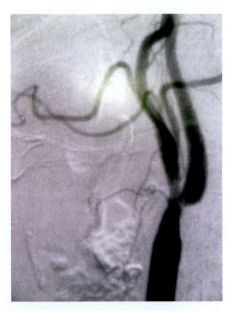

FIGURE 14.3B: Stenosed internal carotid artery

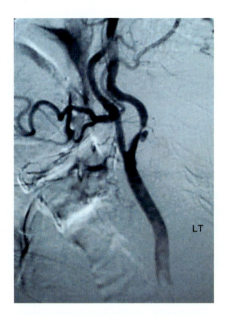

FIGURE 14.3C: Stenosed internal carotid artery with ulcerated plaque

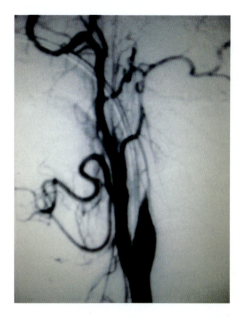

FIGURE 14.3E: Occluded internal carotid artery

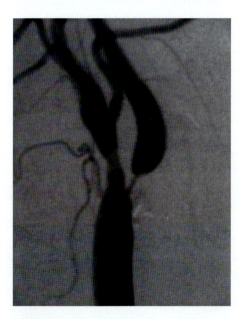

FIGURE 14.3D: Severely stenosed internal carotid artery (string sign)

of catheters and guide wires are available. It is worth noting that contrast angiography involves the risks, e.g. damage to artery secondary to puncture, dissection, plaque-embolization from the aortic arch or carotid bifurcation causing TIA/ stroke (1%), contrast-induced nephropathy and anaphylaxis.

MRA works on the principle of detecting the differences in energy emitted from moving versus stationary protons after application of radiofrequency energy pulses within a magnetic field. The technique of differentiating energy released from stationary and moving protons is called 'time of flight' (TOF) technology. Two dimensional TOF MRA is better in detecting flow-related abnormalities whereas three dimensional TOF is better in detecting structural anatomy including the degree of stenosis. MRI of brain allows assessment of cerebral circulation along with structural assessment of brain parenchyma. Although MRA is quite sensitive, it is not very specific. The assessment of the degree of stenosis can be erroneous as MRA often overestimates the degree of stenosis.

CT angiography (CTA) gives good anatomical detail including information about plaque morphology. However, it does need a significant contrast load and is not readily available. There is not enough data to support its use routinely prior to CEA at present.

Newer non-invasive modalities, e.g. ultrasound, MRA, CTA have replaced catheter angiography. With increasing expertise the patients can be offered CEA on the basis of duplex ultrasound alone. CT or MRI is not indicated routinely in patients requiring CEA. They are required in acute, evolving stroke, patients with atypical neurological features, patient with prior history of head injury or intracranial lesions.

Treatment

The optimal invasive treatment for the prevention of stroke has been a matter of much debate and controversy. The debate earlier was between the best medical treatments alone versus carotid endarterectomy (CEA) along with the best medical treatment. However, over the past 15 years carotid angioplasty and stenting (CAS) has emerged as an alternative treatment modality. It is important to understand: 1. The correct indications of carotid revascularization, 2. What constitutes the optimum carotid intervention.

Indications for Treatment

Following a referral for the internal carotid artery (ICA) stenosis, the patient is assessed and listed for an intervention if he/she satisfies the well-defined criteria. These criteria for intervention are clearer in symptomatic patients compared to the asymptomatic group.

Symptomatic patients: Indications for intervention in symptomatic patients are relatively straightforward. All symptomatic ipsilateral ICA stenotic lesions pose greater risk of subsequent disabling stroke/ death in comparison to asymptomatic ICA stenosis. Initially there were two unsuccessful attempts to prove the benefit of CEA in symptomatic patients.[6,7] This was followed by two landmark randomized controlled trials (RCT) conducted in 1980s which provided a level I grade A evidence in favor of CEA. These were European Carotid Surgery Trial (ECST) and North American Symptomatic Carotid Endarterectomy Trial (NASCET). Although historical, 15 years down the line, these studies remain the "gold standard" in defining indications for CEA in symptomatic patients.

European Carotid Surgery Trial (ECST) was a randomized controlled trial conducted in 80 centers of Europe.[8] The degree of ICA stenosis was determined using the minimum residual lumen compared with the estimated normal lumen at the level of greatest ICA stenosis. Symptomatic patients having 70-99 percent ICA stenosis treated with best medical treatment alone had a significantly higher risk of stroke/death compared to surgery. During the 3-year follow-up, risk of ipsilateral stroke and perioperative death was 10.3 percent in CEA group compared to 16.8 percent in patients on best medical treatment. Risk of death/ stroke from any cause during follow up was 12.3 percent for surgical patients and 21.9 percent in the medical group. Patients with 30 to 69 percent ICA stenosis who had CEA,

did not get any benefit over medical treatment alone when followed for 4 to 5 years. Also in patients with ICA stenosis of 0 to 29 percent, no benefit from CEA was seen.

North American Symptomatic Carotid Surgery Trial (NASCET) analyzed the data from 50 centers in US and Canada.[9] Only those surgeons who had a documented stroke/death-rate of <6 percent after CEAs for at least 50 consecutive cases over a 2-year period contributed to this trial. The degree of ICA stenosis was determined by comparing the diameter of the minimum residual lumen with the diameter at a point well beyond the region of greatest stenosis of the ipsilateral ICA. In severely stenosed ipsilateral ICA, the diameter of the ipsilateral external carotid artery or the contralateral ICA were used for comparison. In patients with 70-99 percent ICA stenosis, CEA was beneficial in comparison to best medical treatment alone. The 30-day stroke morbidity and mortality rate for surgical group was 5.8 percent while in patients treated with best medical treatment this was 11.2 percent. The cumulative risk of any ipsilateral stroke at 2 years was nine percent and 26 percent for surgical and medical patients respectively. The incidence of major or fatal ipsilateral stroke was 2.5 percent for the surgical group and 13.1 percent for patients on best medical treatment alone. In patients with ICA stenosis of 50 to 69 percent, there was some benefit from CEA in men. The women with symptomatic 50-69 percent ICA stenosis benefited only if they had one or more additional features such as age > 70 years, severe hypertension, history of myocardial infarction, or a hemispheric event rather than a retinal event. Symptomatic patients with ICA stenosis of 30 to 49 percent and 0 to 29 percent had no significant difference between surgical and best medical treatment groups.

Since the NASCET method of calculating the degree of stenosis was more accurate, the findings of the trials for symptomatic and asymptomatic ICA stenotic lesions were amalgamated by re-calculating the degree of stenosis using NASCET method in all patients. This data, now referred as Carotid Endarterectomy Trialists Collaboration (CETC) data, is summarized in Table 14.6.

Interestingly it has been shown that the risk of stroke recurrence in the 'near occlusion' group was significantly lower than 90 to 94 percent stenosis group, 11 percent vs 35 percent respectively.[11] Subsets of patients with 94 to 99 percent stenosis in NASCET and ECST pooled data-base had a stroke-risk of 14.1 percent on best medical therapy

Trial	% stenosis	Number of patients	30-day CEA risk	5 years risk		Strokes prevented per 1000 cases
				CEA	Medical	
Symptomatic						
CET	< 30%	1746	-	2.6%	15.7%	None at 5 yrs
CETC	30-49%	1429	6.7%	22.8%	25.5%	26 at 5 yrs
CETC	50-69%	1549	8.4%	20.0%	27.7%	78 at 5 yrs
CETC	70-99%	1095	6.2%	17.1%	32.7%	156 at 5 yrs
CETC	String	262	5.4%	22.4%	22.3%	None at 5 yrs
Asymptomatic						
ACST	60-99%	3120	2.8%	6.4%	11.8%	53 at 5 yrs
ACAS	60-99%	1662	2.3%	5.1%	11.0%	59 at 5 yrs

Table 14.6: Estimate of strokes prevented per 1000 cases[10]

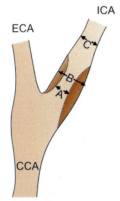

NASCET% ICA Stenosis = C-A/C
ECST% ICA Stenosis =B-A/B

FIGURE 14.4: NASCET and ECST methods for calculating internal carotid artery stenosis

NASCET (%)	ECST (%)
30	65
40	70
50	75
60	80
70	85
80	91
90	97

Table 14.7: Approximate equivalent percentage of ICA stenosis in NASCET and ECST[14]

compared to 10.9 percent with surgery.[12] It is acceptable to offer CEA to patients with 95 to 99 percent stenosis if there is lack of collateral circulation from the contralateral carotid or ipsi/contralateral vertebrobasilar system.

In summary, despite differences in their design pattern, entry and exclusion criteria, methodology of estimating the degree of stenosis and end-points, the main findings of the trials for symptomatic patients have shown that:

1. For high-degree of symptomatic stenosis (70-99%) CEA is beneficial in both sexes.
2. For symptomatic stenosis of 50 to 69 percent, according to NASCET, CEA did offer some benefit to men. For the same degree of stenosis, it did not offer any benefit to patients with diabetes and those with previous TIA rather than stroke. Women with 50 to 69 percent stenosis benefited from surgery if they had one or more additional risk factors. According to ECST for symptomatic 50 to 69 percent stenosis, there was no benefit from CEA in either sex. This major difference in this category between

NASCET and ECST was explained by the different measuring criteria used for estimating the degree of stenosis (Fig. 14.4). ECST method overestimated the degree of stenosis as shown in Table 14.7. Therefore, what was calculated as an ICA stenosis of 50 to 69 percent in ECST was < 50 percent ICA stenosis by NASCET measurement technique. In < 50 percent ICA stenosis there was no difference in either studies.[13]

3. In patients with low-grade stenosis (<30%), whether symptomatic or asymptomatic, surgical treatment was actually harmful by increasing the risk of stroke and death.

Asymptomatic patients: In a general population aged 70 years and above, about 10 percent people have an asymptomatic ICA stenosis of higher than 50 percent. If hypertensives aged above 70 years are considered, this incidence will increase to 25 percent. In an ever increasing aging population in the West, more asymptomatic lesions are likely to be identified. Usually this lesion is found when neck is auscultated, contralateral symptomatic side is scanned or as a work up for other surgical procedures, i.e. coronary artery bypass graft (CABG). This asymptomatic plaque can either remain stable or become problematic. The exact mechanisms responsible for converting a stable plaque to a vulnerable one are not completely understood.

There have been two randomized controlled trials for asymptomatic patients: Asymptomatic Carotid Artery Stenosis study (ACAS) and Asymptomatic Carotid Surgery Trial (ACST). In ACAS there was an absolute risk-reduction of 5.9 percent in surgical patients with ICA stenosis of >60 percent demonstrated by duplex Doppler ultrasound.[15] The operative risk of stroke and/or death was only 2.3 percent. It showed that 20 CEAs were needed to prevent 1 stroke when followed for 5 years. Despite this CEA in asymptomatic patient was cost-effective. ACST included 3120 asymptomatic patients with ICA stenosis > 60 percent as demonstrated by duplex Doppler ultrasound.[16] The 5-year stroke risk in surgical patients was 6.4 percent compared to 11.8 percent for patients in whom surgery was deferred. It showed a clear benefit for the patients aged < 75 years. The efficacy of CEA in women compared to men was one-third due to their higher perioperative risk.

ACAS trial recommended CEA for asymptomatic patient provided the patient was anticipated to live in good health for 2 years or more and the operating surgeon had operative risk of stroke/death < 3 percent. If the operative risk of an individual surgeon exceeds 4 percent, that surgeon should not recommend CEA for asymptomatic lesions. The summary points of ACAS are highlighted in Table 14.8.

The American Heart Association 2005 guidelines for CEA in asymptomatic ICA stenosis based on the risk of operative intervention are summarized in Table 14.9.

If interventionist's peri-procedural stroke/death rate is higher than 2 to 3 percent, it may be more harmful to intervene on an asymptomatic standard-risk patient. Till date there are no reliable methods to identify the asymptomatic lesions with an increased risk of embolization in which the intervention could be justified. It has been suggested[17] that three group of patients will benefit from revascularization procedure:

1. The patients with plaque instability identified with MRA and/or duplex, with or without silent embolic signals.
2. The patients with insufficient collateral circulation detected by transcranial Doppler, transcranial color-coded Doppler and/or magnetic resonance arteriography.
3. The patients with severe metabolic compromise characterized by increased oxygen extraction fraction as measured with positron emission tomography.

The mainstay of the best medical treatment in these trials was Aspirin. Since then, there have been significant additions to the available treatment. Statins, beta-blockers, and clopidogrel are advocated more aggressively in these patients and have been shown to offer significant benefit. Due to more effective and aggressive medical management the risk of ipsilateral TIA/stroke has dropped significantly in non-operated asymptomatic cases with 50 to 75 percent stenosis.[18] Patients who were aged > 79 years, who had < 5 years life-expectancy or who suffered from conditions like unstable angina, atrial fibrillation, severe diabetes, uncontrolled hypertension and renal insufficiency, were

---

Table 14.8: Summary of ACAS trial results

1. No apparent benefit in women (17% relative risk reduction versus 66% for Men)
2. No evidence that CEA reduced the risk of disabling stroke
3. No correlation between the degree of stenosis and late stroke
4. Patients with bilateral disease do not have worse outcome
5. To gain maximum benefit from CEA patients should live at least for 5 years
6. The cost per stroke prevented is extremely high.

Table 14.9: American Heart Association Guidelines (2005) for CEA in asymptomatic stenotic lesions

Patient characteristics	Proven indications	Acceptable indications	Uncertain indications
Surgical risk <3% and life expectancy ≥ 5 year	Ipsilateral ICA stenosis > 60% with/without ulceration and with/without antiplatelet therapy irrespective of contralateral artery status	CEA simultaneous with CABG for > 60% ICA stenosis	Unilateral stenosis > 50%
Surgical risk of 3-5%	None	Ipsilateral ICA stenosis >75% with contralateral ICA occluded or stenosed >75%	ICA stenosis >75% irrespective of contralateral artery status If CABG required: uni/bilateral asymptomatic stenosis >70%
Surgical risk of 5-10%	None	None	If CABG required: uni/bilateral ICA stenosis >70 %

excluded from NASCET and ACAS. Therefore, the findings of these trials cannot be extrapolated to this group. The true benefit of surgery for asymptomatic stenosis can be passed to the patients if the perioperative stroke-rate of the center/surgeon offering surgery is low. Only high-volume surgeons performing > 25 CEA per year with < 6 percent combined perioperative stroke/death-rate participated in the NASCET trial. The complication-rate may be much higher in the hands of surgeons performing fewer cases.

Newer studies such as Transatlantic Asymptomatic Carotid Intervention Trial (TACIT) consisting of a three way randomization of high and low-risk patients with a >70 percent asymptomatic stenosis to: 1. Best medical therapy with antiplatelets, statins, and anti-hypertensives, 2. CEA plus best medical therapy, 3. CAS plus best medical therapy will hopefully give better answers to the objections raised to these historical trials.

THE OPTIMUM INTERVENTION

Best Medical Treatment

Optimal medical treatment includes control of blood pressure, hyperlipidemia, ischemic heart disease and diabetes, cessation of smoking and commencing antiplatelets and statins. Hypertension is the most important treatable risk factor for stroke. A gradual individualized control is necessary. Sudden lowering of blood pressure may be counterproductive as due to the carotid stenosis high level of blood pressure may be required to maintain cerebral perfusion. Lowering of blood pressure reduces the chances of stroke and slows down the progression of atherosclerotic lesion. Similarly lowering the blood lipid by statins not only reduces the rate of progression of carotid stenosis but also exerts a plaque-stabilizing (pleotropic) effect which thereby minimizes the chances of cerebral embolization. Tobacco use increases the risk of stroke in proportion to duration

and amount of smoking. If an average smoker quits smoking for five years, his risk of stroke drops to the level of non-smoker. Use of recreational drugs (cocaine, amphetamines) should be avoided. There are various anti-platelet pharmaceutical agents which help the patients of carotid stenosis (Table 14.10). Warfarin is only used if TIA/stroke is due to embolization from heart usually due to atrial fibrillation.

Carotid Endarterectomy

First successful carotid revascularization was reported by Eastcott, Pickering and Rob in 1954.[19] The durability of carotid endarterectomy (CEA) is backed by level I grade A evidence generated from randomized controlled trials and therefore remains "gold-standard".

Informed Consent

It should be made clear to the patients and their family that CEA is a prophylactic surgery with the sole aim to minimize the chances of disabling or fatal stroke. It does not improve the current state of health. They should be clear that although the long-term stroke risk is lower with surgery, short-term postoperative risk is higher. Treating units should aim for a stroke/death rate of fewer than 5 percent. The possibility of local complications like wound hematoma requiring re-operation and nerve injuries to greater auricular, sensory branches of cervical plexus, glossopharyngeal, recurrent laryngeal nerve, and systemic complications such as myocardial infarction (MI), cerebral hyperperfusion should also be discussed.

Timing of Surgery

Patients with TIA or minor stroke need to be referred, seen and investigated for possible surgery as soon as possible preferably within 2 weeks. But this is unfortunately not

Table 14.10: Antiplatelet agents used in patients of carotid stenosis			
Name	*Mode of action*	*Side-effects*	*Comments*
Aspirin	Cyclooxygenase inhibitor	Gastric irritation, peptic ulcer, GI bleeding, metabolic acidosis, renal insufficiency	Standard treatment, lower dose is as useful as large dose but better tolerance
Dipyridamole	Phospodiesterase inhibitor	Headache	Usually combined with aspirin
Ticlopidine	Inhibits the exposure of fibrinogen binding site of GPIIa/IIIb receptor complex	GI irritation, diarrhea, allergic skin reaction, neutropenia	More effective than aspirin, not used due to severe neutro/ thrombocytopenia especially in first 12 weeks
Clopidogrel	Adenosine diphosphate receptor antagonists	GI irritation and bleeding	An alternative to aspirin but more expensive

possible even in most developed countries. It was initially thought that if a patient has suffered stroke it is better to delay the surgery for an arbitrary time limit of 6 weeks. The supportive reasons for this were two. Firstly, this period allows the ischemic penumbra to be reduced in size thereby delaying the risk of perioperative stroke. Secondly, an early surgery may lead to hyperperfusion and transform the ischemic penumbra into a hemorrhagic one. However, any delay may be risky as there is higher risk of stroke in first 8 weeks after the original presentation. This risk is higher in male, if there is increasing frequency of TIAs in the previous 3 months, coexisting peripheral vascular disease and hemispheric (rather than ocular) TIA, combined ocular and hemispheric symptoms, presence of complicated carotid-plaque morphology (ulceration or echolucency).

Preoperative Medical Treatment

All the patients who are scheduled to have CEA would be on antiplatelet treatment. This may increase the risk of hemorrhage from incision and endarterectomy site. On the other hand if antiplatelet treatment is withheld, the chances of cerebral embolization and thrombosis at endarterectomy site may increase. Aspirin, irrespective of dose (varying from 75-1300 mg) should not be stopped preoperatively. There is uncertainty about clopidogrel. Either alone on its own, or in combination with aspirin it does increase the hemostatic time but there is no significant increase in postoperative hemorrhage.[20] If the patient is on dual antiplatelet therapy, most surgeons still stop clopidogrel 3 to 7 days prior to CEA. Patient receiving anticoagulants (for atrial fibrillation or mechanical valve) should stop warfarin 3 to 5 days preoperatively. To cover this period they should be switched to IV heparin or low-molecular weight heparin. Their International Normalized Ratio (INR) on the day of surgery should be <1.8. Irrespective of level of cholesterol all these patients should be on statins which are continued uninterrupted throughout the perioperative period. Statins are beneficial by dual mechanisms, lowering the cholesterol level as well as exerting pleiotropic effect.

Once it is decided that patient needs CEA, it is worth going through a preoperative checklist to ensure that the correct operation is performed in the right patient for the correct indication. These points are listed in Table 14.11.

Technique of Carotid Endarterectomy

Choice of anesthesia: CEA can be performed either under local anesthesia (LA) or general anesthesia (GA). For local

Table 14.11: Preoperative checklist for CEA

1. What is the reason for surgery especially for asymptomatic lesions?
2. Does any atypical symptom warrants further investigations?
3. The degree of stenosis is appropriate considering the perioperative risk of surgery?
4. Is patient on best medical treatment?
5. If the patient is on antiplatelet therapy does it need to be modified perioperatively?
6. Does the patient need rescanning of carotid artery prior to surgery?
7. Is the operation side marked?
8. Is an informed consent obtained?
9. Does the patient need a bed in ITU/HDU for postoperative care?

anesthesia there are two techniques: cervical plexus block (deep and superficial) or infiltration. Local anesthesia allows conscious cerebral monitoring by talking to the patient and in the event of an inadequate cerebral perfusion a shunt may be inserted. The disadvantage of local anesthesia is that patient has to lie in a slightly uncomfortable position for considerable period of time. Patient anxiety may lead to high catecholamine levels and a higher blood pressure. Initial non-randomized studies suggested that LA was associated with significant reduction in the odds of death, stroke, MI, stroke and death and pulmonary complications within 30 days of the operation. However, these studies were too small to draw a definite conclusion. This led to GALA (general anesthesia vs local anesthesia) trial, one of the largest randomized surgical/anesthetic trial ever performed. This trial recruited 3526 patients at 95 centers in 24 countries.[21] The results suggested that both GA and LA are equally safe irrespective of age or co-existing co-morbidities. Patients with contralateral carotid occlusion have lesser chance of further neurological event if operated under LA. Therefore the decision about type of anesthesia should be taken jointly between the surgeon, anesthetist and the patient.

Position: The operation site is marked preoperatively. Patient lies supine with head extended and rotated away from the operation site. A head ring and sandbag beneath the shoulders stabilize this position. The head end of the table is raised which reduces the venous congestion. It is a good practice to mark the angle of mandible, lower border of mandible, tip of mastoid process, sternal notch and anterior border of sternocleidomastoid muscle. Just one dose of antibiotic is given intravenously (Co-amoxiclav + gentamycin). Usually there is no need to pass a urinary catheter unless patient has symptoms of urinary frequency, takes diuretics and cannot lie comfortably still (when an awake CEA is being done) on operation table.

Incision: Skin incision is usually given along the anterior border of sternocleidomastoid muscle. If the level of carotid bifurcation is marked preoperatively with the help of duplex Doppler, this point should be at the middle of incision. Some surgeons give a transverse skin crease incision in the neck skin crease extending from anterior border of SCM towards Adam's apple. It may be difficult to approach high bifurcation of carotid with the transverse incision. In terms of damage to sensory nerves by these incisions, there is no difference. After incising the platysma, the upper and lower flaps are raised. Below this level there is no difference between two incisions. Both involve incising the deep cervical fascia between the anterior border of SCM and trachea. At this level common facial vein is a constant landmark. This is mobilized, ligated and divided bringing the carotid artery along with the internal jugular vein (IJV) into view. If carotid artery is dissected with an approach posterior to the IJV (retrojugular approach), the division and ligation of common facial vein is not required. Retrojugular approach also minimizes the chances of injury to hypoglossal nerve. CCA is mobilized circumferentially and encircled with sloop or rubber sling. The carotid bifurcation is dissected carefully but not mobilized till the ICA is clamped. Carotid bulb is handled very gently as a friable atherosclerotic plaque may dislodge and embolize leading to stroke. ECA and ICA are dissected and controlled with slings. The ICA should be dissected till a blue hue on the arterial wall is seen which indicates a healthy, plaque-free segment of the artery. Some surgeons block the carotid sinus nerve by injecting 1-2 ml lidocaine which blocks the reflex vagal response causing sinus bradycardia. Surgical exposure of the carotid arteries is shown in Figure 14.5.

Optimal intraoperative antithrombotic regimen: All dissection is completed except mobilization of carotid bulb. Before applying any clamp systemic heparin (70 units/kg body weight) is given. There is no evidence to support this but most surgeons use it to minimize the chances of MI and thrombosis of the ICA stump induced by clamping alone or by clamping and shunting both. Proponents of heparin highlight that the beneficial effect of heparin are not just confined to inhibition of coagulation. Heparin decreases platelet activation, thromboxane release, adhesion to collagen and anti-inflammatory effects which minimize the ischemia-reperfusion injury to endothelial cells. A two minutes time-gap is given to ensure that heparin has circulated in the system. Usually a high dose heparin needs

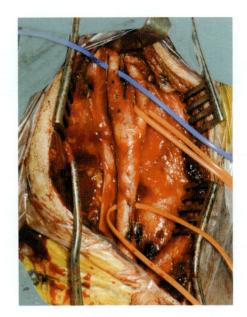

FIGURE 14.5: Surgical exposure of carotid arteries

to be reversed by protamine 1 mg for 100 units of heparin. Because the half-life of heparin is 60-90 minutes, the dose of protamine is commonly calculated to reverse half the original heparin dose given. There is a slight increase in the chance of stroke by reversal of heparin. Patients may develop an allergic reaction to protamine which is higher in those who have used Neutral Protamine Hagedorn (NPH) insulin for diabetes or had prior vasectomy. Protamine should be avoided in these patients. Any allergic reaction should be treated by steroids and antihistamines.

Should the patient be shunted? The best way to assess the safety of cross-clamping is a temporary occlusion of ECA, CCA and ICA (in that order). In patients having CEA under local anesthesia the speech and movement of the contralateral arm and leg are assessed after the clamping. If there is no evidence of weakness or disturbance of consciousness, intracranial circulation is judged to be adequate and operation proceeds without any circulatory support (shunt). If the surgeon prefers GA this technique cannot be employed. Surgeons fall in three categories: some use shunt routinely in all cases, some use it selectively, others never shunt. There are many different types of shunts as shown in Figure 14.6. There is no evidence that one type is better than other. Various pros and cons of deploying a shunt are listed in Table 14.12. If a shunt needs to be employed a longitudinal arteriotomy is made on the posterolateral part of CCA. This is extended to ICA beyond

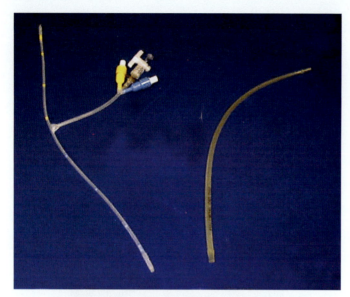

FIGURE 14.6: Carotid shunts (on left: Pruitt-Inhara, on right: Javid)

the diseased intima. The distal end of shunt is placed in the ICA, a back-bleed is allowed to fill the shunt. The proximal part of shunt is now passed into the CCA. With the help of handheld Doppler the flow-signals in shunt are detected to ensure the proper functioning. It is important to remember that having a shunt in place does not mean it is working. About three percent of shunts malfunction, usually due to impaction on distal ICA by kink or coil.

Selective shunters use various techniques to identify the patients who have inadequate collateral or contralateral cerebral circulation. These techniques are enumerated in Table 14.13.

Only stump-pressure monitoring technique is worth mentioning as it is validated by various researchers. There is a relationship between intracranial collateral blood flow and cerebral perfusion pressure. For measuring the stump pressure a green needle (19 gauge) is connected to a plastic tubing which is flushed with saline ensuring that there is no trapped air-bubble in it. This line is connected to the pressure transducer. After waiting for 3 minutes the needle is inserted in carotid bulb. It is ensured that a pulsatile reading is obtained with the needle well-placed intraluminally rather than abutting the arterial wall. ECA and CCA are clamped. This leaves the needle in continuity with a static column of blood which is open to ICA. Even though the needle is inserted proximal to ICA stenosis, pressure will equalise on both sides of the carotid stenosis because there is no blood flow. As soon as the clamp is applied on CCA the pressure starts dropping down and in few minutes it stabilizes. This residual pressure in the carotid bulb (carotid stump pressure) is recorded. If this stabilizes at/above 25 mm Hg or more than 1/3rd of systemic intra-arterial pressure (checked in radial artery), shunt is not required.

Bifurcation endarterectomy: The optimal plane of dissection lies between the diseased intima and circular fibers of the

Table 14.12: Carotid shunting: pros and cons	
Advantages	*Disadvantages*
1. Provides flow to all patients	1. Technically more cumbersome to perform endarterectomy
2. Relieves surgeon of time-pressure	2. More difficult to visualize the distal end-point of endarterectomy
3. Optimizes the training opportunities for the trainee surgeons	3. Disruption of distal intima by shunt
	4. Air/thrombotic embolization

Table 14.13: Methods of identifying inadequate collateral cerebral blood flow		
Methods	*Status*	*Reasons*
1. Ipsilateral jugular venous oxygen tension	Inaccurate	Venous drainage is a mixture of both cerebral hemispheres
2. Intraoperative electro-encephlaogram	Inaccurate	Changes on EEG may be due to GA
3. Carotid stump pressure measurement	Useful	A stump-pressure >25 mm Hg or >1/3rd of systemic pressure indicates acceptable collateral cerebral flow
4. Somatosensory-evoked potential		
5. Transcranial Doppler		
6. Near infrared spectrometry		

arterial media. The endarterectomy performed in this plane leaves a smooth distal tapering end-point of plaque in ICA.

Should it be patched, if yes–what patch to use: On completion of endarterectomy, the closure is performed. Some surgeons close the arteriotomy primarily without patch by using continuous closely placed stitches whereas others patch either selectively or routinely. Primary closure avoids complications associated with patch angioplasty, e.g. patch blowout, pseudoaneurysm formation, prosthetic graft infection. The evidence supports the use of patch to close the arteriotomy especially in women (smaller arteries) and cases of restenosis. Patching increases the size of artery and minimizes the chance of perioperative arterial occlusion and restenosis due to neointimal hyperplasia. Nature of patch material is a matter of personal preference. The available options are knitted Dacron, polytetrafluoroethylene (Fig. 14.7), bovine pericardium, autologous (long saphenous, jugular or cephalic) vein patch. Autologous vein patch minimize the chances of any patch infection. Bovine pericardium has a higher rate of developing a pseudoaneurysm. The results of PTFE and Dacron patches are comparable.

Eversion carotid endarterectomy: Another method called eversion carotid endarterectomy avoids use of any patch. It involves an oblique transaction of ICA at its origin at carotid bifurcation and endarterectomy by everting the ICA, endarterectomy of the carotid bifurcation and of ECA, and reimplantation of the ICA on CCA. Theoretical advantages of this technique include avoidance of longitudinal arteriotomy of the ICA, use of patch and very effective correction of carotid kinks and tortousity.

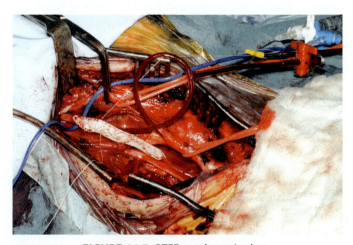

FIGURE 14.7: PTFE patch angioplasty

Once the arteriotomy is closed one should wait to ensure that there is an excellent hemostasis. Some surgeons leave a vacuum drain. The platysma and skin incision is closed using absorbable suture material or skin clips. Skin clips can be removed between 3rd and 5th postoperative day.

Where should patient recover: Usually patient is recovered in high dependency area where invasive intra-arterial blood pressure monitoring and close neurological observations are performed.

Special Scenarios

High Bifurcation

This is expected if the ultrasound examination fails to show the ICA above the stenosis clearly. The strict definition of high disease is when the plaque in ICA extends above a line joining the tip of mastoid process to the lower border of ramus of mandible. This corresponds to the lower border of second cervical vertebra. To tackle high disease, patient should have nasolaryngeal rather than orolaryngeal intubation. This increases the available space between the mandible and mastoid process. Division of posterior belly of digastrics muscle makes access to higher segment of ICA easier. By dividing the branch of ECA which hooks the hypoglossal nerve one brings at least 2 cm or more of the ICA in view. The subluxation of temporomandibular joint has been described as another technique but it increases the joint dysfunction later on in life.

How to Avoid/Minimize Nerve Injuries

In order to avoid nerve injury one must be aware of their anatomy. Figure 14.8 shows the distribution and course of cutaneous and cranial nerves in relation to carotid artery in lateral profile.

The upper extent of incision should stop at least two finger breadths below the lower border of mandible. If for high-bifurcation it needs to be extended, it should be curved posteriorly towards mastoid process running parallel to the lower border of mandible. Diathermy should not be used close to nerves. Apart from the ansa cervicalis no other nerve like structure that traverses the bifurcation should be divided. Dissection of vagus should be performed carefully in the carotid sheath and this nerve should not be caught while applying the carotid clamps. Care should be taken to avoid over-stretching of accessory nerve during the retro-jugular approach to the carotid artery.

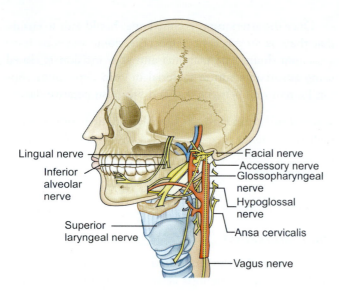

Lingual nerve

Inferior
alveolar
nerve

Superior
laryngeal nerve

Facial nerve
Accessory nerve
Glossopharyngeal
nerve
Hypoglossal
nerve
Ansa cervicalis
Vagus nerve

FIGURE 14.8: Distribution of relevant nerves (lateral profile)

When to Abandon a Planned CEA

If there is a significant delay between the duplex revealing high-grade stenosis and planned CEA, one may find a totally occluded ICA on exploration. Such an occluded ICA should not be re-opened. If ICA above the plaque is hypoplastic and the patient is embolizing from this severely stenosed ICA, ICA should be ligated and no CEA should be performed. If there is no evidence of embolization, one should leave the stenosed ICA well alone. There is no evidence to support either interventions. Either way, the patient should be anticoagulated for 6 months. If the plaque is extending beyond the surgically accessible area, CEA should be abandoned.

How to Manage the Perioperative Neurological Deficits

Carotid thrombosis is the commonest cause of early postoperative neurological deficit. If it occurs in less than 24 hours, the patient should return to operation theater immediately and carotid re-explored. During re-exploration one should be careful not to dislodge friable thrombus into the brain. Patch should be re-opened, and the thrombus removed. Once good back-bleed from ICA is obtained, a shunt should then be inserted. Usually there is an underlying intimal defect which should be repaired and arteriotomy site re-patched. Neurological deficit which develops later could be due to cerebral hemorrhage or hyperperfusion. Urgent CT scan of head will be helpful in this situation. Cerebral hemorrhage is managed by carefully controlling

the blood pressure with the input of specialist stroke physician. Cerebral hyperperfusion is also managed with an accurate control of blood pressure and seizure.

When to Reoperate for Recurrent Stenosis

Restenosis of ICA is attributed to neointimal hyperplasia (within 24 months) or due to recurrent atherosclerosis (> 24 months later). The true incidence is ill-defined due to variable follow-up and diagnostic standards. The reported incidence in the literature is between 2 to 30 percent. A higher recurrence does raise the possibility of a residual disease rather than a true recurrent stenosis. Patch angioplasty reduces the incidence of recurrent stenosis. There is a consensus that symptomatic recurrent stenosis needs to be re-operated. For asymptomatic patients a careful surveillance alone is proposed. There could be restenosis beyond the original endarterectomy site making the dissection more difficult. Therefore, re-do CEA has a higher incidence of cranial nerve injuries, wound hematoma, perioperative stroke and death. Carotid angioplasty offers an alternative to re-do CEA.

How to Manage Infected Prosthetic Patch

Up to 1 percent of patients who had CEA with prosthetic patch angioplasty may develop patch infection. It may present early (within 6 months) or late. Clinically they present as deep wound infection, discharging chronic sinus or false aneurysm. False aneurysm may occasionally rupture. Duplex/angiography/radioisotope-labelled white cell scan may be helpful in diagnosing and planning the re-intervention. Presence of any abscess overlying the carotid incision should raise its suspicion. Mostly the causative microorganisms are either staphylococci or streptococci. The optimal treatment involves patch removal with autologous venous reconstruction with either patch or bypass.

Perioperative Complications

Following CEA the cerebral blood flow is increased. If this is well above the metabolic demand of the brain tissue it may result in cerebral hyperperfusion which is characterized by unilateral headache, face and eye pain, seizures, and focal neurological symptoms related to cerebral edema or intracerebral hemorrhage. Patients who have a high-grade stenosis, malignant hypertension, and poor collateral supply or had recent stroke/TIA are more likely to develop cerebral hyperperfusion. Strict control of arterial blood pressure keeping the systolic pressure below 160 mm of Hg helps these patients.

The main nerve injuries are those to sensory branches of cervical plexus. The loss of sensation in men who shave may be more troublesome. They cut their jaw/neck skin very easily and as they are on anti-platelets it bleeds more easily and profusely. Mostly it recovers in 3-6 months. Damage to unilateral RLN causes hoarseness of voice which also improves with time.

Pseudoaneurysms are rare and are mostly due to breakdown of suture line itself rather than degenerative changes in the patch. Patch infection is another uncommon complication. Eversion endarterectomy avoids use of any patch. Autologous vein patch angioplasty carries a lower chance of infection. If the synthetic patch becomes infected the patient needs to be treated with antibiotics and often requires replacing the synthetic patch with the autologous vein patch.

Carotid Angioplasty and Stenting

First balloon angioplasty for the internal carotid stenosis was performed in 1979 while the first balloon-expandable stent was deployed in the internal carotid artery in 1989.[22,23] Initially carotid angioplasty and stenting (CAS) was performed without cerebral protection devices and had a high risk of cerebral embolization. Carotid angioplasty with stenting using cerebral protection device has evolved as a viable alternative for treating ICA stenosis. Though it is still uncertain whether CAS is as effective and durable as CEA, the proponents argue various potential advantages with CAS, e.g. no incision, no nerve injury, improved cost-effectiveness and possible less cardiovascular co-morbidity. CAS initially evolved to treat 'high-risk' patients who were excluded from NASCET and ECST trials for various reasons or for treating the carotid dissection. The term 'high-risk' is used in the medical literature without specifying the context and is hence confusing. 'High risk' patient for a surgeon could be defined by certain risk-factors which increase the probability of complications in the peri-operative period. These may be classified as preoperative or intra-operative and are summarized in Table 14.14. Pre-operative high risks include certain characteristics either in the carotid artery plaque or in the patient whereas intra-operative risk factors are subdivided according to anatomical, surgical or pathophysiological higher risks.

A number of nonrandomized and randomized controlled trials for CAS have been performed comparing CEA and CAS which are summarized in Table 14.15.

Though there was a significant reduction in the risk of cranial neuropathy 30 days after CAS, CEA had a more favorable outcome in terms of death or any stroke at 30 days, 6 months and 1 year time-points after the procedure.

Randomized controlled trials conducted so far to evaluate CAS had different designs and the results have been heterogeneous. Whilst few trials favored CEA, e.g. EVA-3S, others have favored CAS, e.g. SAPPHIRE. Few other trials have been neutral as they neither favored CAS nor CEA e.g. CAVATAS and SPACE. There have been no uniform criteria about including or excluding the interventionist on the basis of their experience and training. Most trials have included both symptomatic and asymptomatic patients without any sub-analysis of each group. Therefore, the applicability of the results to the patient becomes unpredictable and remains open to the personal bias of the person either analysing the results or offering the treatment. The results of CAS vary according to the patient's age. A subgroup analysis of SPACE trial suggests that the risk of stenting may be higher in patients aged >75 years.[25] Four out of six symptomatic CAS trials were stopped prematurely either because of excess stroke rate after CAS or due to the lack of funding. Due to overall recruitment shortfall, the power calculations of all these trials are significantly compromised and therefore the inferences remain open to criticism.

Table 14.14: High-risk factors	
Preoperative risks	*Intraoperative risks*

1. Plaque-related
  a. Degree of stenosis
  b. Plaque morphology
2. Co-morbidities
  a. Advanced age
  b. Cardiac disease
  c. Others- pulmonary disease, renal disease, diabetes, tracheostomy, neck immobility
	1. Anatomical
	  a. Aortic arch and proximal carotid anatomy
	  b. High carotid bifurcation
	  c. Contralateral recurrent laryngeal nerve dysfunction
	2. Surgical
	  a. Hostile neck
	  b. Recurrent stenosis
	3. Pathophysiological
	  a. Contralateral carotid occlusion

Name of trial	Number of patients	Patients characteristics	Primary end-points	Results (%)	
Leicester	17	Low risk Symptomatic	30-d stroke and/death	CAS	7.0
				CEA	0.0
Wall stent	219	Low risk Symptomatic	1-y stroke and/death	CAS	10.4
				CEA	4.4
SAPPHIRE	334	High risk Symptomatic	30-d stroke and/death	CAS	12.2
				CEA	20.1
Kentucky 1	104	Low risk Symptomatic	30-d stroke and/death	CAS	1.8
				CEA	1.9
Kentucky 2	84	Low risk Asymptomatic	30-d stroke and/death	CAS	0.0
				CEA	0.0
CAVATAS	504	Low risk Symptomatic	30-d stroke and/death	CAS	10.0
				CEA	9.9
SPACE	1183	Low risk Symptomatic	30-d stroke and/death	CAS	6.8
				CEA	6.3
EVA-3S	527	Low risk Symptomatic	30-d stroke and/death	CAS	9.6
				CEA	3.9

Table 14.15: Summary of CAS trials results[24]

Technique of CAS

Prerequisites

A recent non-contrast CT head is mandatory to rule out intracranial hemorrhage. Unlike CEA which is increasingly performed on the basis of duplex Doppler, CAS requires a diagnostic carotid cervical and cerebral angiogram. They also should have ECG and chest X-ray done. Patients are given antiplatelet regimens usually clopidogrel, an adenosine diphosphate inhibitor, and aspirin both for 2-4 days pre-operatively. If possible, the level of platelet inhibition should be checked with an aggregometer with a target of 70-90 percent inhibition. CAS can be done under general or local anesthesia. General anesthesia gives the additional benefit of muscle paralysis and easier control of blood pressure. Peripheral venous access is gained for systemic heparinization and atropine (if necessary for bradycardia).

Procedure

Technique of high-magnification road-mapping which allows superimposition of a stored image of the opacified blood vessel on a blank fluoroscopic image in real-time. Intra-arterial access is obtained via femoral route. One should avoid excessive catheter manipulations into the aortic arch to minimize the chances of detaching atheromatous plaque. Various different types and shapes of catheter help in negotiating the origin of great vessels. Intravenous heparin is given after arterial puncture and a diagnostic angiogram is carried out. This allows size calibration for proper stent diameter and length in regards to the stenosis and native vessel diameters. If the stenosis is too tight initial microwire manipulation and angioplasty may be needed. The stent diameter is over-sized by 10-20 percent to avoid stent-migration/embolization. The stent assembly is passed co-axially through the sheath and across the lesion (Fig. 14.9). If a Monorail stenting assembly is not used, an exchange length guide wire across the lesion is placed all the time with its tip just proximal to the petrous ICA. This allows over-the wire exchange of the stent assembly for an angioplasty balloon or other device, if necessary, without having to cross stenotic lesion twice. Avoidance of repeated crossing minimizes the chances of plaque-embolization. Self-expanding stents are most widely used but even these often require 'post-stenting in-stent angioplasty' known as "touch-up angioplasty" which is done with standard angioplasty balloons. Angioplasty may stretch the nerves in carotid sinus which may cause bradycardia. To counteract this atropine (0.5-1.0 mg) intravenous may be required just prior to angioplasty. A completion angiogram is done. Closure-device is used to minimize the chances of bleeding from the arterial puncture site as these patients are on dual antiplatelet therapy and heparinized. There is no need to reverse the heparin.

To minimize the risk of downstream (cerebral) emboli, embolic protection devices (EPDs) have been used. There are two broad families of these devices: balloon-based or filters. Two specific types of balloon-based protectors are occluders to flow or reversers to flow. The detailed description of each of these is not within the remit of this chapter. However, pros and cons of various EPDs are summarized in Table 14.16.

Postprocedure Care

A detailed neurological examination is carried out. Blood pressure is maintained at a mean arterial pressure of <85 mm Hg. Clopidogrel is continued for 6 weeks to minimize the risk of thromboembolic complications. Aspirin is continued for life. Follow-up carotid duplex is done at 6 months, 1 year and 2 years to assess stent-patency. If in-stent restenosis or development of a tandem lesion is suspected, CT angiography is done.

Complications

The main complications are summarized as in Table 14.17.

It is worrying to note that CAS is increasingly being practised especially for asymptomatic patients despite lacking strong evidence in the current era of evidence-based-medicine. In UK the National Institute for Health and Clinical Excellence (NICE) recommendations (Sept 2006) about CAS with embolic protection device state that:

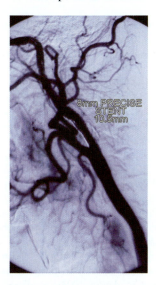

FIGURE 14.9: Carotid angioplasty with stenting

1. Clinicians undertaking CAS should have adequate training.
2. Patients should understand that long-term safety is uncertain.
3. Selection should only be done by involving a multi-disciplinary team consisting of surgeon, radiologist and a neurologist.
4. Preferably only symptomatic patients should be offered CAS.

It is recommended that CAS with embolic protection device should be offered only as a part of a trial because so far insufficient data is available about CAS. Outside the trial it should only be considered if patients are unsuitable for CEA due to medical or surgical contraindications and have high-risk of stroke with medical treatment alone. Irrespective of the modality of treatment offered to these patients, presence of various co-morbidities increases the peri-procedural complication rate. It should be emphasized that for many high-risk patients one must question whether any form of revascularization is preferable to medical therapy alone. Extreme carotid artery elongation and tortousity with co-existing stenotic disease are more appropriately treated with open surgery than with CAS.

SUMMARY POINTS

1. Stroke is the most common cause of disability in western world.
2. Despite advances in management the incidence of stroke is likely to increase over the next 25 years.
3. The majority of strokes are ischemic.
4. The majority of ischemic strokes affect the carotid territory.
5. The largest single cause of ischemic stroke is thromboembolism of the ICA or MCA.
6. Optimal medical care is very important for long-term stroke prevention.

Table 14.16: Advantages and disadvantages of various embolic protection devices concepts ECA= External carotid artery; ICA= Internal carotid artery			
Features	Filters	Occluders	Flow reversers
Embolization during lesion crossing	+++	++	–
Cerebral flow decrease	+	++	+++
ICA protection from emboli	+	++	+++
Ability to perform angiography during protection	+++	–	+++
Embolization through ECA	–	+++	–
Potential spasm/damage to ICA	+++	+++	–
Tolerance	+++	+	+
Ease of use	+++	++	+

Table 14.17: Complications of CAS		
Intraprocedural	*Periprocedural*	*Delayed*
• Thromboembolism • Stent mispositioning • Stent thrombosis • Intra-arterial stent loss • Contrast-related: Anaphylaxis, nephropathy • Puncture-site: Hematoma, pseudoaneurysm • Arterial dissection: Carotid, femoral • Closure device related: Stenosis, embolization	• Cerebral embolization • TIA/stroke • Myocardial infarction • Hemorrhagic events • Hypotension	• In-stent stenosis • Recurrent stenosis • Stent kink/fracture/migration

7. Carotid endarterectomy has an important role in the management of symptomatic patients with severe stenosis.
8. Carotid angioplasty and stenting with the use of cerebral protection device is an alternative for patients with symptomatic stenosis and hostile neck.

REFERENCES

1. Thom T, Hasse N, Rosamond W, et al. Heart disease and stroke statistics—2006 update: a report from the American Heart Association Statistics Committee and Stroke Statistics Subcommittee. Circulation 2006; 113(6): e85-151.
2. Dennis MS, Bamford JM, Sandercock PAG, et al. Incidence of transient ischaemic attacks in Oxfordshire, England, Stroke 1989; 20:333-9.
3. Adhiyaman V, Adhiyaman S. Transient ischaemic attack: 10 minute consultation. BMJ 2009;338:a2343, 949.
4. NICE. The diagnosis and acute management of stroke and transient ischaemic attacks, 2008.
5. Moneta GL, Edwards JM, Chitwood RW, et al. Correlation of North American Symptomatic Carotid Endarterectomy Trial (NASCET) angiographic definition of 70-99% internal carotid artery stenosis with duplex scanning. J Vasc Surg 1993. pp.152-9.
6. Fields WS, Maslenikov V, Meyers JS, et al. Joint study of extracranial arterial occlusion: progress report of prognosis following surgery or nonsurgical treatment for transient cerebral ischaemic attacks and cervical carotid artery lesions. JAMA 1970;211:1993-2003.
7. Shaw DA, Venables GS, Cartlidge NE, et al. Carotid endarterectomy in patients with transient cerebral ischaemia. J Neurol Sci 1984;64:45-53.
8. European Carotid Surgery Trialists' Collaborative Group. Randomised trial of endarterectomy for recently symptomatic carotid stenosis: Final results of the MRC European Carotid Surgery Trial (ECST). Lancet 1998;351:1379-87.
9. Barnett HJM, Taylor DW, Eliasziw M, Fox AJ, et al. Beneficial effect of carotid endarterectomy in symptomatic patients with high-grade carotid stenosis. North American Symptomatic Carotid Endarterectomy Trial Collaborators. N Eng J Med 1991;325:445-53.
10. Naylor AR. Is surgery still generally the first choice intervention in patients with carotid artery disease? Surgeon 2008; 61:6-12.
11. Morgenstern LB, et al. The risks and benefits of carotid endarterectomy in patients with near occlusion of the carotid artery. North American symptomatic carotid endarterectomy (NASCET) group. Neurology 1997;48:911-5.
12. Fox AJ, Eliasziw M, Rothwell PM, et al. Management of patients with carotid artery near occlusion. Am J Neuroradiol 2005;26:2086-94.
13. Shaw DA, Venables GS, Cartlidge NE, et al. Carotid endarterectomy in patients with transient cerebral ischaemia. J Neurol Sci 1984; 64:45-53.
14. Donnan GA, Davis SM, Chambers BR, et al. Surgery for prevention of stroke. Lancet 1998;351:1372-3.
15. Executive Committee for the Asymptomatic Carotid Atherosclerosis Study. Endarterctomy for asymptomatic carotid artery stenosis. JAMA 1995;273:1421-8.
16. Asymptomatic Carotid Surgery Trial Collaborators. The MRC Asymptomatic Carotid Surgery Trial (ACST): Carotid endarterectomy prevents disabling and fatal carotid territory strokes. Lancet 2004;363:1491-1502.
17. Rijbroek A, Wisselink W, Vriens EM, et al. Asymptomatic carotid artery stenosis:past, present and future. Eur Neurol 2006;56:139-54.
18. Abbot A, et al. What should we do with asymptomatic carotid stenosis? Int J Stroke 2007;2:27-39.
19. Eastcott HH, Pickering GW, Rob CG. Reconstruction of internal carotid artery in a patient with intermittent attacks of hemiplegia. Lancet 1954;67(6846):994-6.
20. Payne, et al. Beneficial effects of clopidogrel combined with aspirin in reducing cerebral emboli in patients undergoing carotid endarterectomy. Circulation 2004;109:1476-81.
21. GALA Trial Collaborative Group, Lewis SC, et al. General anaesthesia versus local anaesthesia for carotid surgery: a multicentre, randomised controlled trial. Lancet 2008;372:2132-42.
22. Bockenheimer SA, Mathias K. Percutaneous transluminal angioplasty in arteriosclerotic internal carotid artery stenosis. Am J Neuroradiol 1983;4:791-2.
23. Diethrich EB, Ndiaye M, Reid B. Stenting in the carotid artery: initial experience in 110 patients. J Endovasc Surg 1996;3:42-62.
24. Luebke T, Aleksic M, Brunkwall J. Meta-analysis of randomized trails comparing carotid endarterectomy and endovascular treatment. Eur J Vasc Endovasc Surg 2007;34:470-9.
25. Ringleb PA, Allenberg J, Bruckmann H, et al. 30-day results from SPACE trial of stent protected angioplasty versus carotid endarterectomy in symptomatic patients: a randomised non-inferiority trial. Lancet 2006;368:1239-47.

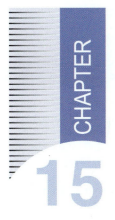

Peripheral Vascular Diseases

MP McMonagle, S Rai, RK Vohra

ETIOLOGY

The predominant lesion in peripheral arterial disease (PAD) is atherosclerosis. An atherosclerotic arterial plaque may progress, leading to chronic lower limb ischemia which may in turn progress to critical ischemia leaving a limb threatened. There are other rare causes of PAD giving rise to similar symptoms which the vascular surgeon needs to be aware of. These include persistent sciatic artery, cystic adventitial disease, popliteal artery entrapment, fibromuscular dysplasia and Buerger's disease. These conditions are summarized in Table 15.1. There are also other rheumatoid and vasculitic conditions that may present to a vascular service but are not covered in this chapter.

ATHEROSCLEROSIS

Atherosclerosis [from the Greek word 'athera', meaning 'lump of porridge' (International Classification of Diseases 10:I70)] is the commonest pathophysiological process leading to cardiovascular disease, including PAD. The resulting vascular lesion, almost ubiquitous in the western world, commonly affects the medium and larger sized arteries including; the coronary arteries, aorta, carotid arteries, mesenteric arteries and lower limb vessels. Histologically, the lesion primarily forms in the tunica intima of the arterial wall and consists of a nodular accumulation of soft, yellowish material at the centers of a harder plaque. It is composed of macrophages with cholesterol crystals and occasional calcified segments.[1]

The development of atherosclerosis is probably multifactorial. It may result from an increase in vascular permeability, perhaps as a response to injury, creating 'vascular leak'. Entry of lipoproteins such as LDL and VLDL (low density lipoproteins and very low density lipoproteins

respectively) particles through the endothelium and into the subendothelial space places them directly at the site of disease. These lipoprotein molecules may undergo further oxidation by endothelial cells to be taken up later by macrophages via 'scavenger' pathways leading to the formation of foam cells, which are pathognomonic of atherosclerosis.[1] The sequence of changes seen in the arterial lesion are outlined in Figure 15.1. Unless otherwise specified, this chapter will deal with the treatment and management of atherosclerosis as a cause of PAD.

PREVALENCE AND EPIDEMIOLOGY

PAD is caused by atherosclerotic occlusion or stenosis of the arteries in the lower limb. It is difficult to quantify the exact prevalence of PAD in the population, as in the majority it is silent and asymptomatic. However, studies, including the Edinburgh Artery Study, have suggested that the prevalence of asymptomatic PAD is 7 to 15 percent with the age-adjusted prevalence being about 12 percent and that the disorder equally affects men and women.[2-5] Using ultrasound criteria for the diagnosis of PAD, the British Regional Heart Study estimated a prevalence of 64 percent between the ages of 56 and 77 years, but only 10 percent of these were symptomatic.[6]

The Edinburgh Artery Study suggests that 7-15 percent of asymptomatic patients will go on to develop intermittent claudication over a 5-year period.[7] More importantly, patients suffering from PAD, even if asymptomatic have a higher risk of other cardiovascular events and death, including acute myocardial infarction (AMI) and stroke.[4] In fact, patients with PAD, even in the absence of a history of AMI and stroke, have approximately the same relative risk of cardiovascular all-cause death as those with a history of

Table 15.1: Summary of the non-atherosclerotic causes of PAD	
Non-atherosclerotic cases of PAD	*Notes*
Persistent sciatic artery	Congenital persistence of the embryonic sciatic artery. May be bilateral (22%). Proximal symptoms and iliofemoral hypoplasia. Prone to aneurysmal degeneration. Cowie's sign positive (absent proximal pulses with present distal pulses)
Cystic adventitial disease (CAD)	Cystic degeneration of the tunica adventitia of the popliteal artery. May be in continuity with the synovium of the knee joint. Presents as claudication. Pulses present, but disappear on knee flexion. Results of angioplasty poor with high complication rate.
Popliteal artery entrapment	May be confused with CAD. Bilateral in 66%. Popliteal artery courses around the medial head of gastronemius (types I-III) or deep to popliteus muscle (type IV). Compression of artery on knee flexion. Prone to aneurysmal degeneration.
Fibromuscular dysplasia	Unknown etiology. More commonly affects the renal and carotid arteries. Classically beaded appearance on angiogram. May affect external iliac artery. Best treated with angioplasty (± stenting). Prone to aneurysmal degeneration.
Buerger's disease (thromboangiitis obliterans)	Classically affects younger males and heavy smokers. Also prevalent amongst people of Middle Eastern and Asian origin. Numerous thrombotic occlusions of small and medium sized arteries (i.e. below knee). Vessels on angiogram are normal to a sudden point of occlusion with numerous, tortuous, cork-screw collaterals. Raynaud's phenomenon also associated. Excellent prognosis with smoking cessation and exercise.

either documented coronary or cerebrovascular disease, regardless of whether the PAD is symptomatic or not.[7,8] There is, however, a direct correlation between the severity of the PAD, as measured by the ankle-brachial index and the risk of cardiovascular events. Patients with critical limb ischemia and a very low ankle-brachial pressure index (ABPI) have an approximate annual mortality of 25 percent.[9-11] Hence, many of the treatments for patients with PAD are not only aimed at ameliorating the symptoms of the disease, but also aim to 'risk-modify' for other cardiovascular events that this population of patients are at higher risk for.

RISK FACTORS FOR PAD

Numerous epidemiological risk factors for the development of atherosclerosis (and thus PAD) have been identified. These include, advancing age, male gender, cigarette smoking, diabetes mellitus, hypertension, abdominal obesity (Table 15.2). It is also important to mention that PAD is also an independent risk factor for other vascular diseases such as coronary artery disease and stroke. The REACH (Reduction of Atherosclerosis for Continued Health) has shown that up to 40 percent of patients with symptomatic PAD also have evidence of coronary artery disease. In addition, this registry has identified numerous other risk factors for atherosclerosis, including diabetes (39%), hypertension (73%), hypercholestolemia (59%) and history of smoking (46%).[12]

AGE AND GENDER

Advancing age and male gender are independent risk factors in the development of atherosclerosis. The traditional lifestyle choices of men over the last century (i.e. diet, lack of exercise, smoking habits), especially in the western world may be the contributing factors. The Framingham Heart Study showed that men have double the risk of PAD compared to women.[13] However, neither the Edinburgh Artery Study nor the Limburg study supported the findings of the Framingham Heart Study.[14,15] Both the Framingham Heart Study and the Edinburgh Artery Study found advancing age to be an independent risk factor in the development of PAD.

SMOKING

Cigarette smoking is the leading contributor to the major mortalities in the Western World, including coronary artery

Table 15.2: Summary of the modifiable and non-modifiable risk factors for the development of PAD	
Non-modifiable	*Modifiable*
Advancing age	Smoking
Male gender	Dyslipidemia
Diabetes mellitus	Hypertension
	Obesity and sedentary lifestyle
	Glucose control
	Hyperhomocystinemia

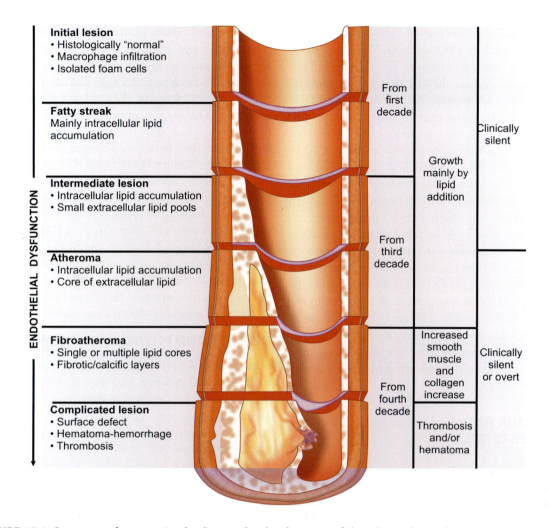

ENDOTHELIAL DYSFUNCTION

Initial lesion
• Histologically "normal"
• Macrophage infiltration
• Isolated foam cells

Fatty streak
Mainly intracellular lipid accumulation

Intermediate lesion
• Intracellular lipid accumulation
• Small extracellular lipid pools

Atheroma
• Intracellular lipid accumulation
• Core of extracellular lipid

Fibroatheroma
• Single or multiple lipid cores
• Fibrotic/calcific layers

Complicated lesion
• Surface defect
• Hematoma-hemorrhage
• Thrombosis

From first decade

From third decade

From fourth decade

Growth mainly by lipid addition

Increased smooth muscle and collagen increase

Thrombosis and/or hematoma

Clinically silent

Clinically silent or overt

FIGURE 15.1: Sequence of progression leading to the development of the atherosclerotic lesion in the arterial wall.
(From en.wikipedia released under GNU Free Documentation License)

disease, stroke, carcinoma (especially lung carcinoma) and respiratory disease. These disease categories form four out of the top five all-cause mortality for the Western World, thus making cigarette smoking perhaps the leading 'preventable' contributor to disease.

Smoking increases the risk of developing PAD by up to about three-fold.[16] Continued smoking in the face of established asymptomatic PAD is much more likely to progress to symptomatic disease compared to non-smokers, with worse clinical outcomes, including critical ischemic events and the risk of major limb amputation.[17] The Framingham Heart Study estimates that up to three quarters of cases of PAD are attributable to smoking.[13]

Although difficult to quantify, smoking cessation produces cardiovascular benefit even in those with established disease. The cardiovascular risk is halved within one year of cessation and is the same as non-smokers after about 5 to 15 years, or earlier in women.[18,19] Furthermore, cessation of smoking after intervention, especially coronary artery disease will significantly improve the medium and long-term outcomes for these patients.[20]

It would appear, therefore, that smoking cessation would be cost-effective with regard to health expenditure. Nicotine-replacement studies have demonstrated up to two-fold success rates in smoking cessation, with perhaps the nasal spray being most effective.[21]

DIABETES

Diabetes is an important independent risk factor in the development of atherosclerosis, which may be modifiable in the form of good glucose control. Lower limb arterial disease in diabetics tends to produce more diffuse and distal (below the knee) arterial disease. The UKPDS (UK Prospective Diabetes Study) showed that type 2 diabetic patients have a 3-5 fold increase risk of developing PAD compared to non-diabetics and that for every 1 percent rise in the HbA1C level, there was an associated 28 percent increase in PAD.[22,23] Diabetic patients also have a 10-16 fold increased lifetime risk of lower limb amputation and those who develop critical limb ischemia tend to have higher failure rates with revascularization attempts.[24,25] The high incidence of peripheral neuropathy contributing to ulceration and infection rates in the diabetic population also contributes to the poorer outcomes for these patients.

Work from the UKPDS has shown that glucose level is an independent risk factor for PAD in both type 1 and type 2 diabetes mellitus and that a reduction of 1 percent in the HbA1C is associated with a 21 percent reduction in complications.[22,26] However, the benefit of good glucose control on the modification of macrovascular disease does not appear to be as beneficial as the effect on microvascular disease.

HYPERLIPIDEMIA AND HYPERCHOLESTEROLEMIA

Hyperlipidemia and hypercholesterolemia are established risk factors for the development of atherosclerosis and coronary artery disease.[1] The Framingham Heart Study suggested that it is also a risk factor for PAD.[13] The post-hoc analysis showed that a fasting cholesterol >7 mmol/L doubled the risk of intermittent claudication. The ratio of LDL to HDL was also identified as an independent variable hence the term dyslipidemia. These findings were supported by the Edinburgh Artery Study.[14]

HYPERTENSION

Hypertension is a common public health problem, affecting up to about 24 percent of the adult population suffering from this condition. The Framingham Heart Study identified hypertension as a risk factor for cardiovascular disease, especially coronary artery disease and stroke, but also as an independent predictor for PAD and intermittent claudication (by about three-fold).[13] Elevated blood pressure (>160/95) is associated with a 2.5 fold increased risk in men and a 4-fold increased risk in women of PAD. Other studies have also shown an increased risk in the incidence of PAD in untreated hypertensives by up to three-fold.[27]

The Framingham Heart Study also demonstrated that treatment of hypertension is associated with a reduction in the stroke rate by 38 percent, reduction in cardiovascular deaths by 14 percent and a reduction in peripheral vascular events by 26 percent. The Blood Pressure Lowering Treatment Trialists' Collaboration group have demonstrated that even modest reductions in blood pressure (10/5 mm Hg) are associated with a reduction in stroke mortality (40%), coronary artery mortality (16%) and all cardiovascular causes (30%).[28] Further evidence was supplied by the UKPDS which showed that for every 10 percent decrease in SBP, there is a 12 percent decrease in cardiovascular risk and a 16 percent decrease in lower limb amputation or PAD-related mortality amongst diabetics.[29] In fact, the blood pressure lowering beneficial effects on cardiovascular outcomes may be more important in the diabetic population, even more than glycemic control, which as mentioned earlier is less involved in the macrovascular changes associated with diabetes.[30,31]

OBESITY AND PHYSICAL EXERCISE

Obesity forms part of an arbitrary 'metabolic syndrome' including dyslipidemia and insulin resistance. Obesity is the dominant feature in this syndrome and is possibly best identified by the waist circumference (>102 cm in men and >88 cm in women).[32] Patients with this syndrome have a 20 percent increased risk of cardiovascular disease.

A sedentary lifestyle is a known risk factor for cardiovascular disease including PAD and the benefit of exercise has long been established in post-MI patients.[33] There are similar benefits seen in PAD (see section on Treatment).

HOMOCYSTEINEMIA

Elevated serum levels of homocysteine are associated with an increased risk of cardiovascular disease and PAD (four-fold increase compared to normal levels), especially early-onset atheroma. Up to one-third of patients with PAD will have raised homocysteine levels.[34,35] One theory postulated, is that homocysteine-induced atheroma formation is secondary to impaired endothelial production of nitric oxide. Furthermore, vascular smooth muscle proliferation has been shown to be suppressed by dietary folic acid and vitamins B_{12} and B_6.[36] Therefore, it would seem reasonable to treat elevated serum homocysteine (>5 mmol/L) with folic acid especially if associated with low levels of B_{12} and folate.

OTHERS

As described earlier in this chapter, the oxidation of lipoproteins plays a role in the development of atherosclerotic plaque formation. Thus, the use of antioxidants such as vitamin C and E may have a beneficial role. One systematic review failed to support their use as modifiers in vascular disease.[37] Similarly, chelation therapy using EDTA (ethylenediamine tetra-acetic acid) as an anti-oxidation agent has also failed to show benefit in the treatment of arterial disease.[38]

CLINICAL MANIFESTATIONS, SEVERITY AND PROGRESSION OF PAD

PAD may be asymptomatic or symptomatic. In symptomatic patients, the clinical manifestations and symptoms of PAD depend on the anatomical location and the extent of the disease. As with any ischemic symptoms, pain is the dominant presentation. In general, disease confined to the aorto-iliac system will give rise to buttock, hip and thigh pain. Patients may also complain of impotence due to lack of blood flow in the internal iliac arteries. Concomitant femoropopliteal disease is quite common and therefore there may be associated calf pain. In general, patients will not get rest pain secondary to aorto-iliac disease, unless also accompanied by severe fem-pop disease. Leriche syndrome is a constellation of symptoms secondary to aortoiliac and femoropopliteal disease, including; sexual impotence, buttock and leg claudication and muscle atrophy (usually the gluteal muscles).

In patients with femoral-popliteal and tibial disease, the classic presenting symptom is intermittent claudication (IC). IC is defined as a muscle cramp-like pain (usually in the calf muscles, but this depends on the site of occlusion) that is brought on by exercise and relieved with rest. This scenario is analogous to cardiac angina, where the arterial supply of blood and oxygen is insufficient to meet the demands of the working muscles (working muscle may require an increase in blood flow by an order of about 10-fold above resting demands). This is non-critical ischemia, in that the tissues at rest have enough blood supply for viability and hence there is little immediate threat of gangrene and limb loss. In fact, the blood demand of resting muscles is so small that the resting blood flow in the common femoral artery is only in the order of 130-150 mL/min.

A crude measurement of the severity of disease in non-critical ischemia is the patient's 'claudication distance'. This is the distance on flat ground that the patient can walk before the symptoms of muscle cramp begin and also the time taken on resting for the pain to subside enough so that walking may be recommenced. A change in the claudication distance also lets the physician know if the disease is improving with treatment (i.e. walking distance is increasing) or deteriorating (decreasing walking distance over time). Rather ironically, although it is the oxygen demand of muscle that leads to claudication, generally this will be well-tolerated when there is a bulky muscle bed, as the muscle groups can generate collaterals to bypass the occlusion that has led to the symptoms in the first place. Collaterals may develop adequately to supply the muscles of the calf with a more proximal occlusion (e.g. SFA occlusion with collaterals from the profunda and geniculate branches). An occlusion within the iliac system may also generate collaterals around it. However, conservative management of an iliac stenosis is often less successful due to the larger muscle bulk in the lower limb distal to the iliac in-flow and hence higher oxygen demand from the exercising muscle.

Critical ischemia is present when the blood supply to the lower limb is severely reduced so that the demands of the resting limb cannot be met. This is characterized by rest pain, which typically starts at the most distal level, i.e. the forefoot with a risk of gangrene, infection and tissue loss. A critically ischemic limb is under immediate threat, where the blood supply to the tissues is not capable of meeting the resting oxygen demand and may manifest as rest pain, tissue loss with wet (infected) or dry (not infected) gangrene. The limb is cool, mottled, dusky and usually pulseless in the affected field with variable amounts of gangrene (Figs 15.2A and B).

Although somewhat arbitrary, the objective pressure at which a limb is considered critical is an ankle systolic pressure of < 50 mm Hg.[39] However, patients with symptoms and signs of critical ischemia may have pressures higher than this.[40] The rest pain and gangrene is usually in the distal arterial tree, hence foot pain and digital gangrene (Fig. 15.3). The limb is under immediate threat and therefore revascularization is imperative. The prognosis is much worse in the patient with critical ischemia, as there is a high-risk of amputation. As atherosclerosis is a systemic illness, these patients are also at a much higher risk of AMI and stroke.

The goals of treatment will depend on the patients level of symptoms. The treatment of patients with asymptomatic disease is controversial, but given the increased risk of AMI and stroke that these patients have, it is certainly reasonable to treat them conservatively with 'risk factor modification' and best medical therapy. This has the potential to reduce progression of their PAD as well as reducing the risk of a serious cardiovascular outcome.

The severity of PAD can be classified according to the symptoms and signs of the disease, and the two most accepted

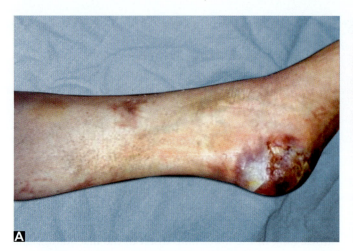
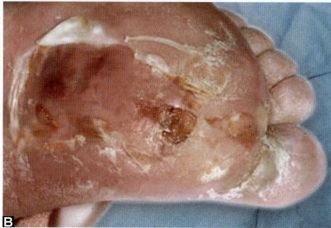

FIGURES 15.2A and B: Critically ischemic leg and foot with gangrene and tissue loss of the heel (A) and deep infection of the forefoot (B). Urgent revascularization is required if the limb is to be salvaged

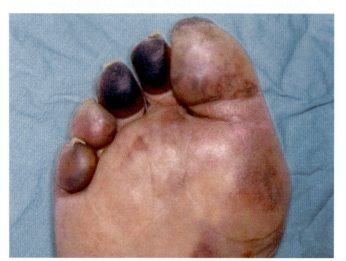

FIGURE 15.3: Forefoot ischemia with mottled skin, poor capillary refill and digital gangrene (dry)

classifications are by Fontaine or Rutherford and these are outlined in detail in Table 15.3. Classifying the disease is less important as therapeutic decisions are made on the patient's symptoms and on whether or not the ischemia present is critical or non-critical, combined with the patient's general overall health (over 50% of the mortality after treatment of PAD is cardiac in origin). In patients suffering from claudication, the aims of treatment are to relieve the exertional symptoms, increase walking capacity and improve the quality of life. These goals are the same for patients with critical ischemia, but also to relieve rest pain, heal tissue loss and ulceration, treat infection and limb salvation.

CLINICAL EXAMINATION

Many of the findings on clinical examination will depend on the site and extent of the disease and also on whether the ischemia is critical or not. An outline of clinical examination and investigations is described in Table 15.4.

INSPECTION

The affected limb will display variable degrees of hypoperfusion depending on the extent and severity of the PAD. In general, there may be a lack of hair growth (subjective and unreliable) with shiny, atrophic-looking skin over the shin and forefoot. The lower limb usually displays varying degrees of pallor, which is usually most severe distally in the foot and toes. The pallor is dependent on the position of the limb. If the severity of the disease is only mild, then the limb may only blanch on raising the leg. With more severe disease, the limb becomes white whilst lying on the flat. This finding is reflected in the Buerger's angle. This is the angle to which the leg must be raised before it becomes white, which is directly related to the perfusion pressure of the limb. The height in centimeters between the sternum (with the patient lying flat) and the heel on elevation of the foot approximates to the perfusion pressure in the foot vessels in mm Hg. An angle of 15 to 30 degrees corresponds with an ischemic leg. Below this would reflect a sub-critical perfusion pressure.

Table 15.3: Classification of the severity of PAD using the Fontaine and Rutherford classification systems

Fontaine classification		Rutherford classification	
I:	Asymptomatic	0:	Asymptomatic
II:	Intermittent claudication	1:	Mild claudication
IIA:	Mild	2:	Moderate claudication
IIB:	Disabling	3:	Severe claudication
III:	Rest pain	4:	Ischemic rest pain
IV:	Non-healing ulceration	5:	Minor tissue loss; non-healing ulceration; focal gangrene
	Gangrene	6:	Major tissue loss
			Extending above TM level

Table 15.4: Physical examination and relevant investigations for PAD

Clinical examination

Inspection	Shiny atrophic skin. Hair loss. Skin color (pallorcyanosis). Underfilled veins (guttering). Gangrene. Tissue loss. 'Sunset foot'
Palpation	Skin temperature (including gradient). Capillary refill (normal <2 seconds). Pulses (aorta, femoral, popliteal, AT, DP, PT)
Auscultation	Bruits (including aorta)
Adjuvant bedside tests	Blood pressure measurement. Hand-held Doppler examination. ABPI measurements. Buerger's angle*. Buerger's test and reactive hyperemia time. Examination pre- and post-exercise.

Investigations

Noninvasive (Bedside and vascular laboratory)	Hand-held Doppler and ABPI, Toe pressures, Continuous wave, Doppler, Segmental pressure studies, Duplex ultrasound.
Noninvasive (specialized)	CT angiography, MR angiography
Invasive (specialized)	Angiography

*May be carried out during 'Inspection'

A pale limb may also display color changes associated with 'reactive hyperemia', and become suffused and red (see 'adjunctive tests'). As the ischemia progresses, pallor may give way to cyanosis indicating a critical degree of deoxygenated blood in the limb, which may in turn progress to black, indicating gangrene.

The veins on the dorsum of the foot may look underfilled, referred to as guttering of the veins. In fact, often after reperfusion of a limb, even if there is not a return of the pulse, the first sign of improved perfusion is 'filling of the veins'. Figure 15.4 shows a typically sub-critically ischemic leg.

Finally on inspection, there may be variable amounts of tissue loss with or without gangrene. Although gangrene is skin and tissue necrosis, ulceration may also develop in the limb with subcritical ischemia as a result of infection or minor trauma. Here, although the blood supply is capable of meeting the resting demands of the limb, it cannot meet the demands necessary for normal tissue healing and repair after trauma and infection. Such tissue loss is an indication

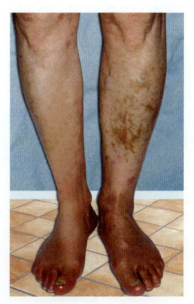

FIGURE 15.4: Typical appearance of subcritical ischemia of the legs with shiny atrophic skin, hairlessness and suffused but poorly perfused feet

for a more aggressive approach to the management of the PAD. Classically, arterial ulceration occurs at the sites of repeated daily minor trauma, most notably 'pressure points', including the heel, between the toes and over the heads of the metatarsals, especially the 1st and 5th (Figs 15.5 and 15.6). Pressure changes in an ischemic foot may manifest early as hypertrophied skin, blistering, ulceration and later frank gangrene. Gangrene may also manifest in an ischemic limb without preceding ulceration as a result of infection. This is especially problematic in diabetic patients.

One must not miss the 'sunset foot' on inspection. Here the foot, in particular the forefoot is cool and slightly cyanosed, but with a red, hyperemic look with demarcation between the critically ischemic forefoot and the better

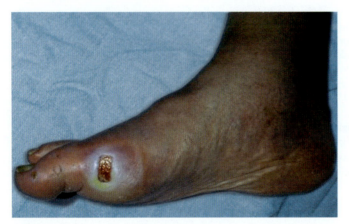

FIGURE 15.5: Pressure ulceration over outer aspect of the head of the first metatarsal

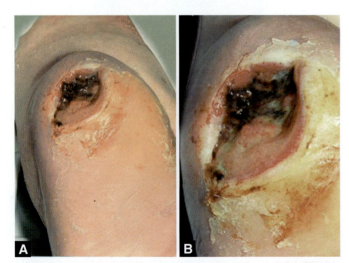

FIGURES 15.6A and B: Severe ulceration secondary to critical ischemia affecting the heel area

perfused proximal foot. This is a sign of critical ischemia, as the microcirculation is maximally dilated with little tolerance for further ischemia and must be investigated and treated aggressively.

PALPATION

The hypoperfused foot is cool and such skin temperature should be compared at the same points along the limb between both legs. A temperature gradient can often be appreciated as the palpating hand moves from the proximal portion of the limb towards the foot (using the dorsum of the fingers). The capillary refill time should also be palpated for by pressing on the tip of the toe or the nail for 2-5 seconds, allowing it to blanch. Upon release of this pressure, count in seconds the time it takes for the skin to return to its pre-palpation color. Perfusion time longer than 2 seconds is considered abnormal.

All pulses should be palpated for, starting proximally with the aorta to exclude aneurysmal disease, and then progressing distally to the femoral artery, popliteal artery and the posterior tibial, anterior tibial and dorsalis pedis arteries. The corresponding arteries on both sides should be compared which may give an indication as to the level of disease in the affected limb. It is important to remember that a patient complaining of intermittent claudication may have palpable pulses at rest which disappear on exercise, if the predominant occluding lesion is proximal iliac artery disease. In this situation, it may be necessary to palpate the pulses after exercise, for example after walking the patient or after tip-toe exercises (in the fairly immobile patient).

AUSCULTATION

After palpation, the aorta, femoral and popliteal arteries should be auscultated for bruits which may indicate a significant stenosis or aneurysmal disease with turbulent flow.

ADJUVANT TESTS

As described above, Buerger's angle should be sought and Buerger's test performed. Buerger's test is essentially pallor on elevation of the limb followed by abnormal rubor on dependency of the limb. A low angle corresponds to severe ischemia. Following this, the hyperemia test should be performed. Whilst lying flat, the patient's legs are elevated by the examiner to determine Buerger's angle. The patient is asked to plantar-dorsiflex the ankles repeatedly to simulate an increased exercise demand on the limb. This should be done for about 20 repititions. Often the limb becomes even more pale, possibly cyanosed and cold as the demand for blood outstrips supply. Immediately following this, the patient is asked to sit over the edge of the bed with the legs in a dependent position. The feet will become erythematous-looking as a result of reactive hyperemia. The time taken for this to occur reflects the severity of the occlusive disease. However, in severe cases, the limb may never become hyperemic-looking as no blood can reach the foot. Also, in chronic, severe PAD, especially in diabetic patients, this hyperemic change may not occur, as the blood vessels have already lost their sympathetic tone and are already maximally dilated.

An exercise challenge may also be used to define the site and severity of an occlusion. This is often suited to the patient with a very proximal occlusion, e.g. aortoiliac disease where there is sufficient blood flow through the lesion, or via collaterals giving palpable pulses at rest and lying flat, but who still give a good history of intermittent claudication. The patient may be asked to take a walk, ideally as close to the distance that brings on symptoms, and the pulses are examined again. Alternatively, with the patient in the examining office, he/she may undergo repeated tip-toe exercises (about 20 repetitions) and then re-examined. With symptomatic proximal aortoiliac disease, there will be a loss or decrease of pulses distal to the occlusion after exercise. A femoral bruit may also become evident. The hand-held Doppler and ABPI measurement may also be performed at rest and subsequently post-exercise challenge (see below).

MEASUREMENT OF DISEASE SEVERITY AND IMAGING

The simplest bed-side test to obtain an estimation of the severity of PAD is the Buerger's test and measurement of Buerger's angle (see last section).

HAND-HELD DOPPLER AND THE ABPI

Pulses that cannot be palpated may be identified by insonation with a hand-held Doppler (4-8 MHz continuous-wave Doppler probe). Usually some evidence of flow can be detected in the arterial tree, even in the presence of severe or critical ischemia. Therefore, insonation of pulses by hand-held Doppler alone is of limited use unless the pressures at which the pulses become audible are also measured. Normally about 90 mm Hg is needed to palpate the DP and PT pulses and about 70 mm Hg for the popliteal pulse. An ankle pressure less than 50 mm Hg is indicative of critical ischemia.

In an artery with normal compliance, the normal 'signal' using the hand-held Doppler probe is described as 'triphasic' in nature. This reflects the systolic pressure, kinetic changes and finally Doppler pressures in the arterial system. Triphasic signals signify a healthy, elastic arterial wall with no significant resistance to flow. With more rigid vessel walls, the signal may become 'biphasic' in nature with the loss of arterial wall elasticity. A monophasic waveform indicates an increased flow resistance proximal to the point of insonation. Although not an absolute indication for intervention, when taken in the correct clinical context this will signify a potentially significant occlusion that may warrant further evaluation. A very dampened and monophasic signal may also be confused with a venous signal, which may be prominent in patients with venous insufficiency or congestive cardiac failure.

The ankle-brachial pressure index (ABPI) is the ratio of the pressure at which the highest foot pulse is measured compared to the brachial pulse (which is considered the perfusion pressure at the heart). The equipment needed to measure the ABPI is shown in Figure 15.7. Ideally the patient should be well-rested and lying supine for about ten minutes in a warm room. It is important that the patient is rested to mitigate any exercise effect on the measurements. Both brachial pressures are measured by placing a standard sphygmomanometer tourniquet on the arm as normal. The cuff must measure at least 2/3 the length of the humerous and be 50 percent wider than the limb diameter to minimize false positive artefact. The cuff is inflated above systolic pressure to obstruct flow in the brachial artery and then slowly deflated whilst the hand-held Doppler probe is kept in position over the brachial pulse at the antecubital fossa. The pressure is recorded at the highest pressure when flow

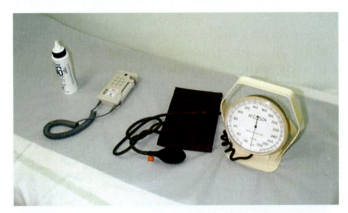

FIGURE 15.7: Equipment used to measure the ABPI, including the hand-held Doppler machine (with ultrasound gel) and a manual sphygmomanometer

resumes in the brachial artery as detected by the probe. This is repeated for both arms and the highest value is taken for calculating the ABPI.

The tourniquet is then placed around the calf of the affected limb. If there is ulceration in this area it should be covered with a simple non-adherent, non-porous material such as cling-wrap to protect the ulcerated area. Again, the same process is repeated by inflating the cuff to occlude the ankle arterial signals with the Doppler probe held in position. The pressures are measured with the Doppler probe over the DP pulse on the dorsum of the foot and PT pulse behind the medial malleolus respectively. As the cuff is deflated, the highest pressure at which a signal is insonated with the Doppler probe, is taken as the systolic pressure for the respective artery. The highest reading, DP or PT is taken to calculate the ABPI. To calculate the ABPI, the highest ankle pressure is divided by the highest brachial pressure. Although more cumbersome, occasionally the peroneal artery is also used. This can be located by placing the Doppler probe just above the lateral malleolus and slowly moving the probe in a cephalad direction along the line of the fibula until the pulse is detected.

The differential pressure gradient between the brachial pulse and the ankle pressures will reflect the severity of perfusion. The normal ABPI is 1.0 – 1.2. Less than 0.9 is considered abnormal and indicates arterial disease. Claudication will occur with an ABPI of less than 0.7 and less than 0.4 is associated with critical ischemia (Table 15.5). An exercise challenge (as described above) may also be performed on patients with normal or close to normal ABPI measurements, but with the clinical suspicion of proximal aortoiliac occlusion. The ABPI is then re-measured immediately on stopping exercise with no rest period and compared to those measured previously with the patient at rest.

Very calcified arteries may give rise to a falsely elevated ABPI as the occlusion pressure of the vessel is abnormally high due to increased arterial wall rigidity. This is typical of long standing diabetes and chronic renal failure and therefore ABPI measurements are less helpful in this group of patients. In fact, it is not unusual to be unable to compress the arteries in the lower limbs due to extensive wall calcification, and hence, the ABPI cannot be measured. Another group of patients with whom the ABPI measured is not reliable is with subclavian artery occlusion (e.g. due to atherosclerosis or thoracic outlet syndrome). Therefore both arms should be measured if there is a clinical suspicion.

Doppler signals may also be employed as part of Buerger's test. The pedal signal is measured with the patient supine and upon elevation of the limb. The angle of the limb at which the signal disappears is the ischemic angle. Obviously the smaller the ischemic angle, the more severe the ischemia.

Toe pressures may be useful in patient with incompressible, calcified arteries or when very distal disease is the likely source of ischemia. Again, a rested patient in a warm room is essential to avoid a false-positive reading. A specific digital occlusion cuff (2-3 cm wide) is placed around the proximal toe with a measuring device attached to the distal portion of the digit (e.g. photoelectric cell or mercury strain gauge plethysmograph). Photoplethysmography via the photoelectric cell is used to detect the disappearance and reappearance of the toe pulse as the cuff is inflated and deflated. The recorded toe pressure is expressed as a ratio to the brachial pressure similar to ABPI and are normally lower (0.8-0.9), but should be greater than 0.7. Critical ischemia may occur with a toe-brachial pressure < 0.3 or an absolute toe pressure of < 30 mm Hg.

CONTINUOUS WAVE DOPPLER

Continuous wave Doppler uses the same principle as the hand-held Doppler except that it uses spectral analysis to study the waveforms created within the vessel. As described above, the resistance in a normal peripheral artery is high and triphasic in character. This triphasic component may be seen on the Doppler machine consisting of the high velocity of systolic forward flow, followed by the early flow reversal at the beginning of diastole (elastic recoil) followed by low velocity late forward flow of late diastole. With increasing stenosis of an artery, the waveform downstream will be 'dampened', becoming biphasic (distal to 50% stenosis) and later monophasic (distal to 70% stenosis) with a lower amplitude antegrade flow with loss of early reversal component. If the peak systolic velocity at the site of a lesion increases by more than 100 percent then the lumen is likely to be narrowed by at least 50 percent.

The waveforms shape and characteristics displayed at a vessel lesion reflect both the degree of stenosis at the lesion as well as the level of resistance further downstream which is also affected by temperature, arterial dilatation, recent exercise and the presence of multi-segmental disease.

Table 15.5: Summary of ABPI readings and their clinical significance	
Normal	1.0–1.2
Claudication	< 0.7
Rest pain	< 0.4

SEGMENTAL PRESSURE STUDIES

Segmental pressures may also be used to map out and localize the site of significant stenosis. In this case, the blood pressure cuff (of an appropriate size) is placed around the leg at various points, including high calf, low thigh and high thigh and repeating the pressure measurements using the continuous wave Doppler as described above to see where the greatest drop in pressure is. A pressure drop of more than 20 mm Hg between two segments is considered significant. The same principle as measuring the ABPI can also be used, in that the three measurements taken during segmental pressure studies may be divided by the brachial pressure in an attempt to localize the greatest pressure drop, and hence, stenosis. If there is a fall in the ratio of greater than 0.2 between two cuff measurements, then this indicates a significant segment of disease.

ARTERIAL DUPLEX ULTRASOUND

Duplex ultrasonography uses a combination of gray-scale imaging, color flow Doppler mapping and pulse Doppler velocity measurements. Therefore, both visualization of the artery and hemodynamic assessment of the blood flow within the vessel is possible in a continuous fashion. Figure 15.8 shows a typical Duplex ultrasound machine that may be employed either in the outpatient setting or vascular laboratory.

Gray-scale imaging (B-mode) converts ultrasonic echoes from tissue into a two-dimensional image, the brightness of which is dependent on the intensity of the reflected signal. This allows the artery and its wall to be seen as well as the

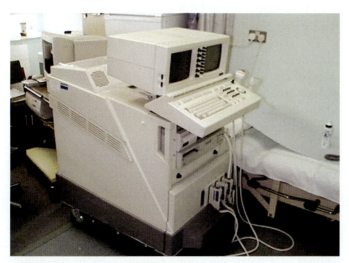

FIGURE 15.8: Typical Duplex Doppler machine used to visualize the arterial tree and flow-velocities

stenosis and character of the plaque. Both color-flow and pulsed Doppler are added to the images to gather information on blood flow within the tissues. Color-flow Doppler will enhance the image further by showing in color where there is blood flow versus non-moving areas such as thrombus. The color of the moving blood will also change with increasing blood flow velocities (e.g. across a stenosis). Hence, a picture of the vessel will be constructed on the computer screen in gray-scale with the flowing blood as a mosaic of colors (changing velocities) in between. This gives a very accurate picture of the diseased segment of artery. As blood flowing towards the probe moves faster than blood flowing away, these will register as differing colors. Traditionally if the image is red, then it is flowing towards the probe and blue if flowing away (Think: BART—Blue Away, Red Towards).

Pulsed (gated) Doppler allows the ultrasound signal to be directed to a specific depth. The change in frequency of the transmitted signal is determined by many factors, including the velocity of the blood flowing across a lesion. Hence, the peak systolic velocity may be measured in the normal proximal artery, across the lesion and distal to the lesion. The increase in velocity across a lesion is proportional to the severity of the stenosis. For example, an increase in velocity of two-fold corresponds to a stenosis of 50 percent. A 2.5 fold increase indicates a stenosis of greater then 50 percent. The distal velocity will in turn be reduced with a dampened waveform. In general, a ratio of 3 or greater is considered a clinically significant stenosis.

Duplex ultrasonography of the aortoiliac system can be difficult, even for experienced ultrasonographers, due to the depth of the vessels and the presence of overlying bowel gas and shadows cast by other pelvic organs. The sensitivity and specificity in this area has been reported as 89 percent and 90 percent respectively.[41] Duplex assessment of the leg vessels is considered more accurate and is comparable to conventional angiography, with a sensitivity and specificity of 84-87 percent and 92-98 percent respectively.[41-43] The calf vessels are more difficult to image compared to the thigh vessels, especially in the presence of proximal disease.[44,45]

ANGIOGRAPHY

Angiography is considered the 'gold standard' in the assessment of arterial disease. Since there are other less invasive techniques for assessment available now, angiography should really be confined to those patients with whom either further intervention is likely or can be

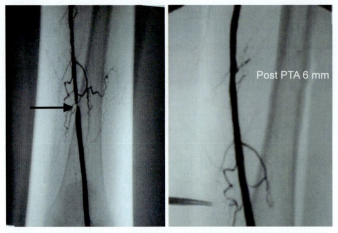

Post PTA 6 mm

FIGURE 15.9: Angiogram pre- and post-angioplasty of distal SFA lesion (arrow)

achieved by angio-catheterization (Fig. 15.9). Hence, there is now a greater tendency to perform both a diagnostic angiogram with a therapeutic procedure (e.g. angioplasty and/or stent insertion) at the same cath-lab visit. With conventional angiography, contrast media is injected directly into the vessel after needle catheterization (usually by the Seldinger technique) and usually via the transfemoral route (lower complication rate: 1.7%). The procedure is invasive with a risk of arterial wall damage and thromboembolism. Other risks include: subintimal dissection, inadvertent venous puncture, nerve trauma, arteriovenous fistula formation, infection, plaque and cholesterol embolization, limb loss and complications from the contrast medium used.

Modern contrast media used are iodine-containing, non-ionic, hypo-osmolar agents (e.g. Omnipaque™). Although safer, these substances still carry a risk of both nephrotoxicity and allergic reaction of about 1/1000 (rash, urticaria and bronchospasm) and even anaphylaxis (1:40,000). The risk of an allergic reaction does not appear to be dose-related and is probably as a result of mast cell degradation (type 1 allergic reaction). The traditional ionic contrast media carried a risk of anaphylactic reaction of 0.01-0.02 percent, but the modern non-ionic, hypoosmolar agents are thought to be much safer. The risk of an allergic reaction is higher if the patient has a history of atopy (especially shell-fish and iodine allergy) and therefore precautions should be taken (e.g. steroid prophylaxis). Treatment of an anaphylactic reaction, should it occur includes; oxygen therapy and airway management as appropriate, intravenous fluids to treat hypotension, intravenous steroid loading, nebulized B-agonists and epinephrine treatment. Further treatment may

include the use of anti-histamines, H1 blockers, H_2 blockers and intravenous glucagon for refractory hypotension.

The nephrotoxicity seen after intravenous contrast injection is usually transient (peaks at about 48 hours post-procedure) and is of little significance in patients with previously normal renal function.[46] The degree of renal impairment seen after contrast administration is related to the extent of the pre-existing renal impairment, the dose of contrast material used and the state of hydration of the patient. Other risk factors include advanced age (>70 years), presence of congestive cardiac failure and concomitant use of other potentially nephrotoxic medications (e.g. nonsteroidal anti-inflammatories, ACE inhibitors). Thus, if possible, prior to angiography, any nephrotoxic agents should be temporarily stopped (but not aspirin) if safe to do so and the smallest dose of a low osmolar, non-ionic agent should be used. In general, good fluid management will mitigate the effects of the contrast material on renal function. If the patient has normal renal function, is generally well and hydrated, then normal oral fluid intake should suffice. If there is evidence of decreased renal function (raised creatinine), then intravenous fluid administration before (at least 6 hours) and after (for at least 12 hours) the injection of contrast should suffice. There is also some evidence that the administration (either orally or intravenously) of N-acetylcysteine has a nephroprotective effect in contrast-induced toxicity, especially with pre-morbid evidence of renal dysfunction.[47] With high creatinine levels > 300 mmol/L then an alternative imaging medium should be strongly considered (e.g. gadolinium, carbon dioxide) and the advice of a nephrologist sought. In all cases the risk/benefit ratio must be weighed up and full informed consent taken from the patient.

Patients taking metformin also need special consideration. A rare toxic side effect of metformin is metabolic acidosis secondary to lactic acid accumulation. As metformin is exclusively cleared by the kidneys, then the administration of contrast media may increase the risk of a lactic acidosis, especially if there is also a degree of renal impairment. As well as taking the precautions outlined above into consideration, the metformin should be stopped up to 48 hours prior to angiography or the patient switched to another diabetic treatment regimen. The advice of a diabetologist may be sought if in doubt.

Other potential side effects of contrast media administration include: nausea and vomiting, flushing and feelings of a warm senzation, metallic taste in the mouth and rarely cardiac arrhythmias and pulmonary edema (rare and dose-related). As the contrast material is iodine-based, it should be avoided in patients suffering from hyperthyroidism. In patients with thyroid carcinoma, the use of iodinated contrast material will preclude the use of radio-iodine therapy for up to eight weeks post-administration.

The intra-arterial injection of contrast gives an outline of the arteries like a 'road-map' and any occlusions or stenosis may be visualized. Most angiographic suites are now computerized, where the contrast-enhanced image is displayed on a computer screen. 'Digital subtraction angiography' (DSA) may therefore be deployed, where a single 'mask image' is taken prior to injection of contrast. After the contrast-enhanced images are taken, the computer 'digitises' these and they are 'subtracted' from the mask image in order to remove unwanted details, such as bony detail, giving a clearer, sharper image of the arterial system. DSA also has the advantages over older, conventional angiography in that generally smaller doses of contrast media are required.

The on-table angiogram should take images of the aorta (from the level of the renal arteries) down the affected limb including the foot and arch vessels. The images above a significant lesion are described as the 'in-flow', whereas the images below a lesion are described as the 'run-off'. Good in-flow and run-off are essential for successful revascularization.

CT ANGIOGRAPHY

CT angiography is a non-catheter based imaging modality and the newer spiral (helical) CT scanners and can process numerous images to give accurate detail as the computer 'reconstructs' them to give 3-dimensional detail. The computer can reconstruct 'maximum intensity projection' (MIP) images as well as subtracts unwanted detail to produce an angiographic-like image of the arterial tree. Detail such as vessel calcification, thrombus deposition and blood flow can also be appreciated on CT angiography. Disadvantages of this technique include the use of high-dose ionizing radiation as well as the need for iodinated contrast agents (same potential risks as standard angiography described above). It is not necessarily available in every center and its accuracy over standard angiography has yet to be defined. Also, heavy calcification of a vessel is difficult to decipher from a stenosis, making a false-positive image more likely. However, it has the advantage in that being noninvasive. This may be important in the older, infirm and immobile patient where catheter-based intervention may be less desirable.

MR ANGIOGRAPHY

Magnetic resonance imaging works by placing the patient in a very strong pulsed magnetic field and creates images from the radiofrequency pulse given off by hydrogen ions as they 'spin' from one axis (while the magnet is switched on) back to their normal axis and alignment (as the magnet is switched off), giving very accurate images.

Arteries and veins as well as flowing blood may be visualized on MRI. Phase-contrast angiography detects differences in the phase of spin of the protons in blood and shows flowing blood as white on the MR image. This can be determined from the stationary tissues (black images) and can help to provide flow quantitation in the vessels. Just like CT angiography, a 3D image can be created. However, turbulence created at the level of a lesion, may give rise to an overestimation of the severity of stenosis, as there will be a 'loss of signal' distal to the turbulence which may look like black and be misinterpreted as an occlusion in the vessel. Attempts to overcome this drawback of MR angiography include the use of gadolinium as a contrast agent. Gadolinium is a para-magnetic element and is used in a 'bolus-chase' technique. A 'time-of-flight' acquisition (or in-flow angiography) is obtained where images of the vessels are taken before and after administration of the gadolinium. There is a difference in the T1 relaxation time of blood versus gadolinium and therefore these images can be subtracted from each other to increase the signal ratio between the moving blood and stationary tissue.

Disadvantages of the use of MR angiography include the overestimation of a lesion as described earlier. Also, contrast material in the venous system, especially in the smaller vessels (i.e. calf vessels) may obscure the images. Many patients cannot undergo MR imaging (e.g. metal implants such as pacemakers) and may find the MRI tunnel too claustrophobic to withstand lying in a narrow space whilst the images are taken (about 10% of patients). MR angiography is less valuable at determining in-stent stenosis and although the stainless steel stents are particularly prone to this problem, the nitinol ones also produce artefact. Although small surgical clips in the tissues are generally safe (but may produce artefact mimicking an occlusion), the presence of intracranial aneurysm clips, cochlear implants or metallic intraocular foreign bodies are a contraindication to its use.

Nephrogenic systemic fibrosis (NSF) is a rare condition which has been linked to the use of gadolinium. Symptoms may start from the day of exposure up to 3 months post-exposure. Symptoms classically begin in the legs and include pain, pruritus, swelling and erythema. It may progress onto thickening of the skin and subcutaneous tissues with fibrosis of the internal organs including the heart, liver, lungs and diaphragm. Patients can suffer contractures, cachexia and death. High risk patients appear to be those with stage 4 and 5 chronic renal disease, acute renal failure and those on dialysis as well as children under the age of 12 months, due to the immature excretion of the kidneys. No cases have been reported in patients with a GFR > 60 ml/min. Just like the use of other contrast agents, patients should be screened for the possibility of deteriorating renal function after which the risk/benefit ratio may be established. If the treating doctor continues with the examination, written informed consent should be sought and the lowest dose of agent to give optimum images should be used.

MANAGEMENT OF PAD

As stated previously, the goals in management will depend on whether the ischemia is critical or non-critical and on the general health of the patient and the ability to withstand invasive procedures especially surgery. Overall, all patients will undergo 'general management' and then the decision with regard to more invasive measures will depend on the degree of ischemia and the patient symptoms. The management of PAD is outlined in Flow chart 15.1.

GENERAL MANAGEMENT

Almost all patients will benefit from such disease modification approaches such as smoking cessation, exercise, good control of diabetes and hypertension as well as BMT.

BMT aims to modify PAD by stabilizing plaque, reducing platelet aggregation and preventing already-developed atherosclerotic lesions from progressing to complications. Even after more invasive treatment such as angioplasty, stent insertion and arterial bypass surgery, all patients should remain on the general conservative measures as well as disease-modifying medications. Such measures will not only potentially modify the course of the PAD and patient symptoms, but more importantly there will be an overall reduction in cardiovascular deaths including fatal MI and stroke.

RISK FACTOR/LIFESTYLE MODIFICATION

Although many of the risk factors for PAD cannot be altered (e.g. gender, advancing age), there are other risk factors that may be improved on, including smoking cessation, strict diabetic control, blood pressure control and lifestyle improvements such as weight loss and exercise.

SMOKING CESSATION

Cessation of smoking is probably the single biggest modifiable risk factor that the patient can undertake. More

Flow chart 15.1: Overview of management of patients diagnosed with PAD. All patients should receive conservative management. Active management will depend on the severity of disease and patient symptoms

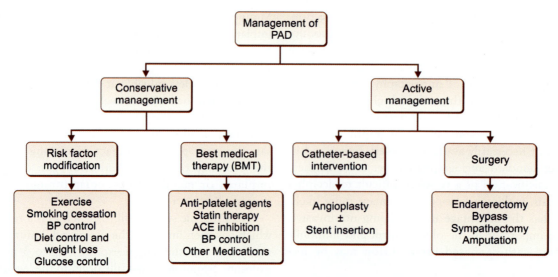

importantly, stopping smoking will reduce the incidence of cardiovascular deaths including AMI and stroke, but may also help in reducing the patient's claudication symptoms. Smoking cessation will also improve the outcomes of any likely intervention.[20] As smoking is highly addictive, many patients find giving up very difficult. Nicotine replacement therapy has been shown to significantly affect smoking cessation habits in motivated patients, improving the odds of quitting by about 1.2-2 fold.[21]

BLOOD PRESSURE CONTROL

The Framingham Heart Study confirmed that hypertension is a predisposing factor for PAD, with BP measurements >160/95 mm Hg increasing the risk by × 2.5 in men and × 4 in women over a 26-year period. Even modest reductions in blood pressure (i.e. 10/5 mm Hg) were associated with a decrease in stroke mortality by 40 percent, decrease in coronary artery disease mortality by 16 percent, decrease in all cause cardiovascular events by 30 percent and a decrease in PAD events by 26 percent. The conclusion from this study was to aim for a blood pressure of less than 140/85 mm Hg in treated individuals.

GLUCOSE CONTROL

This is a little more controversial, as the PAD disease seen in diabetics is already well established over many years of hyperglucosemia and therefore, improving glucose control over a short period of time may not alter the disease course. The major benefits in glucose control in diabetic patients appear to be in the microvascular protection and prevention of neuropathy and secondary foot complications and not for the macrovascular disease.

EXERCISE

Exercise will improve overall cardiorespiratory health as well as a treatment for PAD. A meta-analysis of exercise regimens studies has demonstrated a benefit of walking in patients with PAD by up to 150 percent.[48] This improvement is certainly comparable to other treatments for PAD, including angioplasty and best medical therapy. The benefit of exercise is probably more important for general cardiac health and the recommended exercise routine is walking for up to 30 minutes at least three times per week for six months. This arbitrary routine has never been scrutinized properly. However, the Cochrane review did report that walking to near maximum pain produced best results, which is also supported by other studies.[49]

The conclusion from the Cochrane analysis that a prescribed exercise regimen had better outcomes than angioplasty was also supported by Perkins et al. This study concluded that exercise, especially when disease was confined to the superficial femoral artery, conferred a better outcome with regard to walking distance compared to angioplasty at 1 year. However, there was no difference on follow up at 70 months, perhaps due to reduced compliance in the exercise group.[50] Whyman et al showed that angioplasty was better at six months, but that there was no difference on follow up at 2 years.[51,52] Furthermore, iliac lesions are best treated with angioplasty than exercise alone.[50]

BEST MEDICAL THERAPY

Best medical therapy (BMT) refers to agents that have shown benefit in clinical studies in the treatment of PAD. These agents include: angiotensin converting enzyme inhibitors, statins and antiplatelet agents.

ANGIOTENSIN CONVERTING ENZYME INHIBITORS

The renin-angiotensin system is an important regulator within the cardiovascular system, especially with regard to blood pressure and homeostasis. However, it also exerts important autocrine effects within the vascular tree, where its effects are found in both the endothelium and smooth muscle cells.[53,54] Angiotensin-converting enzyme (ACE) is a membrane-bound dipeptidyl peptidase that converts the inactive angiotensin I (AI) to the active angiotensin II (AII) and inactivates bradykinin. There are two receptors to which AII binds to: AT_1 and AT_2. The AT_1 receptor is primarily found on SMCs and the AT_2 receptor on ECs.[55,56]

During periods of cardiovascular stress, injury and inflammation, levels of ACE increases within vascular tissue. In normal vascular tissue the ratio of AT_1/AT_2 is greater. However, there is a reversal of this ratio in vascular disease with an up-regulation of AT_2.[57,58]

There is good evidence that patients with symptomatic PAD will benefit from ACE inhibitor therapy in addition to good blood pressure control. The HOPE study (Heart Outcomes Prevention Evaluation) conferred the protective effects of ACE inhibition (ramipril) in reducing cardiovascular events in treated patients who had established vascular disease or were considered high-risk (e.g. diabetic patients).[59,60] Interestingly, its benefits were irrespective of blood pressure control and normotensive patients with PAD also had significant reduction in cardiovascular outcomes when treated with ACE inhibition. Evidence from the PROGRESS trial also conferred the positive benefit in normotensive patients treated with an ACE inhibitor. ACE inhibition in diabetic patients also slows the onset of microproteinuria and renal disease, which in itself is an independent risk factor for vascular disease.[61]

Many patients are intolerant of ACE inhibition and instead are more suited to angiotensin-receptor-2 blockade (A2RB). The ONTARGET study was a large randomized controlled trial comparing ACE inhibition with A2RB in patients with established cardiovascular disease of high-risk diabetic patients (evidence of end-organ damage).[62] The results were similar between both groups of patients with regards to efficacy, although hypotensive episodes were more common in the A2RB group. Probably ACE inhibitors should be tried in the first instance and A2RB agents for those intolerant of ACE inhibition.

HMG-CoA REDUCTASE INHIBITORS (STATINS)

HMG-CoA (3-hydroxyl-3-methylglutaryl-coenzyme A) reductase inhibitors, also known as 'statins', have demonstrated enormous benefit in cardiovascular disease. Statins are specific, reversible competitive inhibitors of the enzyme HMG-CoA. This enzyme converts HMG-CoA to mevalonic acid, which is the rate-limiting step in the synthesis of cholesterol.[63] This inhibition leads to a decrease in cholesterol synthesis by the liver, which in turn leads to an up-regulation of low density lipoprotein (LDL) receptors, thus leading to an increased plasma clearance of LDL as well as decreased plasma cholesterol levels.[63] Although the main biochemical effect of statins is a reduction in plasma LDL, it also reduces plasma triglyceride concentrations and increases high density lipoproteins (HDL).[63]

More recently, the non-lipid lowering properties of statins have been described. These further contribute to their favorable cardiovascular profile. These auxiliary pleiotrophic effects include anti-inflammatory properties (especially within the vascular endothelium), improved endothelial function, reduced platelet aggregation, atherosclerotic plaque stabilization, anti-thrombotic activity and anti-proliferative properties.[64]

Hypercholesterolemia undoubtedly contributes to the development of atherosclerosis, including PAD. The Framingham Heart Study demonstrated that a fasting cholesterol level >7 mmol/L doubled the risk of intermittent claudication and that the LDL/HDL ratio was as important

as the actual serum cholesterol level in the prediction of PAD.[65]

Numerous trials have demonstrated the benefit of statins in the medical management of vascular disease. The British Heart Protection Study was a randomized controlled trial (n > 20,000) comparing simvastatin (40 mg) with placebo. Treatment with a statin significantly reduced late cardiovascular deaths and conferred a relative risk reduction for cardiovascular outcomes, including any major coronary event, stroke and the need for revascularization at five years by almost 25 percent. These benefits were irrespective of age (up to about 80 years), gender or cholesterol levels, thus supporting the non-lipid-lowering benefits of statin therapy.[66]

The 4S Trial (Scandinavian Simvastatin Survival Study) and CARE Trial (Cholesterol and Recurrent Events study) studied simvastatin and pravastatin respectively in post-MI patients. These studies conferred a 30-40 percent decrease in fatal and non-fatal cardiovascular events and stroke. The incidence of new-onset or worsening claudication was also lower in the statin-treated groups compared to the placebo treated groups in the 4S Trial.[67,68] Although statins may help to stabilize PAD with improvement in symptoms,[69] the major benefit in using statins in this group of patients is in its cardiovascular and stroke outcomes.[70]

ANTI-PLATELET AGENTS

Aspirin is a non-steroidal anti-inflammatory agent that acts by irreversibly inactivating both cyclooxygenase (COX) enzymes (COX-1 and COX-2). COX-1 is a principal enzyme involved in the platelet aggregation. Once inactivated by aspirin, platelets will remain inactivated for up to 10 days.[71] The primary prostanoid produced by the action of COX-1 is thromboxane A2 (TxA_2). TxA_2 is a potent vasoconstrictor and platelet aggregator. However, low dose aspirin (e.g. 75 mg once daily) will inhibit COX-1 more in platelets than endothelial cells, with higher doses inhibiting the endothelial cell derived PGI_2. As such, aspirin is both an anti-platelet agent and anti-inflammatory agent (albeit weak). PGI_2 inhibits platelet aggregation and disaggregates pre-formed platelet clumps (aspirin will potentially abolish this action). However, endothelial cells can quickly synthesise more PGI_2 after inhibition by aspirin, but platelets fail to synthesize more TxA_2, due to the lack of a cell nucleus (TxA_2 does not recover until the affected cohort of platelets is replaced in about 7-10 days), and thus the net effect of aspirin is platelet inhibition.[72]

The Anti-Platelet Trialists Collaboration Study was one of the original studies to investigate the benefits of anti-platelet agents and cardiovascular disease. It demonstrated a significant reduction in non-fatal MI, non-fatal stroke and all vascular deaths when treated with low-dose aspirin.[73] In the subset of patients with PAD, there was a relative risk reduction in any serious vascular event by 23 percent. Just like with statin therapy, the major benefit with aspirin in patients with PAD is not in its ability to retard the progression of the PAD, but in the reduction of cardiovascular death, non-fatal MI and stroke. However, there is some evidence, albeit weak that anti-platelet therapy may slow down the angiographic evidence of PAD.[74]

The recently published POPADAD Trial was a Scottish trial investigating the role of aspirin and/or antioxidants in high-risk but asymptomatic vascular patients as a primary preventative agent.[75] The study included diabetics and asymptomatic patients with objective evidence of PAD (ABPI <1.0). Interestingly, aspirin did not significantly improve cardiovascular outcomes as compared to placebo in these patients. The findings of the POPADAD Trial were also substantiated by the JPAD Study and thus its role in cardiovascular disease is probably best restricted to symptomatic patients and/or patients with evidence of significant cardiovascular disease.[76]

Dipyridamole is a phosphodiesterase V and adenosine uptake inhibitor and acts both as a vasodilator and anti-platelet agent, although its role as an anti-thrombotic agent is weak when used alone.[77] Dipyridamole interferes with platelet function by increasing the cellular concentration of cyclic AMP. This effect is mediated by inhibition of cyclic nucleotide phosphodiesterase and/or blockade of adenosine uptake. Dipyridamole probably has little use as a single anti-platelet agent, even in those intolerant of aspirin. However it has added benefit in addition to another anti-platelet agent, especially in the management of stroke. The European Stroke Prevention Study suggests that dipyridamole plus aspirin reduces the incidence of stroke in patients with prior stroke or transient ischemic attack.[78]

Ticlopidine and clopidogrel are thienopyridine compounds with both anti-inflammatory and anti-platelet properties. They inhibit platelet activity via the inhibition of the adenosine diphosphate receptor (ADP-selective anti-platelet agent) on the platelet cell membrane (P2Y$_{12}$ receptor).[77] By blocking this receptor, activation of the glycoprotein IIb/IIIa pathway is prevented, which in turn inhibits platelet aggregation and activation.[77] Clopidogrel is a ticlopidine analog and a pro-drug and is seven times more potent than ticlopidine, but with less documented side effects.[79]

In general, clopidogrel is used in the secondary prevention of vascular events, either in combination with other antiplatelet agents or alone, especially in patients intolerant of aspirin. The CHARISMA study suggested that clopidogrel used in combination with aspirin does not offer any advantage over aspirin alone, even in high-risk patients.[80]

The CAPRIE study enrolled >19,000 patients, including stroke, MI and PAD. It demonstrated a small, but statistically significant net benefit of clopidogrel over aspirin for all composite vascular end-points [absolute relative risk (ARR) 0.51%], which translates into a relative risk reduction of 8.7 percent and a number needed to treat (NNT) of 196. However, the largest benefit was in the subset of patients with PAD.[81] Currently, aspirin is the first line anti-platelet agent in the management of PAD, but for those intolerant or after endovascular intervention; clopidogrel is recommended, even in the short term. Recently, concern regarding protein pump inhibitors (PPIs) and clopidogrel have come to light. Clopidogrel is a pro-drug, dependent on the cytochrome P450 enzyme CYP2C19 for activation, which is inhibited by PPIs. Two studies have now reported a higher risk of re-infarction and cardiac events in those on clopidogrel and a PPI (RR of almost 25% in one study!).[82,83] Therefore, patients taking clopidogrel who may also be taking a PPI should have their gastric protection agent changed to a H$_2$ antagonist (although pantoprazole may be safe).

OTHERS

Cilostazol is a cAMP (cyclic adenosine monophosphate) phosphodiesterase (type III) inhibitor. It inhibits platelet aggregation and is a direct arterial vasodilator and is currently approved for the treatment of intermittent claudication with good improvements in both quality of life and walking distances.[84,85] Treatment with 50-100 mg twice daily may improve both the pain-free walking distance as well the maximum walking distance experienced by claudicants. Potential drawbacks of treatment include headache, flushing and diarrhea.

There is little data to support the use of other vasoactive agents in the treatment of symptomatic PAD such as pentoxifylline, inositol nicotinate and cinnarizine. However, the agent naftidrofuryl has shown some significant improvement in pain-free walking distance, although the absolute benefit is small.[86]

ADVANCED MANAGEMENT OF PAD: ENDOVASCULAR TREATMENT AND SURGERY

Advanced management of PAD includes interventional techniques (angioplasty and/or stent insertion) and surgery. Surgery may involve resection of an atherosclerotic lesion (i.e. endarterectomy) with or without patch grafting (to reduce stenosis) and bypass grafting. The results of both are comparable and will be discussed in more detail below.

ENDOVASCULAR TREATMENT

In general, this uses the same techniques as a diagnostic angiogram and should be done at the same time as the diagnostic study in order to minimize patient complications that would occur with two separate studies. The artery is accessed using the Seldinger technique, usually via the common femoral artery, which may be accessed on the ipsilateral or contralateral side of the lesion. Usually, the contralateral limb is preferred. Ultrasound may be used to gain access to the artery if it is poorly palpable and to minimize the risk of cannulating the common femoral vein, injury to the femoral nerve or extravazation of contrast into the subcutaneous tissues. Puncture may be described as 'antegrade' or 'retrograde' access. Antegrade puncture (used on the ipsilateral leg) aims the puncturing needle in the direction of arterial flow and is generally more difficult and also runs the risk of causing a retroperitoneal hematoma if cannulated above the level of the inguinal ligament. Retrograde puncture cannulates the artery against the direction of flow. Occasionally retrograde puncture of the popliteal artery is necessary to gain access to the femoral artery. Transbrachial and occasionally transaxillary access may also be used.

After cannulation, a soft guidewire (PTFE coated), usually with a straight or J-tip (to minimize the risk of intimal damage) is inserted and the catheter is passed over this and the guide-wire removed. The standard size guidewire is 0.035 inches in diameter and 180 or 260 cm long. Generally the tortuous nature of the vessels of the lower limb requires a stiff wire to negotiate the vessels (e.g. Amplatz wire). A sheath (11 cm long, 5-6 Fr) is placed over the guide wire and left *in situ* for further instrumentation with the angiocatheters as well as contrast medium injection via a side-arm. The one-way valve mechanism at the end of the sheath prevents back-flow of blood out through the sheath.

There are a wide variety of angioplasty balloons available (3-10 mm in diameter) and with varying balloon lengths.

Treatment is then dependent on the site and type of lesion as well as the available equipment and experience of the personnel. Endovascular treatment is useful in treating aorto-iliac lesions, fem-pop lesions and below-knee vessel occlusions and each of these will require a different size balloon and variable lengths. Ideally, the balloon should cover the entire length of the lesion for angioplasty, to reduce the number of attempts and potential complications, but clearly in long, complex lesions, this may not be possible. The guide wire is passed beyond the stenosis and the catheter-containing balloon passed along the guidewire and into position. After full heparinization, the balloon is then inflated (up to 3 – 20 atmospheres) for up to 1-3 minutes to widen the occlusion and allow blood flow.

The balloon should be seen to expand fully, thereby expanding the lesion. Occasionally, the balloon is seen as only partially expanded at one section against the hard, calcified plaque and this is described as 'wasting' of the balloon. Generally, the success of the procedure is described by the radiographical findings at the time of treatment and may be 'fully successful' (<50% stenosis remaining after angioplasty) or 'partially successful' (>50% stenosis remaining after treatment). The angioplasty may be tried several times, but vessel wall re-coil, arterial spasm as well as hard, calcified lesions may prevent a successful outcome. Specific complications (other than those already discussed on the section on 'angiogram') include distal embolization (of material from the atherosclerotic lesion, including thrombus or cholesterol) and *de novo* thrombus formation at the site of treatment. The clot formed may have to be removed with a 'suction' catheter. Similarly, for very hard non-compressible lesions, a 'cutting balloon' may be used to induce further trauma in the lesion to 'break it up'.

In general, angioplasty is more successful in larger vessels, such as the iliacs, as small, narrowed arteries (i.e. tibial vessels) have a higher rate of thrombosis and re-stenosis. The technical success rates are better for the treatment of a stenosis as opposed to a total occlusion, due to the difficulty traversing the lesion, but once traversed successfully the patency rates are similar. Following this therefore, long lesions have a higher failure rate from both a technical viewpoint as well as longer term outcomes. Calcified plaques are more difficult to angioplasty and cause more balloon wasting, and are more prone to complications, such as dissection and thrombosis.

As with all vascular lesion treatments, good inflow and run-off are essential to maintain a vessel pressure gradient and hence flow. Females and diabetic patients seem to have worse outcomes also. The MIMIC Trial has compared angioplasty of lower limb arteries (either aortoiliac disease or fem-pop disease) with exercise regimen and BMT without intervention in patients with mild to moderate claudication. After two years, there were significant differences in favor of endovascular treatment with regard to the initial claudication distance, absolute walking distance and ABPI measurements. These improvements were most marked for the group suffering form aortoiliac disease.[87]

SUBINTIMAL ANGIOPLASTY

Subintimal angioplasty is the technique first described by Bolia whereby the lesion undergoes angioplasty in the subintimal plane instead of directly within lumen, where the occluded vessel will not negotiate a guidewire.[88] The lesion is approached by a combined catheter-wire. The intima is deliberately dissected just at the beginning of the atherosclerotic lesion and the catheter-wire combination is manipulated into the subintimal space whereby developing a subintimal plane of dissection. Beyond the lesion, where the intima is healthy, the looped guide wire re-enters the lumen. The balloon may then be passed into this subintimal plane and angioplasty performed. Potential difficulties with this technique include, perforation of the artery and difficulty re-entering the lumen distal to the lesion.

STENTING

Stents have allowed for the treatment of more complex lesions, especially where angioplasty alone has failed to maintain a good vessel caliber. Usually if a stent is required, it is deployed immediately following angioplasty of the lesion. A stent is a metallic structure designed to maintain patency of a vessel at the site of a stenosis by the radial force it generates on the arterial wall. In theory, elastic recoil of the vessel is minimized and hence re-stenosis, although in-stent re-stenosis can occur secondary to neointimal hyperplasia. Several types of stents are in use, including; stainless steel (e.g. Palmaz stent), nitinol (e.g. SMART stent) and cobalt-chromium stent (e.g. Wallstent). Stents may be rigid and therefore 'balloon-expandable' (e.g. Palmaz stent) or flexible and self-expanding (e.g. Wallstent). The stainless steel Palmaz stent has high radial forces to keep a vessel open, but at the expense of flexibility. Nitinol on the other hand, is a nickel-titanium alloy which is also self-expanding, but with the properties of superelasticity and thermal memory and is therefore best suited for very tortuous vessels (e.g. SMART stent; Shape Memory Alloy Recoverable Technology). The Wallstent is designed from numerous intercrossing wires, like a woven mesh and has good radial strength as well as flexibility. All stents are prone to thrombus formation. In order to minimize this, the surface of the stent is electrically charged or polished to minimise activation of the coagulation cascade.

All stents cause trauma to the arterial wall and hence can activate vascular smooth muscle cells and are prone to re-stenosis, in particular from neointimal hyperplasia.[89,90] Many attempts to combat this process have been tried, but to date there have been no great successes in suppressing its formation. Attempts to suppress or limit the neointimal hyperplasia seen after stent placement have been tried using anti-proliferative agents in the form of 'drug-eluting' stents. Drug-eluting stents (DES) are coated with a polymer matrix which acts as a local reservoir for drug delivery as it incorporates the anti-proliferative agent and controls its release at the site of deployment. Commercially available DES incorporate such agents as rapamycin (sirolomus) and paclitaxel (taxol) whose anti-proliferative properties are also exploited in anti-cancer therapy, but other non-commercially available DES have also been tried experimentally including; heparin-coated and steroid-coated stents. These stents have mostly been tried in the coronary circulation, with good short-term and medium-term results, but with questionable long-term results. The SIROCCO trial was a double-blind, randomized trial (n=36) that studied the use of a Rapamycin-coated DES (SMART stent) with bare metal SMART stent for femoro-popliteal disease.[91] Follow up at six months failed to demonstrate any significant difference between the two groups with regards to the mean in-stent stenosis (P=0.29). However, the mean in-stent lumen diameter was larger for the DES treated groups, perhaps indicating more favourable longer term results for DES (P=0.047). Late follow-up (2 years) in this study failed to show any advantage of DES over BMS in PAD, because the rate of in-stent re-stenosis was so low in both groups.[92]

In recent years, the long-term safety of the DES in the coronary circulation was called into question as there were reports of higher rates of death and myocardial infarction over BMS. However, a meta-analysis published in the Lancet has shown that the mortality rates for DES and BMS are similar, with slightly better clinical outcomes for sirolomus-eluting DES over both BMS and paclitaxel-eluting DES.[93,94]

Finally, some stents are described as 'covered stents' (e.g. Wallgraft), where they are covered with synthetic biomaterial material (e.g. PTFE), thus preventing cellular in-growth like in the conventional non-covered stents. These are useful in the treatment of vessel rupture during angioplasty, which is most likely to occur in the iliac vessels (e.g. 6-8 mm diameter, 8-10 cm long covered stent).

SURGERY

As a general rule, surgery is reserved for patients in whom other measures, including endovascular therapy have failed. This isn't entirely true as TASC have recommended that type C and D lesions should undergo surgery instead of endovascular intervention due to the high failure rate and complication rate of the latter. As a general rule, lesions longer than about 10 cm will not be successfully treated by angioplasty and/or stent insertion and therefore bypass surgery is the best option. However, the principle indications for surgery include: limb salvage (often there is multilevel fem-pop-tibial disease), prevention of recurrent peripheral atheroembolization and incapacitating claudication. Good patient selection is important for good surgical outcomes.

Successful bypass surgery depends on many factors including inflow, and run-off (which should be treated or corrected either before or at the time of surgery) and the graft characteristics. In general, a vein graft is best, but its patency will also depend on the vein quality, diameter and length. In general, for infrainguinal bypass, the long saphenous vein (LSV) should be used. Studies have shown that its patency rate is similar to using the larger SFV for bypass at 3 years (60% vs. 64%, respectively).[95] Similarly, there is no difference in patency rates for reversed and non-reversed vein grafts.[96,97] In general, the vein from the same leg should be used, but if this is unsuitable, then vein from the contralateral limb may also be used, remembering that up to 20 percent of patients will eventually go on to develop critical limb ischemia in the contralateral limb which may also need a bypass procedure.[98] In this situation, arm vein may be used, with patency rates of 70 percent and 49 percent at 1 and 3 years respectively, but with higher rates of aneurysm degeneration.[99]

Synthetic grafts are either Dacron or PTFE and are best used for large diameter bypasses, as the patency rates are lower than for vein with smaller, diseased vessels.

DECIDING ON BEST INTERVENTIONAL TREATMENT AND THE ANATOMICAL CONSIDERATIONS

Numerous factors must be taken into account in deciding treatment for PAD, including patient fitness for a procedure especially surgery, how debilitating the symptoms are as well as the anatomical site of the lesion and whether it is amenable to endovascular treatment or surgery. As a general

rule, endovascular treatment is often tried first and surgery reserved for failure of endovascular therapy, or after endovascular therapy where it as used as a 'bridge' to surgery (e.g. to improve in-flow and/or heal an ulcer before undertaking complex open recon-struction).

Anatomically, PAD and its treatment may be divided into lesions above the inguinal ligament (suprainguinal) and lesions below the inguinal ligament (infrainguinal). In practice of course, a treatment may involve both, but this arbitrary division helps in deciding of the problem is primarily an 'in-flow' or a 'run-off' problem or a combination of both.

SUPRAINGUINAL TREATMENT

This is primarily concerned with the treatment of aorta, aorto-iliac and iliac disease. Treatment of aorto-iliac disease has the best long-term outcomes for both endovascular and open surgical treatment, especially if the lesion is short and confined to the iliac segment only with good run-off. An isolated aortic stenosis has excellent technical success rate and long-term patency rates for both angioplasty and stent insertion (90% for both). Surgery is generally not required because of the success of endovascular treatment and is probably confined to more complex situations, such as complete occlusion of the aorta and symptomatic distal thromboembolization. Complications of endovascular treatment include arterial wall dissection, vessel occlusion, distal embolization and vessel rupture. Poor patency rates are generally associated with poor run-off.

The Trans-Atlantic Inter-Society Consensus (TASC) in 2000 generated recommendations to define iliac disease anatomically and morphologically into types A – D which is summarized in Table 15.6. In general, type A lesions are short (<3 cm) and generally amenable to endovascular treatment, whereas a type D lesion is longer and more complex, where endovascular treatment is more likely to fail and hence surgical treatment more appropriate. Simple iliac stenosis has excellent results with balloon angioplasty with excellent patency rates at 1 year (67-80%), 3 years (60-80%) and 5 years (55-80%) compared to 1 year (68%) and 3 years (60%) for complete iliac occlusions. The technical success rate is lower for occlusive disease (83%) over stenosis (88-99%).[100]

The iliac vessels may also be stented, although the results from angioplasty alone are so good that this is usually not required, especially as stenting is associated with a higher complication rate compared to balloon dilatation alone (6.3% vs. 3.6%). Stenting may be reserved for longer, more

Table 15.6: Trans-Atlantic Inter-Society Consensus (TASC) lesions described for the aortoiliac and femoropopliteal segments

Iliac lesions	Femoropopliteal lesions
TASC A Single stenosis <3 cm of CIA or EIA	Single stenosis up to 3 cm not at SFA origin or distal popliteal
TASC B CFA not involved	3-5 cm single stenosis or occlusion
Single stenosis 3-10 cm	≤3 cm Heavily calcified stenosis Multiple lesions ≤3 cm
Two stenosis <5 cm in CIA or EIA	Single or multiple lesions with reduced run-off
Unilateral CIA occlusion	
TASC C Bilateral 5-10 cm stenosis of CIA and/or EIA	Single stenosis or occlusion >5 cm
Unilateral EIA occlusion	Multiple stenosis or occlusion,
Unilateral EIA stenosis extending into CFA	3-5 cm with or without heavy calcification
Bilateral CIA occlusion	
TASC D Diffuse, multilateral stenosis involving CIA,	Complete CFA or SFA occlusions
EIA and CFA (>10 cm)	Complete popliteal and proximal trifurcation occlusions
Unilateral occlusion of CIA and EIA	
Bilateral EIA occlusions	
Diffuse disease of distal aorta and iliacs	
Iliac stenosis and abdominal aortic aneurysm	

complex lesions or when there is residual stenosis after balloon dilatation (i.e. residual luminal diameter reduction of >30 percent and /or residual pressure gradient >10 mm Hg) or a complication of angioplasty (e.g. intimal flap or vessel wall dissection). Stenting is associated with patency rates at 1, 3 and 5 years of 78 to 95 percent, 53 to 95 percent and 72 percent respectively. As with complete occlusion of the iliac vessel, stent placement gives lower success rates of 75 percent and 64 percent at 1 and 3 years, respectively.

If a unilateral lesion is close to the aortic bifurcation, then there is a risk of distorting the contralateral iliac vessel after angioplasty or stent deployment (e.g. plaque fracture and dissection). Therefore, both sides should be stented, with so-called 'kissing stents' (or 'kissing balloons if balloon dilatation alone is carried out) to maintain patency on both sides, where there is partial projection into the distal aorta. Best published evidence has now suggested that the outcomes from balloon angioplasty alone versus angioplasty and stent placement is similar, but more costly in the stent group and therefore, stenting should be carried out on a selective basis.[101]

Occasionally, after needle puncture with on-going retroperitoneal hemorrhage from rupture of the iliac artery on dilatation, a 'covered' stent may need to be deployed to maintain patency and stop the on-going bleeding. In this situation, the internal iliac artery is often sacrificed from circulation as its origin is covered by the stent.[100]

A selection of surgical procedures may be carried out for the treatment of aortoiliac disease, including aorto-bifemoral bypass, femoro-femoral cross over grafting and axillary-femoral bypass grafting (either Ax-unifem or Ax-bifem grafting). These can be done alone or in combination with endovascular treatment. Aortofemoral grafting (either aorto-bifem or aorto-unifem) is the preferred surgical option in low-risk patients. The procedure has high patency rates (95% at 5 years) and may be performed transperitoneally, through a lower midline incision (for aortobifemoral grafting) or retroperitoneal, via an oblique incision (for aorto-unifemoral bypass grafting). Aortoiliac surgery is associated with a higher mortality (1-4%) as cross-clamping or partial cross-clamping is required as well as retroperitoneal dissection and a higher morbidity (including impotence). The proximal anastomosis should be placed as high as possible on the aorta (usually infrarenal) as this is often associated with the least disease. If the patient is also suffering from an abdominal aortic aneurysm, then this may be repaired at the same time (either by in-lay technique or end-to-end anastomosis) with a trouser graft brought down to the femoral vessels. It is also important to remain vigilant for the heavily calcified aorta, which may make an anastomosis technically very difficult, if not impossible. Grafts used are typically Dacron grafts, although the superficial femoral vein may be used for unilateral disease, especially if a concomitant amputation is undertaken on the contralateral side.

Higher risk patients with unilateral disease may have a cross-over graft performed with inflow from the

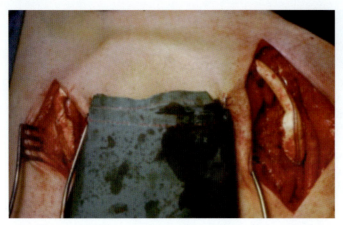

FIGURE 15.10: Both groins dissected to show femoro-femoral cross over graft using PTFE

Table 15.7: 5-year patency rates after bypass surgery and iliac angioplasty	
Aorto-bifemoral bypass	85–90% (15–20% if concurrent distal occlusive disease)
Axillo-bifemoral bypass	70-75%
Femoro-femoral bypass	80-85%
Percutaneous iliac artery angioplasty	80-90%

asymptomatic contralateral artery (iliac or femoral arteries) to below the lesion on the symptomatic leg (iliac or femoral), constituting ilioiliac (anatomical), ilio-femoral (anatomical) or femorofemoral (extra-anatomical) cross-over grafting respectively (Fig. 15.10). Although inferior to aorto-bifemoral grafting, these procedures still carry good 1-year and 5-year patency rates of 90 and 80 percent respectively. In general, an extra-anatomical bypass will have a lower patency rate, but also less morbidity as retroperitoneal dissection is not required. Cross-over grafts are typically Dacron or PTFE (8-10 mm), although vein may also be used. The tunnel may be created either subcutaneously or behind the rectus muscle.

Inflow may also be brought from the subclavian or axillary arteries (axillofemoral bypass) which may be unifemoral or bifemoral for outflow. These extra-anatomical bypass grafts are best reserved for high-risk candidates (ie: there is no intra-abdominal or retroperitoneal exposure required) and are associated with lower patency rates (5-year patency rates of 33-85%) and are therefore not really recommended for patients whose symptoms may be managed by other means or for patients expected to live longer than 5 years. Blood pressure measurement in both arms should be undertaken and ideally the arm with the higher pressure used for inflow. The artery is approached via a mid-infraclavicular incision with separation of the fibers of the pectoralis major muscle. The pectoralis minor may be divided, or the vessel dissected out medial to it. The subclavian vein is retracted downwards to gain access to the artery. The artery must be handled with care as it is quite delicate in this region. A tunneller is used to create a subcutaneous tunnel from the axillary artery to the groin. Typical grafts used are 8-10 mm Dacron or PTFE, which

should be reinforced externally to prevent compression. A general overview of the patency rates for the various treatment options are outlined in Table 15.7.

Aortoiliac endarterectomy is generally not recommended, despite the advantage of avoiding prosthetic material. It is a procedure fraught with danger and equally good results can probably be achieved with endovascular techniques. Iliac endarterectomy, however, may be performed as part of the treatment of infrainguinal disease to improve inflow to the leg.

INFRAINGUINAL TREATMENT

Treatment of infrainguinal disease may be divided into above knee (AK) arteries (common femoral artery, superficial femoral artery, profunda femoris and the AK portion of the popliteal artery) and below knee (BK) arteries (BK popliteal artery, tibio-peroneal stem, anterior tibial artery, posterior tibial artery, peroneal artery, dorsalis pedis artery and the lateral plantar artery).

Above Knee (AK) Arterial Disease

Disease in the common femoral artery (CFA) that is causing a critical stenosis is usually treated by femoral endarterectomy. This may be done is isolation or as part of a more extensive procedure to improve inflow for a more distal bypass. Typically, it is carried out through a vertical incision, gaining access and control of the CFA, SFA and profunda arteries. The artery is opened vertically and the occlusive lesion is dissected in its medial plane using a Watson-Cheyne instrument. Care must be taken to ensure the an intimal flap is not left behind, especially at the distal intima, where the pressure gradient is likely to lift this up and occlude or thrombose the vessel. The procedure may be carried further into the profunda femoris as a 'profundoplasty'. Usually the vessel is then patched to keep it widely patent. Synthetic patch (PTFE or Dacron) may be used, but the close proximity of the superficial veins as they traverse the cribriform fascia to gain access to the CFV make a venous patch more attractive.

An iliac endarterectomy may also be undertaken if this is obstructing inflow. This may be performed via the same incision in the CFA, where the atherosclerotic lesion may be removed with the use of a heavy surgical clip (e.g. Roberts) through a separate, extraperitoneal approach to the iliac artery.

Stenting of the CFA is less successful, as is stenting of the profunda artery, although they may be angioplastied, usually as 'temporising' measures before further treatment. The SFA is amenable to endovascular treatment, although the results are comparable to exercise and conservative measures and therefore may not be indicated for claudication unless very debilitating. The SFA is a smaller artery and more prone to extensive disease compared to the aorto-iliac system, and therefore the success rates for endovascular treatment are less favourable. Patency rates for SFA-AK popliteal artery balloon dilatation at 1, 3 and 5 years are 61, 51 and 48 percent respectively, but about 10 percent higher respectively if the primary failures (about 10% also) are excluded.[100] Stenting the SFA-AK popliteal system has patency rates of 67 percent and 58 percent at 1 and 3 years respectively.[100] Thus it would appear that primary stenting for fem-pop disease yields disappointing results, especially as type D lesions are more likely in this system and therefore poor run-off due to extensive multi-level disease make endovascular treatment more unsuccessful. Stenting should only be carried out as a selective procedure for complicated situations such as significant residual stenosis after balloon dilatation, intimal dissection, etc. Balloon angioplasty and stent insertion may have a more important role to play for CLI as a 'bridge' to further treatment, as the benefits over risk is different for limb salvage. More recent evidence however, suggests that primary placement of a self-expanding stent will yield better results in the intermediate term in 6 and 12 months than balloon dilatation alone.[102] However, this added expense may not make this approach justifiable.

The typical surgical intervention for AK infrainguinal PAD is the femoral-popliteal (AK) bypass procedure. Grafts that may be used include autologous vein or synthetic grafts (Dacron or PTFE). The best results are with autologous vein, usually the long saphenous vein (LSV) which may be reversed or non-reversed. If it is non-reversed, then it may be left in its anatomical bed (*in-situ*) or fully mobilized and placed deeper. By leaving it in its normal anatomical position, its nutrient supply is left fully intact, but the risk of missing a side branch on dissection is higher, thereby resulting in fistula which will need to be repaired. The other advantage of a non-reversed vein is that there is less of a size discrepancy on anastomosis. However, the intact venous valves will obstruct flow in the bypass graft and therefore need to be excised using a valvulotome. This has the disadvantage of causing intimal injury or missing a valve which may later cause obstructive flow and thrombosis of the graft. The use of a reversed vein graft will obviously avoid these risks. Both configurations require the vein to be dissected from its bed and all side branches ligated, taking care not to tie the ligature too close to the base of a side branch which may 'kink' the vein. Any inadvertent tears in the vein are repaired with a 6/0 prolene suture.

Typically the proximal anastomosis is to the CFA (after endarterectomy if needed) and the distal anastomosis to the AK popliteal artery. The AK popliteal artery may be approached from the medial side, making an incision at the lower edge of the vastus medialis muscle, which is felt as a 'groove' by the palpating hand. One may also go a little posterior to this groove, if the long saphenous vein is to be harvested. The fascia is divided below vastus medialis and above the anterior border of sartorius muscle to enter the popliteal fossa. Care must be taken to avoid the saphenous nerve. The space is deepened and widened to gain access to the popliteal artery with care not to damage the popliteal vein and sciatic nerve. After the vein is prepared, a tunneler is used to create a tunnel deep to the sartorius muscle and the distal anastomosis is completed using 5/0 or 6/0 prolene. Just like other procedures, the success of this operation is largely dependent on the inflow and run-off.

The patency results are comparable for both autologous vein and synthetic grafts at two years (75-80%), but the 4-year patency rates were 61 percent and 38 percent for vein and prosthetic grafts respectively.[103] Others have shown 5-year patency rates of 62 percent and 43 percent for vein and prosthetic grafts respectively.[104] Kumar et al compared vein grafts with both Dacron and PTFE synthetic grafts and showed 4-year patency rates of 73, 47 and 54 percent respectively.[105] The patency rates and outcomes are similar for both reversed and non-reversed vein grafts.[106,107] There appears to no advantage of PTFE over Dacron and vice versa, and therefore the choice often comes down to the surgeon's preference.[108,109]

Below Knee (BK) Arterial Disease

This includes disease in the BK popliteal artery, tibio-peroneal trunk (trifurcation disease) and any of the three run-off arteries, AT, PT and peroneal or a combination of these. In general, the patency rates and success rates are lower for BK disease and in general treatment is reserved for critical limb ischemia (rest pain, tissue loss and gangrenous ulceration) or limb salvage as opposed to claudication alone. The principle of balloon angioplasty in this region is to restore axial flow to the foot arch vessels. Smaller balloon diameters (e.g. 5 Fr) can be used for this purpose and vessels down to a diameter of 2-3 mm may be treated, by both transluminal and subintimal techniques. Limb salvage rates of 60 to 88 percent have been reported up to 2-year post-angioplasty, but the success is largely dependent on the 'run-off'.[100] Vessel spasm is more common here and is treated with vasodilators such as GTN and papaverine. Acute arterial damage and thrombosis, which if recognized at the same time, may be treated with suction thrombectomy and anti-coagulation. Stenting in this region is generally unsuccessful as is stenting of the popliteal artery, due to the repeated flexion at the level of the knee joint.

Surgical bypass procedures are also less successful in the BK segment, and therefore are confined to selected patients who either have critical limb ischemia or debilitating claudication who will maintain good post-operative mobility (Fig. 15.11). BK bypasses have a 5-year graft patency rates of 68 percent and 27 percent for venous and synthetic grafts respectively. Furthermore, up to 30 percent of successful BK vein bypass grafts will require further intervention in the future. Often when a BK graft occludes, this may be associated with a worsening of symptoms, due to a combination of factors including: damage to collaterals at the time of surgery, neointimal hyperplasia at the distal anastomosis causing worsening run-off of the limb in general and a loss of pressure gradient after successful bypass resulting in a loss of collateral supply. If possible, the vein graft may be taken from the SFA instead of the CFA to minimize length of graft. If a prosthetic graft is to be used, then an

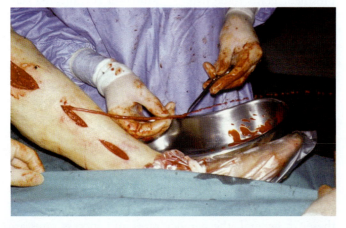

FIGURE 15.11: Lower end of vein graft demonstrating excellent forward flow for anastomosis onto the distal tibial artery

adjuvant venous cuff (e.g. miller cuff, Taylor patch or St Mary's boot) should be constructed to maintain distal patency and reduce the incidence of neointimal hyperplasia and re-stenosis which are believed to result from the compliance mismatch where graft is anastomosed directly onto artery. The use of a vein cuff is associated with higher 2-year patency rates in BK-bypasses (but not AK-bypasses) compared to synthetic grafts without a vein patch (52% vs 29% respectively).

Patency rates for BK bypasses are lower than for AK bypasses. Data from TASC has shown the 1, 3 and 5-year patency rates for tibial bypasses using vein as 85, 80 and 70 percent respectively and 70, 35 and 25 percent respectively for prosthetic grafts.[100] Other evidence has supported this and work by Hunink et al has demonstrated 5-year patency rates for vein graft (AK or BK) of 66 percent, but 47 percent for AK PTFE and 33 percent for BK PTFE.[111]

The approach to the BK vessels for bypass grafting is largely dependent on the target artery, but in general, the incision is made on the medial side. From here the BK popliteal artery, trifurcation, AT and peroneal can be approached. Usually, with the knee slightly flexed with a degree of external rotation of the hip joint, a longitudinal incision is made beginning at the level of the knee joint, just posterior to the medial femoral condyle and running straight downwards about a finger breadth posterior to the medial edge of the tibia. The BK saphenous vein can also be dissected through this incision for use in the bypass. The fascia just posterior to the tibia is then incised and the popliteal fossa entered. Usually the popliteal artery can be accessed deep in the knee recess. However, lower down to the level of the trifurcation may require dissection and division of the upper fibers of soleus muscle. The vessels can then be looped and manipulated, remembering that the popliteal vein usually covers the lower portion of the popliteal artery down to the origin of the AT artery and thus needs to be retracted to gain access. By applying downward traction on the artery with vessel loops at different levels, the AT artery will become more apparent, as it passes anteriorly from the popliteal artery in an attempt to enter the anterior tibial compartment. The interosseous membrane may need to be opened for 2-3 cm to gain further access to the AT, taking care to ligate the small veins and venae comitantes that accompany it.

Inferior to the origin of the AT is the tibioperoneal trunk. The popliteal vein may need to be retracted upwards to adequately expose the peroneal and PT artery, taking care not to damage the posterior tibial nerve which lies close by. If the PT artery is to be exposed further down (i.e.

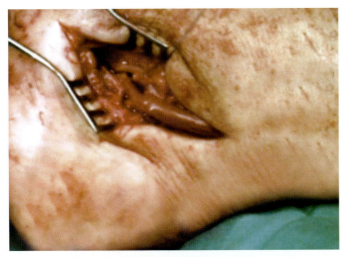

FIGURE 15.12: Vein graft anastomosis onto
the distal posterior tibial artery

PT2 or PT3 level), then a similar longitudinal incision just posterior to the medial edge of the tibia is necessary (Fig. 15.12). On dividing the fascia and separating the gastrocnemius muscle from the tibia, the PT may be exposed as it runs between the muscle and posterior surface of the bone. If the peroneal artery is to be exposed, then dissection deeper behind the tibia will be necessary from the same medical approach. The peroneal artery is seen lying between the soleus muscle and the posterior tibialis muscle in the deep posterior compartment of the leg. The vein for bypass (whether reversed or non-reversed) may be tunnelled subsartorially (if coming from the CFA) as described earlier, or lower down on the SFA (if this has good in-flow). Occasionally, the in-flow is taken from the profunda artery, exposed by a medical incision, about half way along the thigh, but above the sartorius muscle. The vein should then be tunnelled through the popliteal fossa, by blunt finger dissection, so that the distal end may be anastomosed to the BK popliteal artery. If the distal anastomosis is the PT2/PT3, then it may be tunnelled subcutaneously from the BK popliteal fossa to come to rest at the distal anastomosis site.

If the distal anastomosis is to be the AT, in particular AT2 or AT3, then this portion of artery should be approached via an anterolateral incision. Again, the knee joint is flexed, but internal rotation of the hip joint is less amenable. A similar medial exposure of the BK popliteal artery will still be necessary to tunnel the vein from above the knee and through the popliteal fossa. An incision is made on the lateral edge, about half way between the fibula

and tibia, in the natural groove that demarcates the tibialis anterior muscle from extensor digitorum longus muscle. The AT is easily exposed on separation of these two muscles along the natural plane. A tunnel may be created for the graft passing from the medial popliteal exposure to the antero-lateral AT exposure in the anterior compartment. This may be achieved using a blunt clamp to pierce the interosseous membrane, staying close to the tibia bone. The division in the membrane should be carried for a few centimeters cephalad and caudally to avoid kinking or pinching of the vein graft as it pass through.

The peroneal artery may also be approached from the lateral side, and this is probably best reserved for re-operations, where re-exposure medially is too difficult. A segmental fibulectomy is usually necessary. On exposure of the bone, a periosteal elevator is used to remove the periosteum and then using a gigli saw, the section of fibula is removed to allow greater exposure. The peroneal artery lies beneath the removed section of bone. The vein graft is tunnelled to this position as for the AT exposure.

ADJUVANT THERAPY AFTER ENDOVASCULAR TREATMENT

Acute arterial thrombosis is a risk during endovascular treatment in a freshly angioplastied lesion or after stent deployment; therefore the patient should be fully heparinized for the duration of the procedure, with a bolus and repeat if necessary. In more complex cases, or where acute thrombosis occurs, on-going post-procedure heparinization may be necessary.

It goes without saying that BMT should also be continued for these patients, especially aspirin. However, other anti-platelet agents are also used, most notably the platelet GPIIb/IIIa receptor inhibitors (e.g. tirofiban, abciximab), but use of these after treatment of PAD is not widespread. If a stent has been deployed, dual antiplatelet therapy with aspirin and clopidogrel should be undertaken for 4-6 weeks post-procedure to reduce the short-term thrombosis risk.

Numerous other therapies in the suppression of neointimal hyperplasia have been studied, but to date with little clinical success. A recently published trial investigated the efficacy of locally delivered paclitaxel during angioplasty to inhibit re-stenosis during lower limb angioplasty.[94] Both the paclitaxel-coated balloons and paclitaxel dissolved in contrast medium were evaluated in the treatment of patients with femoropopliteal disease. At six-month follow-up, there was a significant difference in the mean late-lumen loss in favor of the paclitaxel-coated angioplasty balloons, but not for the paclitaxel-contrast media. There were also significant benefits in the 6-month target re-vascularization rates for the paclitaxel-coated balloon catheters, but not for the paclitaxel-contrast media.

ADJUVANT THERAPY AFTER SURGERY

All vascular patients should be maintained on BMT after surgery, as this reduces the risk of cardiovascular death (AMI and stroke) and probably 'modifies' further atherosclerosis development which may slow down the disease process in the peripheral vessels. However, it remains an area of some controversy that following a technically successful bypass, whether anything else (i.e. pharmacotherapy) can be done to maintain graft patency. Certainly preoperative platelet inhibition is important in improving patency as it reduces platelet deposition on prosthetic bypass grafts and areas of arterial wall injury.[112] Furthermore, statin therapy appears to improve graft patency and limb salvage rates.[113]

Antiplatelet therapy in combination with warfarin appears to improve graft patency rates in high-risk patients (e.g. limb salvage, poor run-off) over aspirin alone or warfarin alone.[114,115] Anti-coagulation with low molecular weight heparin, treated for three months has also been shown to improve the 1-year patency rates in patients undergoing lower limb bypass surgery for CLI, over dual antiplatelet therapy alone.[116] It would seem reasonable therefore that both anti-platelet therapy and anti-coagulation be used in selected patients at high-risk of graft failure or after limb salvage surgery.

COMPARING ENDOVASCULAR THERAPY WITH SURGERY

Endovascular intervention is often the preferred option over open surgery as it is less invasive. However, not all lesions are amenable to successful balloon dilatation and/or stent insertion. For those lesions that are, there does not appear to be any difference in the patency rates for either technique.[117,118]

The BASIL Trial (n=452) compared angioplasty with bypass surgery in patients with CLI, with the primary end-point of amputation-free survival. After 6 months, there was no difference between the two groups with regard to the 30-day mortality or health-related quality of life. There was no difference with regard to the primary outcome variable at 30 days, 6 months, 1 year or 3 years. The two therapies appeared to be equivalent up to 2 years and post-

hoc analysis of data seems to suggest that surgery is preferable if the patient is expected to survive for 3 years or more.[119] Although there is a tendency to favor surgery, it is reasonable to undergo endovascular therapy first as it is less invasive and to proceed to surgery thereafter if the patient is fit.

GRAFT SURVEILLANCE

The general patency rates of various bypass techniques are summarized in Table 15.7. The role of graft surveillance is controversial. However, up to 30 percent of vein bypass grafts will develop a stenosis requiring treatment. Clinical examination is poor at detecting a stenosis as often the graft has become completely occluded when clinically detectable. Therefore, graft surveillance is generally recommended using duplex ultrasound and many vascular centers have protocols in place to detect a re-stenosis early so that it can be treated, before a complete occlusion occurs, which is more difficult to treat. In general, a peak systolic ratio >3 (i.e. 70% stenosis) is considered significant to warrant further treatment. Significant improvements in patency rates have been reported with a surveillance program.[120]

OTHER TREATMENTS

For many patients with critical limb ischemia, the disease is considered 'unreconstructable' and symptoms are treated with a variety of analgesics (e.g. NSAIDs, opiates) and other neuromodulator agents such as gabapentin and amitriptyline.

Other vasodilators may be tried in an attempt to 'open up' small vessels and improve overall circulation in the resting limb. The prostacyclin (PGI_2) analog iloprost has a short half-life (about 30 minutes) and may be given by intravenous infusion. It has antiplatelet and vasodilatory properties and has been shown to have lower mortality rates and lower amputation rates at 6 months when used for CLI.[121]

Lumbar sympathectomy is another way to abolish sympathetic-control over vasoconstriction thereby leaving vasodilatation as the dominant effect. This may be done by chemical means (chemical sympathectomy), whereby sclerosant is injected translumbar into the sympathetic chain on the affected side, or by open surgery (surgical sympathectomy), where the lumbar sympathetic chain is excised via a retroperitoneal approach, often with mixed results with regard to pain relief and ulcer healing.[87] A sympathectomy is less likely to work in the diabetic population, as many of these already have an 'auto-sympathectomy' secondary to diabetic autonomic neuropathy and therefore, the blood vessels may already be maximally dilated despite the critical level of ischemia.

Numerous other therapies exist including: spinal cord stimulation, hyperbaric oxygen, topical wound oxygen therapy and intermittent compression therapy. Many of these have not gained wide acceptance in clinical practice or are not readily available commercially.

AMPUTATION

In many patients with non-reconstructable disease or failed treatment of critical limb ischemia, an amputation may be necessary. Other indications may include deep necrosis and/ or infection of the foot, especially over a pressure area (e.g. non-healing ulcer of the heel), or a flexion contracture of the limb that is not correctable.

In general, the lowest level of amputation should be chosen and amputation sites are generally either below knee amputation (BKA) or above knee amputation (AKA). A BKA will generally allow the patient to ambulate on an artificial limb as the knee joint is preserved. Also, general movement and transfer are better due to longer limb preservation. The independent ambulatory rates with prosthesis are summarized in Table 15.8. An AKA if necessary is much more difficult to ambulate and the energy demand is much higher for these patients to try to walk. Energy required for walking increase by about 50 percent after a unilateral BKA, but by up to 100 percent after an AKA.

Occasionally, an AKA is selected instead of a BKA, even if a BKA is feasible. This is usually in the patient who is already wheelchair bound, as to leave a BKA stump will only result in a painful contracture and /or a pressure ulceration on the stump secondary to sitting in the chair. Also, an AKA wound is more likely to heal than a BKA wound and this must be taken into account before surgery so as to avoid infection and necrosis of the stump (Figs 15.13 and 15.14). In general a popliteal pressure of 70 mm Hg is required to heal a BKA. Advice from a rehabilitation specialist should be sought with regard to a patient's potential to rehabilitate and ambulate successfully. However, it must also be remembered, that due to underlying generalized atherosclerotic disease, survival after amputation is greatly reduced being approximately 75, 50 and 35 percent at 1, 3 and 5 years post-amputation, respectively.

Table 15.8: Independent (prosthetic) ambulation rates after various amputations		
Unilateral	BKA	66-80%
	AKA	35-50%
Bilateral	BKA	45%
	AKA	10%

REFERENCES

1. Ross R. The pathogenesis of atherosclerosis: a perspective for the 1990s. Nature 1993;362:801-9.
2. Criqui MH, Fronek A, Barrett-Connor E, Klauber MR, Gabriel S, Goodman D. The prevalence of peripheral arterial disease in a defined population. Circulation 1985;71:510-5.
3. Hiatt WR, Hoag S, Hamman RF. Effect of diagnostic criteria on the prevalence of peripheral arterial disease: the San Luis Diabetes Study. Circulation 1995;91:1472-9.

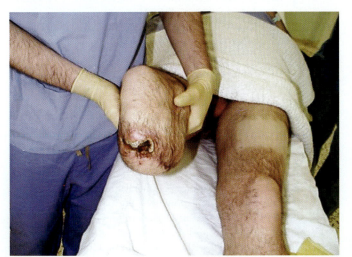

FIGURE 15.13: Infected BK stump

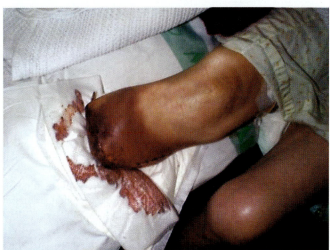

FIGURE 15.14: Necrosis of BKA flaps needing revision to an AKA

4. Fowkes F. Edinburgh Artery Study: prevalence of asymptomatic and symptomatic peripheral arterial disease in the general population. Int J Epidemiol 1991;20:384-92.

5. Newman AB. Ankle-arm index as a marker of atherosclerotic disease in the Cardiovascular Health Study. Cardiovascular Heart Study (CHS) Collaborative Research Group. Circulation 1993;88:837-45.

6. Leng GC. Femoral atherosclerosis in an older British Population: prevalence and risk factors. Atherosclerosis 2000;152:167-74.

7. Leng GC. Incidence, natural history and cardiovascular events in symptomatic and asymptomatic peripheral arterial disease in the general population. Int J Epidemiol 1996;25:1172-81.

8. Newman AB, Shemanski L, Manolio TA, et al. Ankle-arm index as a predictor of cardiovascular disease and mortality in the Cardiovascular Health Study. Arterioscler Thromb Vasc Biol 1999;19:538-45.

9. McKenna M, Wolfson S, Kuller L. The ratio of ankle and arm arterial pressure as an independent predictor of mortality. Atherosclerosis 1991;87:119-28.

10. Vogt MT, McKenna M, Anderson SJ, Wolfson SK, Kuller LH. The relationship between ankle-arm index and mortality in older men and women. J Am Geriatr Soc 1999;12:142-7.

11. Dormandy JA, Heeck L, Vig S. The fate of patients with critical leg ischemia. Semin Vasc Surg 1999;12:142-7.

12. Cacoub CC, Abola MT, Baumgartner I, Bhatt DL, et al. Cardiovascular risk factor control and outcomes in peripheral artery disease patients in the Reduction of Atherothrombosis for Continued Health (REACH) Registry. Atherosclerosis 2009;e86-92.

13. Maurabito JM, D'Agostino RB, Silbershatz H, et al. Intermittent claudication. A risk profile from the Framingham Heart Study. Circulation 1997;96:44-9.

14. Fowkes F. Edinburgh Artery Study: prevalence of asymptomatic and symptomatic peripheral arterial disease in the general population. Int J Epidemiol 1991;20:384-92.

15. Hooi JD. Incidence of and risk factors for asymptomatic peripheral arterial occlusive disease: a longitudinal study. Am J Epidemiol 2001;153:666-72.

16. Hiatt WR, Hoag S, Hamman RF. Effect of diagnostic criteria on the prevalence of peripheral arterial disease. The San Luis Valley Diabetes Study. Circulation 1995;91:1472-9.

17. Hirsch AT. The role of tobacco cessation, antiplatelet and lipid-lowering therapies in the treatment of peripheral arterial disease. Vasc Med 1997;2:243-51.

18. Doll R, Peto R, Wheatley K, Gray R, Sutherland I. Mortality in relation to smoking: 40 years' observations on male British doctors. Br Med J 1994;309:901-11.

19. Rosenberg L, Palmer JR, Shapiro S. Decline in the risk of myocardial infarction among women who stop smoking. N Eng J Med 1990;322:213-7.

20. Cavender JB, Rogers WJ, Fisher LD, et al. Effects of smoking on survival and morbidity in patients randomised to medical or surgical therapy in the coronary artery surgery study (CASS): 10-year follow-up. J Am Coll Cardiol. 1992;20:287-94.

21. Silagy C. Meta-analysis on efficacy of nicotine replacement therapies in smoking cessation. Lancet 1994;343:139-42.

22. UK Prospective Diabetes Study (UKPDS) Group. Intensive blood glucose control with sulphonylureas or insulin compared with conventional treatment and risk of complications in patients with type 2 diabetes (UKPDS 33). Lancet 1998;352:837-53.

23. Adler A. UKPDS 59: hyperglycemia and other potentially modifiable risk factors for peripheral arterial disease in type 2 diabetes. Diabetes Care 2002;25:894-9.

24. Fowkes FG. Epidemiological research on peripheral vascular disease. J Clin Epidemiol 2001;54:863-8.

25. da Silva A. The management and outcome of critical limb ischemia in diabetic patients: results of a national survey. Audit committee of the Vascular Surgical Society of Great Britain and Ireland. Diabetic Med 1996;13:726-8.

26. Stratton IM, Adler AI, Neil HAW, et al. Association of glycemia with macrovascular and microvascular complications of type 2 diabetes (UKPDS 35): prospective observational study. Br Med J. 2000;321:405-12.

27. Hiatt WR. Medical treatment of peripheral arterial disease and claudication. N Engl J Med 2001;344:1608-21.

28. Neal B, MacMahon S, Chapman N. Effects of ACE inhibitors, calcium antagonists, and other blood-pressure-lowering drugs: results of prospectively designed overviews of randomised trials. Blood Pressure Lowering Treatment Trialists' Collaboration. Lancet 2000;356:1955-64.

29. Adler A. Association of systolic blood pressure with macrovascular and microvascular complications of type 2 diabetes (UKPDS 36): prospective observational study. Br Med J 2000; 321:412-19.

30. Hansson L. Effects of intensive blood-pressure lowering and low-dose aspirin in patients with hypertension: principal results of the Hypertension Optimal Treatment (HOT) randomised trial. HOT Study Group. Lancet 1998; 351:1755-62.

31. Beckman J, Creager M, Libby P. Diabetes and atherosclerosis: epidemiology, pathophysiology and management. JAMA 2002; 287:2570-81.

32. Khunti K, Davies M. Metabolic syndrome. BMJ 2005; 331:1153-4.

33. Housley E. Physical activity and risk of peripheral arterial disease in the general population: Edinburgh Artery Study. J Epidemiol Community Health 1993; 47:475-80.

34. Cheng SW, Ting AC, Wong J. Fasting total plasma homocysteine and atherosclerotic peripheral vascular disease. Ann Vasc Surg 1997; 11:217-23.

35. Graham IM, Daly LE, Refsum HM, et al. Plasma homocysteine as a risk factor for vascular disease: the European Concerted Action Project. JAMA 1997; 277:1775-81.

36. Rauwerda JA, de Jong SC. Homocysteinemia and vascular disease. Critical Ischemia 1999; 9:53-7.

37. Kleijnen J, Mackerras D. Vitamin E for intermittent claudication. In: The Cochrane Library, issue 1. Chichester: John Wiley & Sons, 2005.

38. Ernst E. Chelation therapy for peripheral arterial occlusive disease: a systematic review. Circulation 1997; 96:1031-3.

39. Second European Consensus Document on Chronic Critical Leg Ischemia. Eur J Vasc Surg 1992; 6:1-4.

40. Thompson MM, Sayers RD, Varty K, et al. Chronic critical leg ischemia must be redefined. Eur J Vasc Surg 1993; 7:420-6.

41. Kohler TR, Nance DR, Cramer MM, Vandenburghe N, Strandness DE Jr. Duplex scanning for the diagnosis of aortoiliac and femoropopliteal disease: a prospective study. Circulation 1987; 76:1074-80.

42. Cossman DV, Ellison JE, Wagner WH, et al. Comparison of contrast arteriography to arterial mapping with color-flow duplex imaging in the lower extremities. J Vasc Surg 1989; 10:522-9.

43. Moneta GL, Yeager RA, Antonovic R, et al. Accuracy of lower extremity arterial duplex mapping. J Vasc Surg 1992; 15:275-84.

44. Larch E, Minar E, Ahmadi R, et al. Value of color duplex sonography for evaluation of tibioperoneal arteries in patients with femoropopliteal obstruction: a prospective comparison with antegrade intra-arterial digital subtraction angiography. J Vasc Surg 1997; 25:629-36.

45. Grassbaugh JA, Nelson PR, Rzucidlo EM, et al. Blinded comparison of preoperative duplex ultrasound scanning and contrast angiography for planning revascularization at the level of the tibia. J Vasc Surg 2003; 37:1186-90.

46. Waybill MM, Waybill PN. Contrast media-induced Nephrotoxicity: identification of patients at risk and algorithms for prevention. J Vasc Intervent Radiol 2001;12:3-9.

47. N-acetylcysteine and contrast-induced nephropathy in primary angioplasty. N Engl J Med 2006;354:2773-82.

48. Gardner AW, Poehlman ET. Exercise rehabilitation programs for the treatment of claudication pain. A meta-analysis. JAMA 1995; 274:975-80.

49. Leng GC, Fowler B, Ernst E. Exercise for the treatment of intermittent claudication. Cochrane Database Syst Rev 2000(2); CD000990.

50. Perkins JM, Collin J, Creasy TS, Fletcher EW, Morris PJ. Exercise training versus angioplasty for stable claudication. Long and medium term results of a prospective, randomised trial. Eur J Vasc Endovasc Surg 1996; 11:409-13.

51. Whyman MR, Fowkes FG, Kerracher EM, et al. Randomised controlled trial of percutaneous transluminal angioplasty for intermittent claudication. Eur J Vasc Endovasc Surg 1996; 12:167-72.

52. Whyman MR, Fowkes FG, Kerracher EM, et al. Is intermittent claudication improved by percutaneous transluminal angioplasty? A randomized controlled trial. J Vasc Endovasc Surg 1997; 26:551-7.

53. Dzau VJ. Evolving concepts of the renin-angiotensin system. Focus on renal and vascular mechanisms. Am J Hypertens 1988;1:334-7s.

54. Dzau VJ. Implications of local angiotensin production in cardiovascular physiology and pharmacology. Am J Cardiol 1987; 59:59-65A.

55. Griendling KK, Lassegue B, Murphy TJ, Alexander RW. Angiotensin II receptor pharmacology. Adv Pharmacol 1994;28:269-306.

56. Griendling KK, Murphy TJ, Alexander RW. Molecular biology of the renin angiotensin system. Circulation 1993;87:1816-28.

57. Rakugi H, Wang DS, Dzau VJ, Pratt RE. Potential importance of tissue angiotensin converting enzyme (ACE) inhibition in preventing neointimal formation. Circulation 1994;90(1):449-55.

58. Rakugi H, Kim DK, Krieger JE, Wang DS, Dzau VJ, Pratt RE. Induction of angiotensin converting enzyme (ACE) in the neointima after vascular injury. Possible role of restenosis. J Clin Invest 1994;93(1). 339-46.

59. Yusuf S, Sleight P, Pogue J, Bosch J, Davies R, Dagenais G. Effects of an angiotensin-converting- enzyme-inhibitor, ramipril, on cardiovascular events in high-risk patients. The Heart Outcomes Prevention Evaluation (HOPE) Study Investigators. NEJM 2000; 342:154-53.

60. Heart Outcomes Prevention Evaluation (HOPE) Study Investigtors. Effects of ramipril on cardiovascular outcomes in people with diabetes mellitus: results of the HOPE Study and MICRO-HOPE Substudy. Lancet 2000;355:253-9.

61. PROGRESS Collaborative Group. Randomised trial of perindopril-based blood pressure-lowering regimen among 6,105 individuals with previous stroke or transient ischemic attack. Lancet 2001;358:1033-41.

62. Telmisartan, ramipril, or both in patients at high-risk for vascular events. ONTARGET Investigators, Yusuf S, Teo KK, Pogue J, Dyal L, et al. NEJM 2008;358:1547-59.

63. Mahley RW, Bersot TP. Drug therapy for hypercholesterolemia and dyslipidemia. In: Goodman & Gilman's The Pharmacological Basis of Therapeutics: Brunton LL, Lazo JS, Parker KL, (Eds). (11th edn). McGraw-Hill. Philadelphia, PA, 2006.

64. Laws PE, Spark JI, Cowled PA, Fitridge RA. The role of statins in vascular disease. Eur J Vasc Endovasc Surg 2004;27:6-16.

65. Kannel WB. Intermittent claudication. Incidence in the Framingham Study. Circulation 1970;41:875-83.

66. Heart Protection Study Collaborative Group. MRC/BHF Heart Protection Study of Cholesterol-lowering with simvastatin in 20,536 high-risk individuals. Lancet 2002;360:7-22.

67. Scandinavian Simvastatin Survival Study (4S). Randomised trial of cholesterol Lowering in 4444 patients with coronary heart disease. Lancet 1994;244:1383-9.

68. Sacks FM. The effect of pravastatin on coronary events after myocardial infarction in patients with average cholesterol levels. Cholesterol and Recurrent Events Trial Investigators. N Engl J Med 1996;335:1001-9.

69. Pederson TR, Kjekshus J, Pyorala K, et al. Effect of simvastatin on ischemic signs and symptoms in the 4S study. Am J Cardiol 1998;81:333-5.

70. Leng GC, Price JF, Jepson RG. Lipid-lowering for lower limb atherosclerosis. Cochrane Database Syst Rev 2000(2); CD000123.

71. Smyth EM, Burke A, Fitzgerald GA. Lipid-derived autocoids: eicosanoids and platelet-activating factor. In: Goodman & Gilman's The Pharmacological Basis of Therapeutics (11th edn). Brunton LL, Lazo JS, Parker KL, (Eds). McGraw-Hill. Philadelphia, PA.

72. Cheng Y, Austin SC, Rocca B, Koller BH, Coffman TM, Grosser T, et al. Role of prostacyclin in the cardiovascular response to thromboxane A_2. Science 2002;296:539-41.

73. Antiplatelet Trialists' Collaboration. Collaborative overview of randomised trials of antiplatelet therapy. Prevention of death, myocardial infarction, and stroke by prolonged antiplatelet therapy in various categories of patients. Br Med J 1994;308:81-106.

74. Goldhaber SZ. Low-dose aspirin and subsequent peripheral arterial surgery in the physicians' Health Study. Lancet 1992;340:143-5.

75. Belch J, MacCuish A, Campbell I, Cobbe S, Taylor R, et al. The prevention of progression of arterial disease and diabetes (POPADAD) trial: factorial randomised placebo controlled trial of aspirin and antioxidants in patients with diabetes and asymptomatic peripheral arterial disease. BMJ 2008; 337:1840.

76. Ogawa H, Nakayama M, Morimoto T, et al. Low-dose aspirin for the primary prevention of atherosclerotic events in patients with type 2 diabetes: a randomized controlled trial. JAMA 2008;300: 2134-41.

77. Majerus PW, Tollefsen DM. Blood coagulation and anticoagulant, thrombolytic and antiplatelet drugs. In: Goodman & Gilman's The Pharmacological Basis of Therapeutics. Brunton LL, Lazo JS, Parker KL, (Eds). 11th Edition. McGraw-Hill. Philadelphia, PA.

78. Diener HC, Cunha L, Forbes C, Sivenius J, Smets P, Lowenthal A. European Stroke Prevention Study 2. Dipyridamole and acetylsalicylic acid in the secondary prevention of stroke. J Neurol Sci 1996;143:1-13.

79. Hollopeter G, Jantzen HM, Vincent D, Li G, England L, Ramakrishnan V, et al. Identification of the platelet ADP receptor targeted by antithrombotic drugs. Nature 2001;409:202-7.

80. Bhatt DL, Fox KA, Hacke W, Berger PB. Clopidogrel and aspirin versus aspirin alone For the prevention of atherothrombotic events. CHARISMA Investigators. N Engl J Med 2006; 354:1706-17.

81. CAPRIE Steering Committee. A randomised, blinded, trial of clopidogrel versus aspirin in patients at risk of ischemic events (CAPRIE). Lancet 1996;348:1329-39.

82. Juurlink DN, Gomes T, Ko DT, et al. A population-based study of the drug interaction between proton pump inhibitors and clopidogrel. CMAJ 2009;180:713-8.

83. Ho MP, Maddox TM, Wang Li, Fihn SD, et al. Risk of adverse outcomes associated with concomitant use of clopidogrel and proton pump inhibitors following acute coronary syndromes. JAMA 2009;301:937-44.

84. Dawson DL, Cutler BS, Meissner MH, Strandness DE Jr. Cilostazol has beneficial effects in treatment of intermittent claudication: results from a multicenter, randomized, prospective, double-blind trial. Circulation 1998;98:678-86.

85. Money SR, Herd JA, Isaacsohn JL, et al. Effect of cilostazol on walking distances in patients with intermittent claudication caused by peripheral vascular disease. J Vasc Surg 1998;27:267-74.

86. Lehert P, Comte S, Gamand S, Brown TM. Naftidrofuryl in intermittent claudication: a retrospective analysis. J Cardiovasc Pharmacol 1994;23(suppl 3):S48-S52.

87. Greenhalgh RM, Belch JJ, Brown LC, Gaines PA, et al. The adjuvant benefit of angioplasty in patients with mild to moderate intermittent claudication (MIMIC) managed by supervised exercise, smoking cessation advice and best medical therapy: results from two randomised trials for stenotic femoropopliteal and aortoiliac arterial disease. Eur J Vasc Endovasc Surg 2008;36:680-8.

88. Bolia A, Miles K, Brennan J, Bell P. Percutaneous transluminal angioplasty of occlusions of the femoral and popliteal arteries by subintimal dissection. Cardiovasc Intervent Radiol 1990;13: 357-63.

89. Palmaz JC, Tio FO, Schatz RA, et al. Early endothelialization of balloon expandable stents: experimental observations. J Intervent Radiol 1988;3:119-24.

90. Fischman DL, Leon MB, Baim DS, et al. A randomised comparison of coronary stent placement and balloon angioplasty in the treatment of coronary artery disease. Stent Restenosis Study Investigators. N Engl J Med 1994;331:496-501.

91. Duda SH, Pusich B, Richter G, et al. Sirolimus eluting stents for the treatment of obstructive superficial femoral artery disease: 6-month results. Circulation 2002;106:1505-9.

92. Duda SH, Bosiers M, Lammer J, et al. Drug-eluting and bare nitinol stents for the treatment of atherosclerotic lesions in the superficial femoral artery: long-term results from the SIROCCO trial. J Endovasc Ther 2006;13:701-10.

93. Stettler C, Wandel S, Allemann S, et al. Outcomes associated with drug-eluting and bare-metal stents: a collaborative network analysis. Lancet 2007;370: 937-48.

94. Tepe G, Zeller T, Albrecht T, Heller S, et al. Local delivery of paclitaxel to inhibit restenosis during angioplasty of the leg. N Engl J Med 2008;358:689-99.

95. Schulman ML, Badhey MR, Yatco R. Superficial femoral-popliteal veins and reversed saphenous veins as primary femoropopliteal bypass grafts: a randomized comparative study. J Vasc Surg 1987;6:1-10.

96. Wengerter KR, Veith FJ, Gupta SK, et al. Prospective randomized multicenter comparison of in situ and reversed vein infrapopliteal bypasses. J Vasc Surg 1991;13:189-97.

97. Moody AP, Edwards PR, Harris PL. In situ versus reversed femoropopliteal vein grafts. Long-term follow-up of a prospective, randomized trial. Br J Surg 1992;79:750-2.

98. Tarry WC, Walsh DB, Birkmeyer NJ, et al. Fate of the contralateral leg after infrainguinal bypass. J Vasc Surg 1998;27:1039-47.

99. Holzenbein TJ, Pomposelli FB Jr, Miller A, et al. Results of a policy with arm veins used as the first alternative to an unavailable ipsilateral greater saphenous vein for infrainguinal bypass. J vasc Surg 1996;23:130-40.

100. Trans-Atlantic Inter-Society Consensus (TASC) Working Group. Management of peripheral arterial disease (PAD). J Vasc Surg 2000;31:S1-S296.

101. Tetteroo E, Van der Graaf T, Bosch JL, et al. Randomised comparison of primary stent placement versus primary angioplasty followed by selective stent placement in patients with iliac-artery occlusive disease. Dutch Iliac Stent Trial Study Group. Lancet 1998;1153-9.

102. Schillinger M, Sabeti S, Loewe C, et al. Balloon angioplasty versus implantation of nitinol stents in the superficial femoral artery. N Engl J Med 2006;354:1879-88.

103. Veith FJ, Gupta SK, Ascer E, et al. Six-year prospective multicenter randomized comparison of autologous saphenous vein and expanded polytetrafluoroethylene grafts in infrainguinal arterial reconstructions. J Vasc Surg 1986;3:104-14.

104. Michaels JA. Choice of material for above-knee femoropopliteal bypass graft. Br J Surg 2003;90:57-8.

105. Kumar KP, Crinnon JN, Ashley S, Gough MJ. Vein, PTFE or Dacron for above knee femoropopliteal bypass. Int Angiol 1995;14:200-5.

106. Harris PL, Veith FJ, Shanik GD, et al. Prospective randomized comparison of in situ and reversed infrapopliteal vein grafts. Br J Surg 1993;80:173-6.

107. Watlet J, Soury P, Menard JF, et al. Femoro-popliteal bypass: *in situ* or reversed vein grafts? Ten-year results of a randomized prospective study. Ann Vasc Surg 1997;510-19.

108. Abbott WM, Green RM, Matsumoto T, et al. Prosthetic above-knee femoropopliteal bypass grafting: results of a multicenter randomized prospective trial. Above-Knee Femoropopliteal Study Group. J Vasc Surg 1997;25:19-28.

109. Robinson BI, Fletcher JP, Tomlinson P, et al. A prospective randomized multicenter comparison of expanded polytetra-

fluoroethylene and gelatine-sealed knitted Dacron grafts for femoropopliteal bypass. Cardiovasc Surg 1999;7:214-18.

110. Stonebridge PA, Prescott RJ, Ruckley CV. Randomized trial comparing infrainguinal polytetrafluoroethylene bypass grafting with and without vein interposition cuff at the distal anastomosis. The Joint Vascular Research Group. J Vasc Surg 1997;26:543-50.

111. Hunink MG, Wong JB, Donaldson MC, Meyerovitz MF, Harrington DP. Patency results of percutaneous and surgical revascularization for femoropopliteal arterial disease. Med Decis Making 1994;14:71-81.

112. Antiplatelet Trialists' Collaboration. Collaborative overview of randomised trials of antiplatelet therapy. II. Maintenance of vascular graft or arterial patency by antiplatelet therapy. Br Med J 1994;308:159-68.

113. Henke PK, Blackburn S, Proctor MC, et al. Patients undergoing infrainguinal bypass to treat atherosclerotic vascular disease are under prescribed cardio protective medications: effect on graft patency, limb salvage and mortality. J Vasc Surg 2004;39:357-65.

114. Sarac TP, Huber TS, Back MR, et al. Wafarin improves the outcome of infrainguinal vein bypass grafting at high-risk for failure. J Vasc Surg 1998;28:446-57.

115. Arfvidsson B, Lundgren F, Drott C, Schersten T, Lundholm K. Influence of coumarin treatment on patency and limb salvage after peripheral arterial reconstructive surgery. Am J Surg 1990;159-60.

116. Edmonson RA, Cohen AT, Das SK, Wagner MB, Kakkar VV. Low-molecular-weight heparin versus aspirin and dipyridamole after femoropopliteal bypass grafting. Lancet 1994;344:914-8.

117. Wolf GL, Wilson SE, Cross AP, Deupree RH, Stason WB. Surgery or balloon angioplasty for peripheral vascular disease: a randomized clinical trial. J Vasc Intervent Radiol 1993;4:639-48.

118. Holm J, Arfvidsson B, Jivegard L, et al. Chronic lower limb ischemia. A prospective randomised controlled study comparing the 1-year results of vascular surgery and percutaneous transluminal angioplasty (PTA). Eur J Vasc Surg 1991;5:517-22.

119. Adam DJ, Beard JD, Cleveland T, et al. Bypass versus angioplasty in severe ischemia of the leg (BASIL): Multicenter, randomised controlled trial. Lancet 2005;366:1925-34.

120. Lundell A, Lindblad B, Bergqvist D, Hansen F. Femoropopliteal-cural graft patency is improved by an intensive surveillance program: a prospective randomised study. J Vasc Surg 1995;21:26-33.

121. Loosemore TM, Chalmers TC, Dormady JA. A meta-analysis of randomized placebo control trials in Fontaine stages III and IV peripheral occlusive arterial disease. Int Angiol 1994;13:133-42.

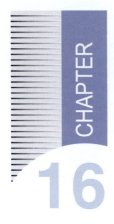

CHAPTER

16

Abdominal Aortic Diseases

Nav Yash Gupta

Although it is true that the art and science of vascular surgery has many basic universal tenants, from a practical standpoint variances in specific disease patterns, the set up for delivery of health care, and the availability of resources and devices specific to vascular and endovascular procedures necessitates that the practice of vascular surgery be tailored to locations such as India and other developing countries.

Vascular surgery, as a separate specialty, has been slow to develop in India. This is related to several factors including the fact that the disease processes are not well recognized and remain under-diagnosed. In addition, most peripheral vascular procedures have traditionally been performed by cardiothoracic surgeons and many endovascular procedures currently are often performed by interventional radiologists in India. Only a few centers provide dedicated training in the field of vascular surgery and endovascular techniques, which have become an integral part of the treatment options for vascular diseases in most western countries. These techniques have not been widely disseminated in India.

ANATOMY AND EXPOSURE

The aortic root originates at the ventricular outflow tract of the heart and includes the aortic valve, the sinuses of Valsalva and the left and right coronary arteries. The aorta ends at the aortic bifurcation in the abdomen and divides into the right and left common iliac arteries, approximately at the level of the second lumbar vertebral body. The ascending aorta curves posterior and to the left as the aortic arch, and the brachiocephalic vessels originate from the aortic arch. They include the brachiocephalic (innominate), left common carotid and left subclavian arteries. The descending thoracic aorta begins just beyond the left subclavian artery

and ends at the 12th intercostal space. The descending thoracic aorta gives off intercostal, bronchial and esophageal arteries. The artery of Adamkiewicz, which is the main source of blood supply to the lower part of the anterior spinal artery, has a variable origin but generally branches from an intercostal artery that originates between the 9th and 12th intercostal spaces. This artery supplies much of the blood flow to the spinal cord. The aorta exits the thorax and enters the abdomen through the aortic hiatus.

Exposure of the brachiocephalic vessels is usually accomplished through a median sternotomy approach. A limited or "mini" sternotomy can also provide exposure to all these vessels other than the first portion of the left subclavian artery. The mini-sternotomy requires a partial median sternotomy and then a transverse transaction of the sternum at the third intercostal space. Exposure of the left subclavian artery for reconstruction of traumatic injuries requires a left anterolateral thoracotomy through the fourth intercostal space. If it is anticipated that distal control of the left subclavian artery will be required a supraclavicular incision is often added.

Wide exposure of the thoracoabdominal aorta is best accomplished via a thoracoabdominal incision going through the fourth or fifth intercostal space. The patient is positioned in a right lateral decubitus position with the aid of a beanbag and support of the left upper extremity on a cushioned stand. The level of the rib interspace incision is determined by the extent to which the aorta needs to be exposed and if access is only required to the distal thoracic aorta this can be done through the seventh or eighth intercostal space.

In the abdomen the visceral vessels originate including the celiac and superior mesenteric arteries. The renal arteries originate below the superior mesenteric artery, and then the inferior mesenteric artery comes off below this level. The aorta ends at the aortic bifurcation in the abdomen and divides into the right and left common iliac arteries, approximately at the level of the second lumbar vertebral body. The common iliac arteries divide into the internal and external iliac arteries and the external iliac artery becomes the common femoral artery at the level of the inguinal ligament.

Small arteries arising from the supraceliac aorta include the inferior phrenic and left adrenal arteries. Main branches of the abdominal aorta include the celiac trunk which branches into the left gastric, splenic and common hepatic arteries. The superior mesenteric artery arises more inferiorly and the renal arteries traverse in a posterolateral direction. The left renal vein crosses anteriorly over the aorta and exposure of the proximal renal arteries at this level requires mobilization of the left renal vein including ligation and division of draining venous tributaries.

Exposure of the infrarenal aorta can be accomplished via a midline transperitoneal approach with retraction of the small bowel to the right side and mobilization of the third and fourth portions of the duodenum. This segment of the aorta can also be exposed through an oblique incision in the left subcostal region with division of the left rectus, oblique and transversus muscles. Medial visceral rotation is then performed by mobilization of the spleen, pancreas and left colon with or without mobilization of the left kidney.

CONGENITAL ANOMALIES

Aortic anomalies generally involve various branching patterns of the brachiocephalic vessels. The most common branching pattern is the brachiocephalic followed by the left common carotid and then the left subclavian artery (75%). A bovine arch describes the pattern in which the brachiocephalic and left common carotid arteries share a common origin off the aortic arch (20%), prior to the left subclavian artery. Infrequently (3%) there are separate origins for the brachiocephalic, left common carotid, left vertebral and left subclavian arteries.

Other more rare anomalies are associated with an anomalous aortic arch and can result in a partial or complete ring around the trachea or esophagus with symptoms related to compression. A right sided aortic arch and a left ligamentum arteriosum associated with a left retroesophageal subclavian artery can result in an esophageal diverticulum known as Kommerell's diverticulum. Another anomaly involves an aberrant right subclavian artery which arises from the descending thoracic aorta (0.5%), distal to the left subclavian artery. The right subclavian artery then traverses posterior to the trachea and esophagus which can result in compression of the esophagus by the aberrant blood vessel and cause dysphagia (dysphagia lusoria).

Although patent ductus arteriosus is the most common vascular anomaly (5-10% of all congenital heart disease) coarctation, which refers to a narrowing of the aortic wall lumen, accounts for 5 to 8 percent of congenital heart disease. This most commonly occurs distal to the ligamentum, but it can occur just proximal to a patent ductus arteriosus. Chronic coarctation results in extensive formation of collateral intercostals arteries, proximal hypertension, and rib notching. Traditionally these patients are treated with resection of the aortic isthmus and primary anastomosis. More recently balloon angioplasty has emerged as an alternative treatment, although the long-term results are unknown.

Abdominal aortic coarctation and hypoplasia is an uncommon entity and may be focal or diffuse in nature. The cause of abdominal aortic coarctation may be related to intrauterine developmental events. Often multiple renal arteries are seen in these patients and the majority of these patients have associated renal artery stenosis which can lead to renovascular hypertension from activation of the renin-angiotensin system. Splanchnic artery occlusive disease is less commonly associated with this disease process and may not be as clinically relevant as renal artery stenosis because of the extensive mesenteric collateral network. Treatment can be medical to manage the hypertension, as well as operative approaches tailored to the specific disease process of the patient. Again, more recently percutaneous balloon angioplasty has been advocated by some, but is not widely accepted as an appropriate treatment for this disease process.

VENOUS ANOMALIES

The most common venous anomaly is a persistent left superior vena cava, which drains into the right atrium through an enlarged orifice of the coronary sinus. This anomaly can be important to recognize during surgical procedures requiring central venous access. The most common anomaly of the inferior vena cava is an interruption of its course in the abdomen with drainage to the heart via the azygos or hemiazygos venous system. Anatomic variants of the left renal vein are estimated to be present in up to 10 percent of patients and the most common variants include a retroaortic vein and a circumaortic venous collar encircling the aorta. If these variants are not recognized at the time of aortic dissection the result can be a significant venous injury and substantial hemorrhage.

AORTIC DISEASE

Atherosclerotic aortic disease is generally divided into occlusive disease and aneurysmal disease. We owe our current treatment concepts and understanding of the treatment of aortic disease to various pioneers including Rudolph Matas who in the 1880s described the technique of endoaneurysmorrhaphy in which the aneurysm sac is actually opened and the contents evacuated. Alexis Carrel is credited with perfecting the technique of repairing a blood vessel and performing an end to end anastomosis using suture and the triangulation technique. He also described patch angioplasty to prevent luminal narrowing of a longitudinal arteriotomy. Rene Leriche, a student of Carrel's, described aortoiliac occlusive disease and in an article published in 1940 he described the constellation of symptoms seen typically in men with severe aortoiliac occlusive disease: absent femoral pulses, lower extremity muscle atrophy and impotence.

Charles Dubost performed the first aneurysm resection and replacement with an aortic homograft in 1951 in France. In the late 1950s Arthur Vorhees worked extensively on developing appropriate synthetic substitutes and in 1957 Charles DeBakey described successful treatment of aortic aneurysms using replacement with a knitted Dacron graft. The description of endovascular treatment of aortic aneurysms by Juan Parodi in 1991 revolutionized the treatment of abdominal aortic aneurysms.

AORTOILIAC OCCLUSIVE DISEASE

Overview

Risk factors for development of atherosclerotic disease in general include tobacco abuse, diabetes mellitus, hypertension and dyslipidemia. In addition advanced age, male gender and a family history seem to be nonmodifiable risk factors for developing atherosclerotic disease. There is some evidence to suggest that race, hypercoagulable states and chronic renal insufficiency also play a role. Atherosclerotic disease of the abdominal aorta and iliac arteries is a common cause of lower extremity ischemia in middle-aged and elderly patients in Western society however, its prevalence in India in not known. Claudication is pain or discomfort that occurs in large muscle groups with exercise. This discomfort is typically reproducible and resolves with rest. Because of the level of occlusion, aortoiliac occlusive disease usually results in claudication of the more proximal muscles groups including the buttocks, hips and thighs, although these patients can also complain of calf claudication. In male patients, limitation of blood flow to the internal iliac artery circulation can result in impotence. The constellation of symptoms in men including diminished femoral pulses, buttock claudication, muscle atrophy and impotence is known as Leriche syndrome.

Although claudication is a common symptom in these patients, because of the extensive collateral circulation that can develop around chronic aortoiliac occlusive disease, they rarely present with rest pain or ischemic tissue loss and gangrene. Rest pain is a sign of advanced ischemia that typically occurs in the forefoot across the metatarsal heads. Often patients describe this pain as occurring at night when they are in a recumbent position and it may be relieved by dangling the affected extremity in a dependant position. Typically multilevel occlusive disease such as that affecting the aortoiliac segment as well as the femoropopliteal segment can result in rest pain and tissue loss. In addition, embolization of atherosclerotic plaque from the diseased aorta can result in painful patches of ischemic tissue in the digits although the perfusion to the feet at baseline may appear to be adequate. In these patients studies such as CT angiography may confirm a more proximal source of atheroemboli.

The disease process usually affects the distal abdominal aorta and the proximal common iliac arteries, but it can progress to complete occlusion of the aorta with preservation of flow into the renal arteries. The suprarenal aorta, renal and visceral vessels are less commonly involved.

Diagnosis

The importance of the history and physical exam cannot be understated. Symptoms suggestive of claudication combined with diminished or absent femoral pulses suggests aortoiliac occlusive disease. As noted previously, tissue loss is uncommon and at rest the legs may appear quite well perfused, however, muscle atrophy may be seen and in male patients a history of impotence can also aid in the diagnosis.

Segmental Doppler pressures are usually noted to be abnormal at all levels including the high thigh level. Measuring ankle pressures at rest and after a period of exercise may help unmask the more proximal inflow disease. The ankle pressures are noted to drop significantly after the exercise. If available, Doppler waveform analysis or pulse volume recordings (PVR) can also help in the diagnosis, although these are not essential.

Surgical Treatment

Treatment varies depending on the severity of the symptoms and the comorbidities of the patient. Consensus guidelines for management of patients with aortoiliac occlusive disease include the Trans-Atlantic Inter-Society Consensus Document on the Management of Peripheral Arterial Disease (TASC) published in the year 2000[1,2] and the Inter-Society Consensus for the Management of Peripheral Arterial Disease (TASC II) published in the year 2007.[3] Patients with severe, diffuse aortoiliac occlusive disease or complete occlusion of the aorta (Fig. 16.1) are best treated with aortobifemoral bypass. This is an involved operation using a bifurcated prosthetic graft (knitted Dacron or ePTFE) requiring either an end to end or end to side anastomosis between the infrarenal aorta and the graft, and an end to side anastomosis between the graft and the femoral arteries in the groin, which may need to be endarterectomized if there is significant plaque at this level as well. This procedure requires appropriate patient selection, a skilled surgeon and adequate anesthetic and postoperative support, initially in an intensive care setting. The mortality rate associated with this procedure in the literature ranges from 2-4 percent, with an excellent 5-year patency rate of over 90 percent.[4] Generally speaking correction of the proximal (aortoiliac) occlusive disease is sufficient to result in resolution of symptoms, unless the patient has extensive tissue loss in which case an outflow procedure such as a femoropopliteal bypass may need to be

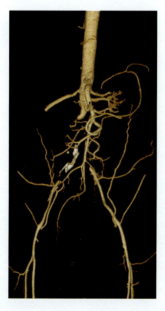

FIGURE 16.1: 3D CTA image showing occlusion of the aorta below the renal arteries with reconstitution of the iliac arteries

added at the same time. This adds to the length of the procedure and potentially the morbidity and mortality associated with it. If the patient is considered too high-risk for a transabdominal aortic procedure an alternative may be an axillary-femoral or bifemoral procedure for bilateral occlusive disease. If only a single iliac artery is involved, a cross-over femoral-femoral bypass may be an acceptable option. These bypasses can be performed with 8 mm externally supported ePTFE grafts or 7 mm Dacron grafts. Another reasonable option may be a unilateral ilio-femoral bypass performed via a retroperitoneal incision but it is critical to ensure that there is adequate inflow from the aorta into the native iliac artery.

Endovascular Treatment

Percutaneous endoluminal treatment of atherosclerotic disease of blood vessels was introduced by Dotter in 1963, however, this technique did not gain widespread acceptance until 1976 when Gruntzig introduced the angioplasty balloon made of polyvinyl chloride. With the rapid evolution of the technology, stents and endovascular techniques, endoluminal treatment of atherosclerotic occlusive disease has become an important modality in the treatment of this disease process.

Stents

Often balloon angioplasty alone is not sufficient to treat these chronic atherosclerotic occlusive lesions. In this situation stents may be used. A stent provides a mechanical scaffold within the diseased segment of the blood vessel to maintain patency. Stents should be relatively flexible and durable with a small profile prior to deployment so they can be introduced into the vascular system percutaneously with the aid of a sheath. A sheath is first introduced into the blood vessel to protect it, minimize blood loss and help with introduction of wires, catheters, balloons and stents into the vascular system. Fluoroscopic imaging, preferably digital subtraction imaging, is generally required for proper positioning of balloons and deployment of stents. Stents are categorized as self-expanding and balloon-expandable. Self-expanding stents are usually constrained within a delivery sheath and after introduction into the vascular system over a guide wide the constraining sheath is withdrawn allowing the stent to expand within the vessel. Although these stents are more flexible than balloon-expandable ones, they have lower radial force against the blood vessel. Some self-expanding stents are made of nitinol (a nickel-titanium alloy) which has a unique temperature associated memory and while the stent can be constrained at cool temperatures, when it is exposed to warm body temperature it assumes the original coil spring shape that it had when it was manufactured at elevated temperatures. Balloon-expandable stents are initially mounted onto a balloon and once positioned within the diseased segment of the blood vessel the stent is deployed by inflating the balloon. These stents can generally be expanded to larger diameters with larger balloons. They have better radial force against the blood vessel but tend to be more rigid and less suited for tortuous blood vessel segments.

Stents can be used to treat occlusive disease in the aorta, common and external iliac arteries. Generally speaking focal atherosclerotic lesions can be adequately treated with balloon angioplasty alone. However, if there is a residual stenosis, or an intimal tear with a flap or dissection, a stent may be indicated. A residual stenosis is considered hemodynamically significant if there is a greater than 10 mm Hg pressure gradient across the area of stenosis. Short segment complete occlusions of the iliac arteries can also be treated endovascularly if the lesion can be traversed with a wire and the true lumen of the blood vessel re-entered beyond the occlusion. In this scenario a stent is generally necessary, however, pre-dilation of the occluded area may ease passage of the stent. If the level of disease is in the very proximal common iliac segment, this essentially represents aortic disease that extends into the iliacs. In this situation, treating just one of the iliac arteries may result in compromise of the lumen of the contralateral iliac artery by plaque being pushed over to that side. A reasonable option in this case would be to treat both proximal common iliac arteries with stents (Figs 16.2A and B). Although the patency of endoluminal treatment of aortoiliac disease has improved in the past several years the long-term patency is limited by the development of intimal hyperplasia leading to re-stenosis. The advantages of endovascular therapy include a high technical success rate with a low morbidity and mortality. Endovascular procedures in the more proximal arterial beds appear to be more durable than those in the distal arteries and often even if the initial endovascular therapy fails the possibility of reintervention, either endovascular or operative, remains an option in these patients. Review of the literature suggests that the primary and secondary patency rates for the treatment of complex aortoiliac occlusive disease range from 69 to 76 percent and 85 to 96 percent respectively, at 2 years.[5-7]

AORTIC ANEURYSMAL DISEASE

Overview

Aneurysms of the abdominal aorta are relatively common in the Western world with an increasing incidence and probably less common in Asian and African populations. The incidence of aortic aneurysmal disease in India is unknown however, the disease entity does exist and the true incidence is probably underestimated. An aneurysm is

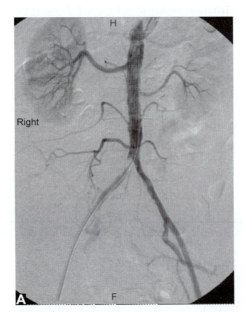
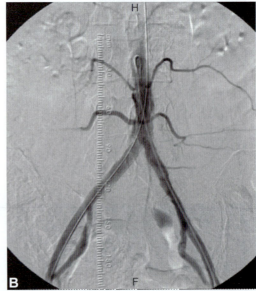

FIGURES 16.2A and B: Digital subtraction angiograms showing bilateral iliac occlusive disease pre- (A) and post- (B) iliac stenting

defined as a focal dilatation of an artery to at least 1.5 times its normal diameter. Most abdominal aortic aneurysms (AAAs) are true aneurysms that include all three layers of the arterial wall and are atherosclerotic in origin. False or pseudoaneurysms of the abdominal aorta can occur and are related to trauma or infection, or can occur at anastomotic sites from prior surgical procedures. The aneurysms can be fusiform in nature with diffuse dilation, or saccular in nature with an abrupt out-pouching of the vessel. The majority of AAAs are infrarenal (over 90%) and patients with an AAA are more likely to have aneurysms of other blood vessels. It is estimated that up to 15 percent of patients with an AAA have popliteal artery aneurysms and 40 to 50 percent of patients with a popliteal artery aneurysm have an AAA. In addition, the majority (50-60%) of patients with a popliteal artery aneurysm will have a contralateral popliteal artery aneurysm.

Pathophysiology

Most (90%) AAAs are associated with atherosclerotic disease of the aorta. Risk factors associated with development of aortic aneurysms include hypertension, tobacco abuse, advanced age, and being male (Table 16.1). Men significantly outnumber women by a factor of 4 to 1, or higher.[8,9] Studies in the past decade have indicated that a decreased amount of elastin and collagen as well as increased levels of matrix-metalloproteinase (MMP)-2 and MMP-9, which may promote arterial wall degeneration, also play a role in development of aneurysms. Rarer causes of AAA formation include various connective tissue disorders (Marfan's syndrome, Ehlers-Danlos syndrome), cystic medial necrosis, and syphilis.

The natural history of an AAA is growth over time and, if left untreated, eventual rupture. The growth rate of an AAA in a particular patient can not be predicted, however, on average most AAAs expand by about 3-4 mm per year. The growth rate can be explained by the law of Laplace which essentially describes the relationship between the tangential stress (T) which causes disruption of the wall, and the radius (R) and transmural pressure (P):

$$T = P \times R$$

Table 16.1: Risk factors for development of aortic aneurysms

- Tobacco use
- Hypertension
- Dyslipidemia
- Male gender
- Family history

As a general principle, the larger the aneurysm diameter, the higher the risk of rupture. AAAs less that 5 cm in maximal diameter have a low risk of rupture of less than 2 percent per year. Once an AAA gets to 7 cm or greater in diameter the risk of rupture is estimated to be 20 to 30 percent per year. Women tend to rupture at slightly smaller sizes compared to men.

Diagnosis and Clinical Findings

Most aneurysms are asymptomatic until the aortic wall begins to disrupt. Unfortunately once an AAA causes symptoms with abdominal or back pain, the patient is usually quite critical and most patients in this situation do not survive and may not even make it to the hospital because of the large volume of blood loss and subsequent cardiovascular collapse. In a patient with severe abdominal or back pain, hypotension and abdominal distention or possibly a pulsatile abdominal mass a ruptured AAA should be suspected and these patients should be rushed to the operating theater for an urgent laparotomy. In this situation the rupture may be contained in the retroperitoneum but will eventually progress to free intraperitoneal rupture if not treated. In some instances the AAA may cause symptoms such as distal embolization of thrombus to the lower extremities, thrombosis of the aneurysm with acute arterial insufficiency of the lower extremities, or pain prior to rupture. In the elective setting the diagnosis can be made by palpation of a pulsatile abdominal mass on physical exam if the aneurysm is of a significant size. These patients should be examined for possible iliac, femoral or popliteal artery aneurysms as well. To properly determine the size of the aneurysm and the anatomical relationship to the renal arteries and visceral vessels imaging techniques such as ultrasonography and computed tomography (CT) are useful. For screening purposes and follow-up of known aortic aneurysms B-mode ultrasonography is sufficient, however a trained technician or physician should perform the test to get accurate information. This imaging modality is relatively inexpensive and does not involve any radiation. Limitations of ultrasound include poor visualization secondary to bowel gas and somewhat imprecise measurements of aneurysm size. CT can give more detailed information regarding the size and extent of the aneurysm, its relationship to the renal and visceral vessels and the iliac arteries and assess for the presence of retroperitoneal hemorrhage. Contrast-enhanced CT scans can give very detailed information regarding the patency of branch vessels and can allow for detailed measurements that are needed for endovascular treatment of aneurysms (Fig. 16.3). Aortography has limitations in the detection of aortic aneurysms and evaluation of the true diameter of the aneurysm because many aneurysms are filled with chronic laminated thrombus that lines the walls of the aneurysm sac to varying degrees. The iodinated contrast agent flows only in the lumen of the blood vessel and this can significantly underestimate the size of the aneurysm. Several studies including the UK Small Aneurysms Trial[10] and the US-based Aneurysm Detection and Management (ADAM) trial[11] have demonstrated that yearly surveillance is adequate for AAAs up to 4.5 cm in diameter and surveillance at 6-month intervals should be performed for AAAs measuring between 4.5 cm and 5.5 cm in diameter. New recommendations in the United States suggest a screening ultrasound for AAA for all men over the age of 65 years of age who have smoked or for men and women who have a family history of aneurysms. This may be impractical in countries such as India where health care resources are scarce and health insurance coverage for the majority of the population is nonexistent. In patients that present with symptoms the test of choice is a rapid CT scan with contrast if the patient is hemodynamically stable. If the patient is unstable then the diagnosis is made based on history and presentation and the patient should be rapidly transported to the operating room for repair of the AAA. Although CT scanning can confirm the diagnosis of a ruptured AAA with retroperitoneal hemorrhage, there are no other specific CT scan findings that have been shown to accurately predict "impending" rupture.[12]

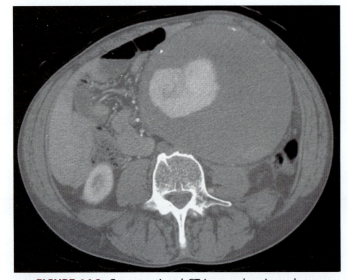

FIGURE 16.3: Cross-sectional CT image showing a large abdominal aortic aneurysm

Treatment

The decision for treatment of aortic aneurysmal disease can be complex because of factors such as the anatomy of the aneurysm, patient comorbidities and life expectancy, and the risk of the operative procedure. In general, infra-renal AAAs should be considered for elective repair at a diameter size of 5 cm in women and 5.5 cm in men. A rapid aneurysm growth rate of over 5 mm in a 6 month period has also been suggested as reason to proceed with aneurysm repair. Other factors that mandate repair (Table 16.2) in the appropriate clinical setting include symptomatic aneurysms, need for concomitant iliac or thoracic aneurysm repair, mycotic aneurysms and significant saccular aneurysms (Fig. 16.4). A thorough medical and surgical history allows for a more complete preoperative evaluation of the patient as well as appropriate surgical planning. Preoperative evaluation should include a thorough cardiopulmonary evaluation. Underlying cardiac dysfunction is the leading cause of mortality after AAA repair[13] and patients with severe coronary artery disease (CAD), unstable angina, a diminished ejection fraction in the range of 25 to 30 percent, severe valvular heart disease (aortic valve area < 1 cm^2) and congestive heart failure are considered very high risk for operative repair. These patients may benefit from preoperative cardiac stress testing and intraoperative use of transesophageal echocardiography (TEE) may help guide management in the operating room. Perioperative heart rate control with beta blockade may be of benefit and several randomized, controlled studies have demonstrated that beta-blockade in high risk patients reduces cardiac morbidity and death.[14,15] Other factors that adversely affect outcomes after AAA repair include chronic renal insufficiency with a serum creatinine of greater than 2.5 mg/dL and severe pulmonary dysfunction.[16-18] Smoking is probably the most important risk factor for development of aortic aneurysms and also predisposes to aneurysm expansion and rupture. Patients that are smokers should be strongly encouraged to cease smoking for at least 2 weeks prior to elective aneurysm

Table 16.2: Indications for repair of aortic aneurysms
Aortic aneurysm ≥ 5.5 cm in diameter in men
Aortic aneurysm ≥ 5 cm in diameter in women
Aneurysm expansion rate of ≥ 1cm per year
Symptomatic aneurysm
Need for concomitant iliac or thoracic aneurysm repair
Mycotic aneurysm
Saccular aneurysm

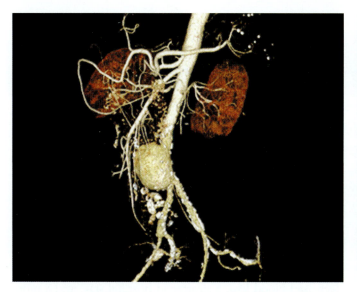

FIGURE 16.4: 3D CTA showing a saccular aneurysm of the distal abdominal aorta

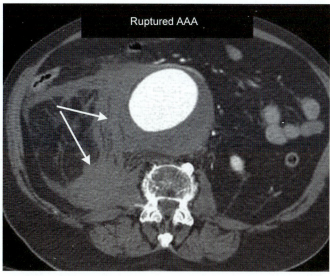

FIGURE 16.5: Cross-sectional CT image showing a ruptured abdominal aortic aneurysm. Note the large retroperitoneal hematoma (arrows)

repair. Patients with significant co-morbidities should only undergo repair after optimizing their medical status and in the setting of adequate anesthetic support and perioperative intensive care monitoring. Patients with ruptured AAA (Fig. 16.5) should be rapidly transported to the operating room for operative repair. Aggressive resuscitation should be avoided in these patients and their abdomen should be prepped prior to induction of anesthesia as they may become profoundly hypotensive upon induction of anesthesia. Rapid proximal control of the aorta in the supraceliac position is recommended. Endovascular repair should only be attempted if there is an adequate setup including equipment, imaging and endovascular devices readily available. Studies have demonstrated that higher surgeon volume is associated with lower mortality in patients with ruptured AAA.[19] Hence rapid transport of these critically ill patients to a higher volume center is probably warranted.

Open Repair

Traditional open surgical repair of AAAs involves either a midline transperitoneal incision or a left sided retroperitoneal incision with medial rotation of the visceral contents. A retroperitoneal approach may be more suitable when the aneurysm extends to the juxtarenal segment or when the visceral vessels have to be addressed. The more normal infrarenal aortic neck and the common iliac arteries

are exposed and prepared for clamping. The level of clamp application may vary depending on the extent of the aneurysm and the amount calcification in the wall of the vessel and the burden of atheromatous debris. After a systemic bolus of heparin the vessels are clamped, the aneurysm incised, laminated thrombus contents evacuated, back-bleeding from lumbar vessels and the inferior mesenteric artery controlled and either a straight tube or bifurcated Dacron or ePTFE graft is sewn in place using permanent monofilament suture. The proximal anastomosis should be performed as close to the renal arteries as is practical to avoid leaving a long segment of native infrarenal aorta that may degenerate and become aneurysmal over time. If, for purposes of exposure, the left renal vein has to be divided, it should be divided as close to the inferior vena cava as possible to allow for collateral venous drainage of the kidney via the gonadal, adrenal and lumbar veins. Significant aneurysmal disease of the iliac arteries generally requires placement of a bifurcated graft with the iliac limbs anastomosed to relatively healthy, nonaneurysmal iliac arteries. If the iliac arteries are healthy and nonaneurysmal a tube graft can be sewn in place. It is important to maintain blood supply to the left colon and pelvis to avoid sexual dysfunction, buttock claudication, colonic ischemia and, rarely, spinal cord ischemia. In most patients the inferior mesenteric artery (IMA) can be ligated with impunity, however, in certain circumstances such as the presence of significant visceral occlusive disease or when hypogastric circulation cannot be directly maintained, consideration should be given to reimplantation of the IMA into the graft. This is aided by preserving a small island of native tissue around the orifice of the IMA (Carrel patch) to facilitate reimplantation. The residual aneurysm sac is then closed over the graft to protect the visceral contents and exclude the graft from the peritoneal contents (Figs 16.6A to C) This can also aid in hemostasis. The operative mortality for elective repair of infrarenal AAAs is under 5 percent in good risk patients.[20-23] If there is associated intra-abdominal pathology it is generally left alone unless it is of a life-threatening nature. Repair of gastrointestinal or genitourinary pathology is avoided to prevent bacterial contamination of the prosthetic graft. If there is a colonic malignancy causing obstruction, significant bleeding or perforation, then it should be treated, generally with a diverting colostomy, prior to aneurysm repair. In most other circumstances aneurysm repair takes precedence.

Endovascular Repair

The development of endovascular techniques has led to the treatment of AAAs with endoluminally placed stent-grafts (Endovascular Aortic Aneurysm Repair—EVAR) and this modality is now gradually replacing open surgery for treatment of AAAs (Figs 16.7A and B). In the United States more than half of all AAAs are repaired endovascularly, however long-term durability is not well established. Although a significant number of AAAs are repaired with stent-grafts in Western countries, this technology has not gained widespread application in India and other developing countries. Several reasons can account for this including

the need for sophisticated imaging equipment, expense of procuring the stent-graft itself and knowledge of the sophisticated wire and catheter techniques required to safely accomplish EVAR. Although in its infancy in India, EVAR could become much more widespread if surgeons are taught the endovascular skills and patients are not forced to bear the entire cost of these expensive devices. It is now well established that EVAR is associated with a lower peri-operative mortality (<2%) compared to open aneurysm repair (4-6%). The mortality rate for EVAR was noted to be significantly lower than for open repair in the DREAM and the EVAR -1 trials, which were both prospective, randomized trials. Specifically the inhospital mortality rates in the DREAM and EVAR-1 trials for EVAR were 1.2 percent and 1.7 percent compared to 4.6 percent and 6 percent for open repair, respectively.[24,25] Other benefits of EVAR include decreased blood loss, a shortened hospital stay, and a more rapid return to normal activities. Open aneurysm repair requires general anesthesia, however, it has been demonstrated that EVAR can be safely performed under regional and local anesthesia. EVAR requires an adequate segment of non-aneurismal vessel at the proximal and distal fixation sites.[26] Various devices are commercially available on the market and there are advantages and disadvantages to each device. Some provide suprarenal fixation and others provide infrarenal fixation. Most of the devices are modular but there are variances in radial force and fabric as well as the range of sizes available such that often the specific device and sizes are chosen by the physician based on the particular anatomy and measurements of the patient's aorta from CT imaging. The rapid advance of technology in this area holds the promise to significantly expand the future possibilities for endovascular repair of the majority of patients with aneurysms. If the common iliac artery is aneurysmal

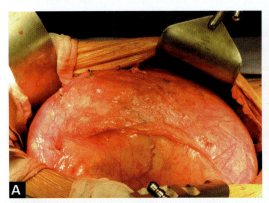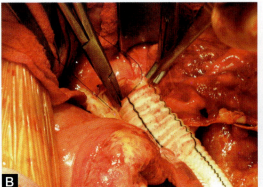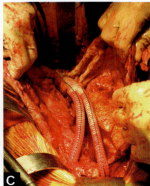

FIGURES 16.6A to C: Midline abdominal exposure of a large abdominal aortic aneurysm (A). Proximal anastomosis of the Dacron graft is performed with monofilament suture (B). The graft has been sewn in place and flow restored to the lower extremities (C)

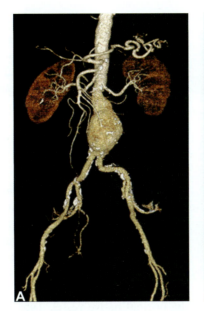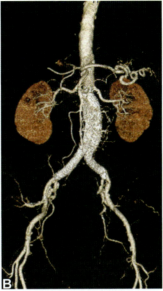

FIGURES 16.7A and B: 3D CTA of AAA pre- (A) and post- (B) placement of a modular bifurcated stent graft

extension of the endograft to the external iliac artery is required. This involves exclusion of the hypogastric artery and several studies have shown that unilateral exclusion of a hypogastric artery is well tolerated.[27,28] Bilateral hypogastric artery occlusion can result in severe buttock claudication and erectile dysfunction and in rare instances severe pelvic or colonic ischemia. The disadvantage of EVAR is that a small percentage of patients can have problems with sealing of the stent-graft against the normal blood vessel resulting in continued perfusion of the sac and pressure (endoleak) leading to growth of the sac over time, and potentially even rupture if left untreated. In addition there can be issues with access vessel injury, graft limb occlusion and graft migration or disruption. Because of these issues patients require regular follow-up and imaging studies such as CT angiography to detect any problems. The 30-day re-intervention rate is higher following EVAR (15-20%)[29] than with open surgical repair. Most of the problems can be treated via an endovascular means. Follow up can be an issue in non-compliant patients or in patients that live a significant distance from the treatment center. There is also a monetary cost associated with the required follow-up imaging studies and there is the potential for progressive renal dysfunction secondary to the contrast agents used in the CT or angiographic imaging studies.

Paravisceral and Thoracoabdominal Aortic Aneurysms

When the aneurysmal aorta also involves the para-visceral or thoracic aorta this presents a challenging situation both from a technical standpoint as well as perioperative care and management. Endovascular and hybrid (open and endovascular) techniques for repair of these types of aneurysms are evolving and these techniques have been employed to treat descending thoracic aortic aneurysms and traumatic aortic transaction.[30] More complex thoracoabdominal aortic aneurysms are best treated with open repair. These aneurysms are best approached with a left sided retroperitoneal incision and medial rotation of the visceral contents to expose an adequate amount of the normal suprarenal or supraceliac aorta. The complications associated with paravisceral aortic aneurysm repair are similar to those seen with infrarenal AAA repair except that the incidence of complications is higher in patients with paravisceral aneurysms. This is related to the need for suprarenal or supraceliac aortic clamping which is associated with a period of renal and/or visceral ischemia as well as increased cardiac stress. Complications include renal insufficiency, cardiac ischemia, respiratory failure, spinal cord ischemia and mesenteric ischemia. These patients are also more likely to develop intraoperative coagulopathy and postoperative bleeding complications requiring re-exploration. As would be expected, the mortality rate associated with this repair is also higher (5-20%).[31]

Perioperative Care of Patients

Open aneurysm repair is performed under general anesthesia with muscle relaxants to allow for adequate retraction of the abdominal wall. Placement of an epidural catheter for infusion of analgesic medication after surgery may assist not only in pain control but also in a shorter time on the ventilator and early mobilization of the patient. EVAR can safely be performed under general, local or regional anesthesia.

Blood loss during open aneurysm repair can be significant. Preoperative donation of autologous blood by the patient for elective operations may be of benefit especially in countries where banked blood supply is limited. In addition return of autologous blood to the patient intra-operatively using various blood cell salvage devices can preserve resources and minimize the need for banked blood transfusion. Use of transesophageal echocardiography can prove to be helpful in unstable patients or those who have a severely diminished cardiac reserve. It is critical to maintain body temperature during the aneurysm repair procedure to prevent acidosis, coagulopathy and diminished cardiac function. In this regard, use of intravenous fluid warmers and forced air warming blankets are helpful. Nasogastric tube decompression is often performed after open aneurysm repair because of the laparotomy and presumed ileus, however some studies have indicated that this is not necessary and may even be detrimental to the patient from a pulmonary standpoint.[32] Appropriate and adequate pain management after surgery can minimize cardiac and respiratory complications and allow for early extubation and mobilization. Deep venous thrombosis (DVT) prophylaxis is appropriate in this group of patients and can be performed with unfractionated heparin or low-molecular-weight heparin administered subcutaneously.

Long-Term Care of Patients

With open repair the concerns include incisional ventral hernia formation and bowel obstruction. Over time if the anastomosis disrupts paraanastomotic pseudoaneurysms can develop. These pseudoaneurysms can be difficult to treat, especially if they occur in the paravisceral segment of the abdominal aorta, and infection may predispose to development these false aneurysms. True aneurysms occur more frequently and can involve the suprarenal or para-

visceral aorta, the iliac arteries, as well as the femoral and popliteal arteries. For this reason patients should be seen at regular intervals for follow up with imaging studies. Graft infection is an extremely rare but devastating complication of aneurysm repair.[33] If a bifurcated graft is used then limb occlusion can occur and seems to be more common in women and in situations where the graft limb extends to the femoral artery. Limb occlusion can occur with both open and endovascular repair, however, there are certain complications that are unique to endovascular repair. The most frequent of these complications is endoleak where there is persistent blood flow into the aneurysm sac around the endograft. It is estimated to occur in as many as 25 percent of patients undergoing EVAR.[34] Endoleaks are classified based on the source of blood flow into the aneurysm sac (Fig. 16.8). Type I endoleaks occur when there is an incomplete seal between the endograft material and the normal native vessel. Type IA describes a seal problem proximally and Type IB describes a lack of appropriate seal distally. In this situation there is still significant pressurized blood entering the sac and the natural progression is that the sac will continue to enlarge and eventually rupture if left untreated. Once detected these endoleaks should be fixed, either endovascularly or via an open procedure. Type II endoleaks occur because of retrograde flow into the sac either from lumbar arteries or the inferior mesenteric artery, or both. Although these types of endoleaks are much more common, they rarely need to be treated and usually resolve spontaneously. Type III endoleaks refer to blood flow into the sac from modular junctions (various components of the endograft that overlap with each other). These should be treated when detected. Type IV endoleaks are related to

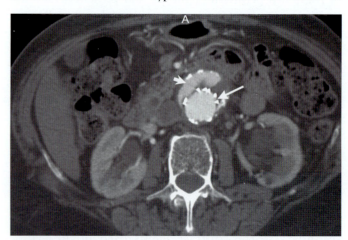

FIGURE 16.8: Cross-sectional CT image showing an endograft (arrow) in the aneurysm sac with persistent flow in the aneurysm sac demonstrating an endoleak (arrowhead)

graft material porosity and these resolve without treatment. Another concern with EVAR is graft migration, either during deployment of the endograft, or detected in subsequent follow up imaging studies. If the migration results in an endoleak it should be treated. For many of the above reasons patients with endograft implanted should be followed with routine imaging studies, typically a contrast enhanced CT scan, to detect problems. Some studies have shown the utility of color Duplex ultrasonography in the detection of endoleaks, however at this time CT imaging remains the gold standard.

Inflammatory Aneurysm

Inflammatory aneurysms are rare and typically have a thickened aortic wall and a dense fibrous ring around the aneurysm. The etiology of inflammatory aneurysms is poorly understood and possibilities include infection, autoimmune response, or lymphatic obstruction. Patients may present with flank pain and weight loss and the erythrocyte sedimentation rate is elevated in the majority of patients. On CT imaging the periaortic inflammatory tissue can be well visualized. Repair of these aneurysms can be technically challenging. Because of the fibrotic process nearby structures such as the duodenum, left renal vein, vena cava and ureters are often stuck to the aneurysm and can be easily injured in the process of mobilization. In fact, it is best to avoid extensive mobilization of the duodenum if possible. Pre-operative placement of ureteral stents can help identify the ureters and prevent injury. EVAR may be a preferred approach if feasible. Following repair the inflammatory process is noted to subside.

Aortocaval Fistula

Aortic aneurysms have been reported to perforate into the inferior vena cava or iliac vein in a small percentage of patients estimated to occur in about 2 to 4 percent of all ruptured aneurysms. The mortality rate is estimated at about 30 percent. Patients can present with high-output cardiac failure as well as signs of venous hypertension including lower extremity edema, hematuria and rectal bleeding. Hypoperfusion of the lower extremities with cyanosis can also be seen. On exam these patients may have a palpable abdominal mass with a very loud murmur. Surgical treatment is required in these patients and closure of the fistula is best accomplished from within the aneurysm sac. There is a high risk of bleeding and air embolism and maneuvers that can assist with control of the venous bleeding during closure include manual compression with sponge sticks or

use of a large balloon catheter. Following repair of the fistula the aneurysm is repaired in the standard fashion.

Primary Aortoenteric Fistula

Primary aortoenteric fistula is quite rare. Patients can present with gastrointestinal bleeding and abdominal pain. The majority of these patients have an AAA and the patients can present with repeated episodes of sudden gastrointestinal bleeding or exsanguinating hemorrhage. CT scan may aid in the diagnosis, and upper endoscopy should include the 3rd and 4th portions of the duodenum as the fistula often involves this portion of the bowel. The recommended treatment is extra-anatomic bypass and repair of the intestinal defect, however, if the patient is unstable an in situ repair with an ePTFE graft can be performed. In this situation a pedicle of omentum may be used to buttress the vascular anastomosis. Post-operative antibiotic treatment should be initiated.

Primary Mycotic Abdominal Aortic Aneurysm

This is another rare entity and can result from primary aortitis, septic emboli or an adjacent infection that spreads to the aorta. Typical organisms include salmonella and staphylococcus. CT scan can aid in the diagnosis with findings such as periaortic inflammation, rapid expansion or development of an aneurysm and rupture. The treatment approach is similar to that for aortoenteric fistula. As expected, EVAR is not a definitive treatment for this disease process as it does not treat the infected tissue and reports in the literature describe a poor outcome for treatment of mycotic AAAs solely with EVAR.[35]

Horseshoe Kidney

This is an uncommon anomaly but when noted in the presence of an AAA appropriate planning is required to avoid renal ischemia. The kidney mass may be fused anterior to the aorta and often the ureters are displaced inferiorly. The isthmus of the kidney does not need to be divided and is generally avoided as it could result in injury to the renal collecting system. In this case the isthmus can be mobilized and the graft tunneled beneath it. In addition multiple anomalous renal arteries may arise from the aorta and preservation of these arteries is essential with reimplantation into the graft. A retroperitoneal approach may facilitate management of the multiple renal arteries as the majority of the renal tissue can be displaced anteriorly. Endovascular repair is usually not feasible in this setting unless there are single main renal arteries originating above the aneurysm.

Iliac Artery Aneurysms

Most iliac artery aneurysms are atherosclerotic in origin and occur in conjunction with aortic aneurysms and are generally repaired at the same time. Isolated iliac aneurysms are rare and most iliac aneurysms occur in older males. Because of their pelvic location iliac aneurysms may not be palpable on routine physical exam but compression of adjacent structures including the bladder, rectum, lumbosacral nerves and pelvic veins can often result in symptoms such as flank and groin pain. These aneurysms can remain undetected until imaging studies are performed and the operative mortality rate with ruptured iliac aneurysms is quite high. Small isolated iliac aneurysms measuring less than 3.5 cm in diameter can generally be observed while larger aneurysms should be repaired. When iliac aneurysmal disease is seen in association with an AAA the disease is treated concomitant with repair of the AAA.

Femoral and Popliteal Artery Aneurysms

The most common peripheral artery aneurysms are popliteal and femoral artery aneurysms and they are atherosclerotic in nature. These aneurysms are often bilateral in up to 50 percent of patients and these patients often have an associated aortic aneurysm.

True femoral artery aneurysms can result in thromboembolic complications or rupture if they become large, and are generally repaired when they become larger than 2 cm. Repair usually involves an interposition prosthetic graft and all attempts are made to preserve the profunda femoral artery. False (pseudo) aneurysms of the femoral artery can occur secondary to percutaneous interventions such as catheterization and these may thrombose spontaneously, however, if they persist they can be treated with open surgical repair or ultrasound guided Thrombin injection of the active pseudoaneurysm cavity. Pseudoaneuryms of the femoral artery can also occur at the site of disruption of a graft to native artery anastomosis. Mycotic (infected) femoral artery aneurysms can occur in IV drug users or at the anastomotic site of a prosthetic graft to the native vessel. Repair in this situation may require resection, debridement, and replacement with autogenous tissue such as a vein graft, or possibly an extra-anatomic bypass.

Complications arising from popliteal artery aneurysms are thromboembolic in nature and can eventually result in limb loss. Rarely large aneurysms can cause symptoms related to compression of the adjacent structures such as the tibial nerve and the popliteal vein. Most of these patients are male and over 50 percent have bilateral disease. Diagnosis can be made on careful physical exam and confirmed with Duplex imaging. Conventional contrast angiography helps with operative planning. Aneurysms larger than 2 cm in diameter and those with a significant amount of laminated mural thrombus should be considered for repair. Traditionally open surgical repair is performed with ligation of the aneurysm and bypass using saphenous vein from either a posterior or medial approach. More recently endovascular repair with covered stent-grafts has been performed in selected patients with decent proximal and distal landing zones and patent, relatively un-diseased tibial runoff vessels. Long-term antiplatelet therapy may help preserve potency of these stent-grafts.

REFERENCES

1. TASC. Management of peripheral arterial disease (PAD). TransAtlantic Inter-Society Consensus (TASC). Eur J Vasc Endovasc Surg 2000;19(Suppl A):Si-xxviii. S1-250.
2. TASC. Management of peripheral arterial disease (PAD) TransAtlantic Inter-Society Consensus (TASC). J Vasc Surg 2000;31(1 part 2):S1-287.
3. Norgren L, Hiatt WR, Dormandy JA, Nehler MR, Harris KA, Fowkes FG. Inter-Society Consensus for the Management of Peripheral Arterial Disease (TASC II). J Vasc Surg 2007;45(suppl S):S5-67.
4. de Vries SO, Hunink MG. Results of aortic bifurcation grafts for aortoiliac occlusive disease: a meta-analysis. J Vasc Surg 1997;26:558-69.
5. Dyet JF, Gaines PA, Nicholson AA, Cleveland T, Cook AM, Wilkinson AR, et al. Treatment of chronic iliac artery occlusions by means of percutaneous endovascular stent placement. J Vasc Interv Radiol 1997;8:349-53.
6. Henry M, Amor M, Ethevenot G, Henry I, Mentre B, Tzvetanov K. Percutaneous endoluminal treatment of iliac occlusions: a long-term follow-up in 105 patients. J Endovasc Surg 1998;5:228-35.
7. Kashyap V, Pavkov M, Bena J, Sarac T, O'Hara P, Lyden S, et al. The management of severe aortoiliac occlusive disease: Endovascular therapy rivals open reconstruction. J Vasc Surg 2008;48:1451-7.
8. Vardulaki KA, Walker NM, Day NE, Duffy SW, Ashton HA, Scott RA. Quantifying the risks of hypertension, age, sex, and smoking in patients with abdominal aortic aneurysm. Br J Surg 2000;87:195-200.
9. Johnston KW. Influence of sex on the results of abdominal aortic aneurysm repair. J Vasc Surg 1994;20:914-23; discussion 923-6.

10. United Kingdom Small Aneurysm Trail Participants. Long-term outcomes of immediate repair compared with surveillance of small abdominal aortic aneurysms. N Engl J Med 2002;346:1445-52.

11. Lederle FA, Johnson GR, Wilson SE, Chute EP, Hyn RJ, Makaroun MS, et al. The aneurysm detection and management study screening program: validation cohort and final results. Aneurysm Detection and Management Veterans Affairs Cooperative Study Investigators. Arch Intern Med 2000;160:1425-30.

12. Boules TN, Compton CN, Stanziale SF, Sheehan MK, Dillavou ED, Gupta N, et al. Can computed tomography scan findings predict (impending aneurysm rupture? Vasc and Endovasc Surg 2006; 40(1): 41-7.

13. Roger VL, Ballard DJ, Hallett JW Jr, Osmundson PJ, Gersh BJ. Influence of coronary artery disease on morbidity and mortality after aortic aneurysmectomy: a population-based study, 1971-1987. J Am Coll Cardiol 1989;14:1245-52.

14. Auerbach AD, Goldman L. Beta-Blockers and reduction of cardiac events in noncardiac surgery: clinical applications. JAMA 2002;287:1445-7.

15. Yang H, Raymer K, Butler R, Parlow J, Roberts R. The effects of perioperative beta-blockade: results of the Metoprolol after Vascular Surgery (MaVS) study, a randomized controlled trial. Am Heart J 2006;152:983-90.

16. Johnston KW. Multicenter prospective study of nonruptured abdominal aortic aneurysm. Part II. Variables predicting morbidity and mortality. J Vasc Surg 1989;9:437-47.

17. Axelrod DA, Henke PK, Wakefield TW, Stanley JC, Jacobs LA, Graham LM, et al. Impact of chronic obstructive pulmonary disease on elective and emergency abdominal aortic aneurysm repair. J Vasc Surg 2001;33:72-6.

18. Upchurch GR Jr, Proctor MC, Henke PK, Zajkowski P, Riles EM, Ascher MS, et al. Predictors of severe morbidity and death after elective abdominal aortic aneurysmectomy in patients with chronic obstructive pulmonary disease. J Vasc Surg 2003;37:594-9.

19. Cho JS, Kim JY, Rhee RY, Gupta N, Marone LK, Dillavou ED, Makaroun MS. Contemporary results of open repair of ruptured abdominal aortic aneurysms: Effect of surgeon volume on mortality. J Vasc Surg 2008;48:10-8.

20. Brewster DC, Cronenwett JL, Hallett JW Jr, Johnston KW, Krupski WC, Matsumura JS. Guidelines for the treatment of abdominal aortic aneurysms. Report of a subcommittee of the Joint Council of the American Association for Vascular Surgery and Society for Vascular Surgery. J Vasc Surg 2003;37:1106-17.

21. Conrad MF, Crawford RS, Pedraza JD, Brewster DC, Lamuraglia GM, Corey M, et al. Long-term durability of open abdominal aortic aneurysm repair. J Vasc Surg 2007;46:669-75.

22. Ernst CB. Abdominal aortic aneurysm. N Engl J Med 1993;328:1167-72.

23. Hirsch AT, Haskal ZJ, Hertzer NR, Bakal CW, Creager MA, Halperin JL. ACC/AHA 2005 practice guidelines for the management of patients with peripheral arterial disease (lower extremity, renal, mesenteric and abdominal aortic). Circulation 2006;113:1474-1547.

24. Prissen M, Verhoeven EL, Buth J, Cuypers PW, van Sambeek MR, Balm R, et al. Dutch Randomized Endovascular Aneurysm Management (DREAM) trial group. A randomized trial comparing conventional and endovascular repair of abdominal aortic aneurysms. N Engl J Med 2004;351:1607-18.

25. Greenhalgh RM, Brown LC, Kwong GP, Powell JT, Thompson SG. Comparison of endovascular aneurysm repair with open reapir in patients with abdominal aortic aneurysm (EVAR trial 1), 30-day operative mortality results: randomized controlled trial. Lancet 2004;364:843-8.

26. Dillavou ED, Muluk SC, Rhee RY, Tzeng E, Woody JD, Gupta N, Makaroun MS. Does hostile neck anatomy preclude successful endovascular aortic aneurysm repair? J Vasc Surg 2003; 38: 657-63.

27. Schoder M, Zaunbauer L, Holzenbein T, Fleischman D, Cejna M, Kretschmer G, et al. Internal iliac artery embolization before endovascular repair of abdominal aortic aneurysms: Frequency, efficacy, and clinical results. Am J Roentgenol 2001;177:599-605.

28. Cynamon J, Lerer D, Veith FJ, Taragin BH, Wahl SI, Lautin JL, et al. Hypogastric artery coil embolization prior to endoluminal repair of aneurysms and fistulas: buttock claudication, a recognized but possibly preventable complication. J Vasc Interv Radiol 2000;11:573-7.

29. Wilt TJ, Lederle FA, MacDonald R, Jonk YC, Rector TS, Kane RL. Comparison of endovascular and open surgical repairs for abdominal aortic aneurysm. Evidence report. Rockville, MD: AHRQ Publication No. 06-E017; 2006.

30. Go MR, Barbato JE, Dillavou ED, Gupta N, Rhee RY, Makaroun MS, Cho JS. Thoracic endovascular aortic repair for traumatic aortic transaction. J Vasc Surg 2007; 46: 928-33.

31. Sarac TP, Clair DG, Hertzer NR, Greenberg RK, Krajewski LP, O'Hara PJ, Ouriel K. Contemporary results of juxtarenal aneurysm repair. J Vasc Surg 2002;36:1104-11.

32. Goueffic Y, Rozec B, Sonnard A, Patra P, Blanloeil Y. Evidence for early nasogastric tube removal after infrarenal aortic surgery: a randomized trial. J Vasc Surg 2005;42:654-9.

33. Lehnert T, Gruber HE, Maeder N, Allenberg JR. Management of primary aortic graft infection by extra-anatomic bypass reconstruction. Eur J Vasc Endovasc Surg 1993;7:301-7.

34. Hobo R, Buth J. Secondary interventions following endovascular abdominal aortic aneurysm repair using current endografts. A EUROSTAR report. J Vasc Surg 2006;43:896-902.

35. Kan CD, Lee HL, Yang YJ. Outcome after endovascular stent graft treatment for mycotic aortic aneurysm: A systematic review. J Vasc Surg 2007;46:906-12.

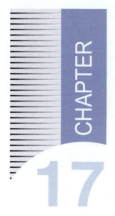
Gastrointestinal Endoscopy: A Bird's Eye View

Ananya Das

Gastrointestinal endoscopy has rapidly evolved over the last few decades with rapid progress in technology, and scope of diagnostic and therapeutic interventions and also, with dissemination of technology.

In India, gastrointestinal endoscopy had a phenomenal growth; in the late seventies, flexible endoscopy was confined only to select tertiary care hospitals in few metropolitan cities but today, basic endoscopic facilities are available even in subdivisional towns in most parts of the country. Such rapid dissemination has not been able to keep pace with the limited training facilities available to interested physicians and surgeons in India with the result that many doctors performing endoscopic procedures are often not well trained. However, it should also be noted that in larger cities, the facilities for diagnostic and therapeutic endoscopic procedures are quite readily available and some of these endoscopic centers have been recognized nationally and internationally as centers of excellence. It is to be noted that, the first ever report of a natural orifice transluminal endoscopic surgery or NOTES procedure came from a reputed institute in Hyderabad, India. Of late, there has been a trend to develop and test newer endoscopic technologies in Indian institutions before commercially marketing in the western countries.

Modern flexible endoscopes are based on **charge-coupled device (CCD)** chips and uses digital imaging technology to obtain digital color images of the gastrointestinal mucosa (Fig. 17.1). Older fiberoptic scopes are much les costly but generate inferior quality images and these endoscopes are mechanically less durable. However, many low-volume centers in India still use fiberoptic endoscopes.

In the following paragraphs a brief review of commonly performed endoscopic procedures are summarized in an organ and disease specific format (Figs 17.2A to D).

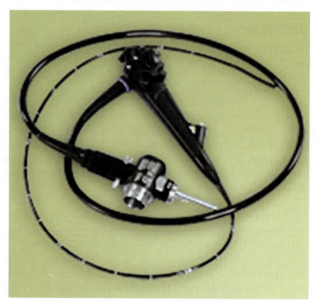

FIGURE 17.1: A video gastroscope which is used for endoscopic procedures in the upper gastrointestinal tract

ESOPHAGUS

The esophagus is routinely examined during diagnostic esophagogastro-duodenoscopy (EGD). Gastroesophageal reflux disease (GERD), particularly with suboptimal response to proton pump inhibitor based therapy is a very common indication for diagnostic EGD. Dysphagia, particularly experienced with solid food and with a progressive course is an alarm symptom and should be promptly evaluated by EGD. Commonly performed therapeutic procedures are esophageal dilation using both boogie and balloon dilators. Caustic strictures are quite common in certain parts of the country because of ingestion of lye and other caustic chemicals. Initial endoscopic

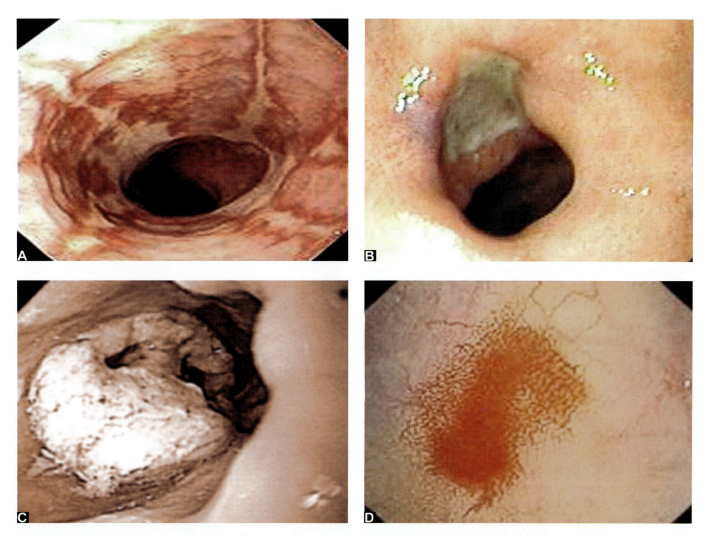

FIGURES 17.2A to D: Endoscopic images of commonly seen upper gastrointestinal pathology: (A) Erosive esophagitis due to reflux, (B) A duodenal ulcer of peptic etiology, (C) A squamous cell esophageal cancer with partial luminal obstruction by the ulcerated mass, (D) An angio-ectasia (arteriovascular malformation) commonly seen in the small intestine as a bleeding lesion

evaluation in such patients, usually in the first 24 hours, is indicated for grading of severity and extent of injury. The treatment of caustic esophageal strictures is often complicated by frequent recurrence and may benefit by endoscopic injection of steroid at the site of the stricture. Esophageal varies, often acutely bleeding, are frequently encountered in patients with chronic liver disease, and endoscopic treatment of varices are commonly performed by Indian endoscopists. Although current data is overwhelmingly in favor of variceal banding in terms of safety and efficacy, esophageal sclerotherapy is much more

prevalent primarily for economic reasons. Complication of GERD, such as, Barrett's is uncommon in India when compared to western countries.

STOMACH

Peptic ulcer is very common in certain parts of the country and EGD is most commonly performed for evaluation of dyspepsia. Functional dyspepsia, often with gastroparetic symptoms of bloating and early satiety, is widely prevalent in the population and is difficult to distinguish from organic dyspepsia and judicious use of diagnostic endoscopy is critical in appropriate work-up of these patients. *H. pylori* infection is highly prevalent in India and many practitioners check and treat *H. pylori* often without clear clinical indications. Gastric varices are common in India and in addition to cirrhosis are also seen in patients of noncirrhotic portal hypertensive diseases such as, extrahepatic portal vein obstruction. Gastric outlet obstruction is frequently seen as complications of peptic ulcer disease and often requires endoscopic therapy, such as balloon dilation.

SMALL INTESTINE

With the advent of newer enteroscopic techniques such as balloon assisted enteroscopy, endoscopic evaluation of small intestine is quickly shifting from radiological studies to direct endoscopic evaluation. With the use of balloons, incorporated on the endoscopes and overtubes in case of double-balloon endoscopes, the mechanical hurdle of looping and consequent nonprogression has been greatly reduced and a good portion of the small intestine can be accessed by enteroscopy performed either via the oral or rectal route (Fig. 17.3). No-specific intestinal ulcerations of indeterminate etiology are the cause of bleeding in the majority of patients presenting with overt obscure gastrointestinal bleeding. Besides intestinal bleeding, infectious disorders such as intestinal tuberculosis are common clinical indications for enteroscopy. Availability of wireless capsule endoscopy is still very limited outside teaching hospitals and cost-effectiveness of capsule endoscopy in the Indian scenario is very limited (Fig. 17.4). In a recent study from central India, the diagnostic yield of

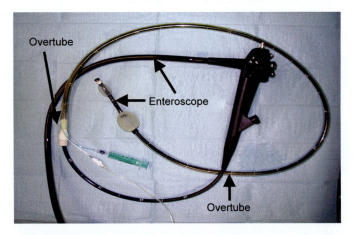

FIGURE 17.3: A double balloon enteroscope with two inflatable balloons on the endoscope and the overtube

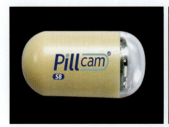 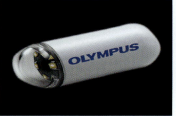

FIGURE 17.4: Two commercially available wireless capsule endoscopes

capsule endoscopy was reported to be similar to western studies.

LARGE INTESTINE

Neoplastic diseases of colon are distinctly less common in the Indian subcontinent and unlike western countries screening colonoscopy is not routinely indicated. It has its fair share of chronic inflammatory bowel disease often requiring endoscopic diagnostic and therapeutic intervention. There are some reports of increasing prevalence of inflammatory bowel disorders such as Crohn's disease in certain segments of the Indian society. Anorectal disorders are quite common and endoscopists routinely practice procedures, such as, endoscopic treatment of hemorrhoids.

BILIOPANCREATIC SYSTEM

Most parts of the country have very high prevalence of gallstone disease and gallbladder cancer is quite common (Figs 17.5A to C). Although many physicians practice diagnostic ERCP, in most communities only a few select endoscopists perform therapeutic ERCP. They often perform endoscopic sphincterotomy and placement of bile duct stents. Biliary ascariasis is a unique disorder often seen in the Indian subcontinent requiring ERCP and endoscopic removal of degenerated round worms. With the dissemination of laparoscopic cholecystectomy, to smaller cities and towns, bile duct injury is commonly encountered and prompt endoscopic therapy with placement of biliary prosthesis is crucial. Pancreatic endotherapy, such as, pancreatic sphincterotomy, or pseudocyst drainage are less commonly performed. Invasive surgical procedures are still mainstay in the treatment of many biliopancreatic disorders, which are typically treated in the west by endoscopic or at least by minimally invasive surgery.

Endoscopic ultrasonography (Figs 17.6 and 17.7) is distinctly uncommonly performed in India primarily because

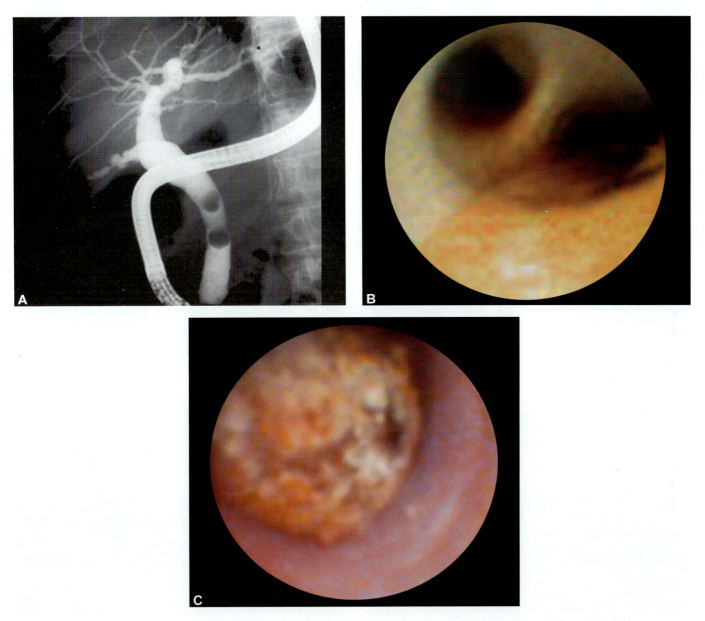

FIGURES 17.5A to C: (A) Retrograde cholangiogram showing two bile duct stones shown as filing defects, (B) Cholangioscopy (Spyglass©, Boston Scientific, Boston, MA) is a useful technique to visualize the endoluminal aspect of the biliary tree (B) for direct visualization of pathologic lesions, such as, stone (C) or tumor

of expensive equipments and lack of trained physicians. There is a perception that practice of advanced but expensive technologies such as EUS may be not be economically viable in most regions of the country.

Gastrointestinal cancer in India has a distinctly different incidence patterns in India compared to the west. Esophageal squamous cell cancer is very common and northern parts of the country falls in the so-called esophageal cancer belt with some districts in the northeastern states having one of the highest incidence rates of this deadly cancer. In absence of established endoscopic screening program, most esophageal cancers are diagnosed late in their clinical course and with very limited opportunity for curative treatment. Utilization of palliative measures such endoscopic stent

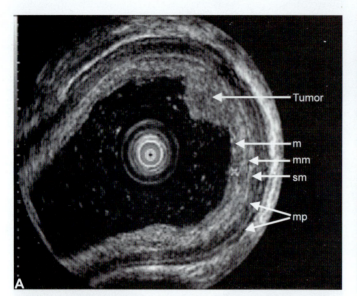 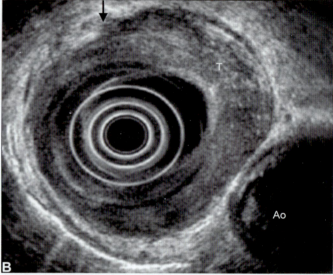

FIGURES 17.6A and B: (A) Endoscopic ultrasonographic image obtained by a high frequency catheter probe of an early esophageal cancer limited to mucosa and amenable to endoscopic resection. m represents: mucosa; mm: muscularis mucosae; sm: submucosal; and mp: muscularis propria, (B) EUS image of a locally advanced esophageal cancer that has progressed through the muscularis propria into periesophageal tissue (T3 category tumor). The tissue plain between the tumor and the descending aorta (Ao) remains intact

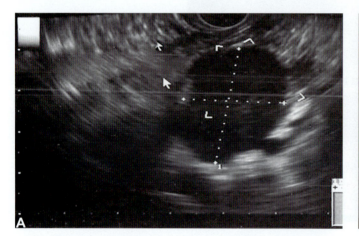 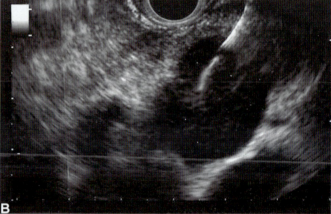

FIGURES 17.7A and B: (A) EUS image of a malignant appearing celiac lymph node in a patient with esophageal cancer, (B) EUS guided fine-needle aspiration is being performed for confirmation of nodal metastasis

therapy and endoscopic gastrostomies are uncommonly offered to these patients. With the initial reports of radio-frequency based endoscopic ablative therapy of early squamous cell cancer and precancerous high grade dysplasia, there may be an opportunity for institution of endoscopic screening programs in high incidence areas of the country. Late diagnosis is typical for other common cancers as well

viz gastric and gallbladder cancer and the access to endoscopic palliation is very limited and is often not pursued for financial reasons. As mentioned, colorectal cancer in uncommon although in some reports increasing incidence has been reported in more affluent segments of the society.

Most diagnostic endoscopic procedures in India are done without or with minimal sedation. Concept of conscious sedation is limited and usually done with rudimentary monitoring of patients during sedation. Paradoxically, profofol based deep sedation is increasingly being used in many nursing homes and hospitals but often without appropriate supervision by trained personnel.

As most of the healthcare in India is based on out of pocket expense, economic considerations are paramount in making medical decisions. Endoscopic diagnosis and treatment is necessarily expensive and in most parts of the country is viewed as being out of the realm of basic medical care. More than 80% of the endoscopic facilities are provided by the private health care sector and endoscopic diagnostic facilities are often rudimentary or nonexistent in governmental health sector. Although exposure to endoscopy is available during postgraduate training in both medical and surgical residencies, hands on training in flexible endoscopies are usually limited to postdoctoral courses (DM, MCh or the DNB) available only in a few select institutions across the country. A further period of focused training for 1 to 2 years is generally recommended to achieve the level of competence expected of advanced therapeutic endoscopists. While many physicians choose to incorporate gastrointestinal endoscopy in their clinical practice, limited opportunity for hands on training remains an important bottle neck and, most physicians' training experience comprise attending conferences with endoscopy workshops, interaction with industry representatives and often learning by self-training. Efforts at improving and standardizing the training and practice of GI endoscopy in India are desperate need of the hour and will require active and dynamic involvement of the leading professional societies such as, Indian Society of Gastroenterology and Society of Gastrointestinal Endoscopy of India.

In summary, gastrointestinal endoscopy has become a cornerstone of treatment of most gastrointestinal and liver disorders and similar to other countries has seen rapid dissemination in India over the last few decades. In order to optimize the application of gastrointestinal endoscopy in delivering cost-effective health care, increasing recognition of the importance of this particular discipline of Medicine by physicians, health care institutions, government and the society as a whole will be required.

Obstetrical Problems for Surgeons

18

Koji Matsuo, Norichika Ushioda

PHYSIOLOGICAL CHANGES IN PREGNANCY

Cardiovascular System

- Blood pressure, decreased in second trimester.
- Heart rate, 17 percent increased.
- Cardiac output, 43 percent increased.
- Stroke volume, 27 percent increased.
- Systemic vascular resistance, 21 percent decreased.

Pulmonary Function

- Respiratory alkalosis.
- Respiratory rate, unchanged.
- Residual volume, 20 percent decreased.
- Functional residual capacity, 20 percent decreased.
- Tidal volume, 39 percent increased.
- Minute ventilation, 42 percent increased.
- Arterial blood gases: pH, unchanged, pO_2, 7 mm Hg increased, pCO_2, 7 mm Hg decreased.

Renal Function

- Glomerular filtration rate, 40-50 percent increased.
- Renal plasma flow, 50-75 percent increased.
- Creatinine, 0.3 mg/dl decreased.
- Blood urea nitrogen, 50 percent decreased.
- Urinary protein, up to 250-300 mg/dl.

Hematologic Laboratory Values

- Hemoglobin, 1.5-2.0 g/dl decreased, hematocrit, 4-6 percent decreased.
- Leukocyte count, $3.5 \times 10^3/mm^3$ increased.
- Platelet, slightly decreased.
- Sedimentation rate, increased.
- Fibrinogen, 0.1-2.0 g/dl increased.
- Coagulation times, unchanged.

Serum Chemistries

- Sodium, 2-4 mmol/L decreased: Potassium 0.2-0.3 mmol/L decreased.
- Total protein, 1.0 g/dl decreased: Albumin, 1.0 g/dl decreased.
- Fasting glucose, 10 percent decreased: Total calcium, 10 percent decreased.
- Iron, 35 percent decreased: Iron binding capacity, 40-50 percent increased: Ferritin, 40-50 ug/L decreased.
- Total cholesterol, 60-80 mg/dl increased: Triglyceride, 100 mg/dl increased.

Liver, Biliary and Pancreatic Enzymes

- Transaminase, GOT/GPT, unchanged.
- LDH, slightly increased.
- CPK, 25-30 percent decreased.
- Amylase, 50-100 percent increased, lipase, 50 percent decreased.

Thyroid Function

- TSH, unchanged.
- Total T4, 5 mg/dl increased: Free T4, unchanged.
- T3, 50 percent increased, T3 resin uptake, 25-35 percent decreased.

ACUTE ABDOMINAL PAIN IN PREGNANCY

Differential Diagnosis

Obstetrical Diseases

Abortion*, ectopic pregnancy*, preterm labor†, labor onset†, abruption placenta†, pre-eclampsia†, acute fatty liver†, HELLP syndrome†, postpartum endometritis

Gynecologic Diseases

Torsion/rupture of ovarian cyst*, pelvic inflammatory disease*, degenerative myoma†

Non-Ob-Gyn Diseases

Appendicitis, urolithiasis, pancreatitis, ileus, pyelonephritis, cholelithiasis/cholecystitis, peptic ulcer disease, diverculitits, gastroentelitis, inflammatory bowel disease.

Ectopic Pregnancy

Etiology

- Common cite: Ampulla (55%), isthmus (25%), and fimbria (17%).
- **Prior ectopic pregnancy**, previous tubal surgery (e.g. tubal ligation), history of pelvic inflammatory disease, multiple sexual partners, exposure to DES *in utero* are risk factors.
- Increasing incidence: 4.5/1000 in 1970, 19.7 in 1000 in 1992.

Signs and Symptoms

- Mild pain and vaginal spotting are symptoms before the rupture of ectopic pregnancies.
- Time of rupture: 8-12 weeks in ampullary pregnancy: 6-8 weeks in isthmic pregnancy.
- Localized or diffuse tenderness is present in over 80 percent.
- Vaginal bleeding is present in 75 percent.
- Syncope, dizziness, lightheadness is present in 33-50 percent.
- Unilateral adnexal mass is palpated in 33-50 percent.

Diagnosis

- Pregnancy test is mandatory to make a diagnosis in acute abdominal pain in female.
- In suspicious case, β-hCG titer must be monitored. In normal pregnancy, β-hCG should be doubled every 48-

hours. An increase of 50 percent or less in a 48-hours is associated with a nonviable pregnancy.

- Among cases with β-hCG levels of more than 2000 mIU/ml, transvaginal ultrasonography identifies an intrauterine gestational sac in all those with viable intrauterine pregnancies.
- Among cases with β-hCG levels of less than 2000 mIU/ml, 48-hours β-hCG monitoring should be performed, and suction curettage should be perfomed in abnormal increase pattern.
- Transvaginal ultrasound shows no gestational sac in the uterus: Heterogeneous hyperechoic lesion in adnexa-fluid collection in cul-de-sac in bleeding case.
- An intrauterine **pregnancy** is visible on transabdominal ultrasonography once chorionic gonadotropin levels have reached 6,000-6,500 mIU/ml.
- Laparoscopy remains the gold standard for the diagnosis of **ectopic pregnancy although the need has declined.**
- Culdocentesis shows nonclotting blood.

Treatment

Medical management

- Methotrexate (MTX), potassium chloride, hyperosmolar glucose, dactinomycin, prostaglandins, and mifepristone are drug agents. MTX has extensively studied.
- MTX regimen is: 50 mg/mm^2 intramuscularly weekly until the decline of β-hCG is more than 15 percent of initial β-hCG in 4-7days.
- Diameter of gestational sac of 2 cm or less, absence of fetal heart rate, and absence of bleeding in peritoneal cavity is favorable **predictors of the success of MTX therapy.**

Surgical management

- In cases of unstable hemodynamics, active peritoneal bleeding, nonresponse to medical management, surgical treatment is performed.
- Diameter of 3 cm or less, unruptured, and easily access are favorable to laparoscopic surgery.
- Interstitial pregnancies require a corneal wedge resection. Cervical pregnancies may be associated with massive bleeding and may mandate hysterectomy.

Spontaneous Abortion

Etiology

- 50 percent of spontaneous abortion occurs during the first trimester. 30-40 percent of cases are a result of

---

*Common in first trimester,
†Common in second to third trimester

subclinical, and 10-20 percent of cases are a result of clinical loss. 0.4-1 percent of women are habitual aborters.

Clinical Findings of Spontaneous Abortion

- Threatened abortion: The cervix remains closed—slight bleeding with or without crampy.
- Inevitable abortion: Abdominal pain, bleeding, and open cervix, impending abortion.
- Incomplete abortion: Abdominal cramps and relatively severe bleeding are present. Products of contraception have partly passed from uterine cavity. In cases of active continuous bleeding, curettage is performed.
- Complete abortion: Entire of conceptus has passed from uterine cavity. Bleeding and pain are not evident once passed.
- Missed abortion: No fetal heart with remained gestational sac in uterus.
- Blighted ovum: No fetus in gestational sac in uterus.

Preterm Labor (PTL)

- PTL occurs in 7-8 percent of all pregnancies.
- Cervical length shorter than 2.5 cm before 32 weeks is high risk of PTL.
- Fetal fibronectin is strong predictor: Negative result promises that PTL will not occur in next 2 weeks.
- Management is stated with IV fluid. Tocolytics prolong up to 48 hours of gestational week: $MgSO_4$, ritodrine, indomethacin, nifedipine, terbutaline.
- Contraindication of tocolysis includes: Chorioamnionitis, severe pre-eclampsia, abruptio placenta, persistent fetal distress.
- Betamethasone is used to decrease neonatal respiratory distress and intraventricular hemorrhage before 34 weeks.

Abruptio Placenta

Etiology

- Frequency is 1-3 percent of all pregnancies.
- Risk factors include: Maternal cocaine use, smoking, pre-eclampsia.

Signs and Symptoms

- Tender uterus with hyperstimulation of uterine contraction.
- Genital bleeding (not all the cases).

- Cardiotocogram shows nonreassuring fetal heart rate pattern.

Diagnosis

- Ultrasound shows retroplacental hematoma but it is not seen in all the cases.
- Work-up for DIC is mandatory: CBC with platelet, PT/PTT, fibrinogen, and FDP.

Managements

- In mild case, careful monitoring on labor and delivery.
- In moderate to severe case, an amniotomy and induction/augmentation of labor is performed. Blood products are supplied with necessary. Cesarean delivery should be prepared in any circumstances of emergency.

Torsion/Rupture of Ovarian Cyst

- Most commonly occur between 6-14 weeks.
- Typically abruption onset of unilateral lower abdominal pain.
- Shock and peritonitis may occur.
- Transvaginal ultrasonography is performed to evaluate blood flow.
- Diagnosis is made by surgery.
- Prompt surgical intervention is mandatory: Salpingo-oophorectomy or untwist of ovary.

Pyelonephritis

Etiology

- Frequency is 1-2 percent all pregnancies. *E. coli* is present in 85 percent of cases.
- Asymptomatic bacteriuria is one of the main causes: 25-30 percent will be pyelonephritis.
- 85 percent of patients are right side, while 15 percent are left side.
- One of the main causes of maternal sepsis in pregnancy.

Diagnosis

- Fever, CVA tenderness, and flank pain.
- Urinarysis with culture and sensitivity.

Management

- Admission with IV antibiotics.
- In patients hemodynamically stable: Cefadyl 2g IV, QTD, or ampicillin 2g IV every 4 hour.

- In patients with high fever, chills, and tachycardia, gentamicin is added to ampicillin.

Pancreatitis in Pregnancy

- Frequency in pregnancy is 0.01-0.1 percent while 0.5 percent for nonpregnant patients.
- Relatively common in the third trimester and postpartum.
- Majority of cases are related with gallstone.
- Abortion and preterm labor could be triggered.
- In severe pancreatitis, surgical intervention reduces the risk of maternal mortality.

Appendicitis in Pregnancy

Etiology

- Frequency is not changed from the general population (1/2000 pregnancies).
- Once peritonitis occurs due to the rupture of appendix, the rate of fetal loss is significantly increased (15%). Abortion and preterm labor is also increased.
- Maternal mortality is significantly increased compared to nonpregnant patients: Less than 0.1 percent for nonpregnant patients, 2 percent for the first trimester, 7.3 percent for the third trimester, and 5 percent for perforated cases.

Diagnosis

- Diagnosis of appendicitis in pregnancy is often difficult due to these factors:
  - Leukocytosis is common in pregnancy
  - Nausea and vomiting are common in pregnancy
  - The appendix moves upward and laterally in pregnancy
  - Abdominal signs of appendicitis are atypical in pregnancy.

Management

- Once appendicitis is suspected, surgical treatment is treatment of choice.
- Cesarean section is not necessary just in the presence of appendicitis.
- Antibiotics are not necessary in uncomplicated appendicitis.

Cholelithiasis/Cholecystitis

Etiology

- Pregnancy is the state of intrahepatic and bile duct cholestatsis due to excessive estrogen and progesterone (same mechanism in oral contraceptive pills).
- Asymptomatic gallstone is 2-4 percent of frequency in pregnancy.
- Prevalence of gallstone in pregnancy is increased due to cholestatsis.
- Acute cholecystitis is 0.3 percent of frequency in pregnancy.

Diagnosis

- Diagnosis of cholecystitis in pregnancy is difficult due to following reasons:
  - Nausea, vomiting, and anorexia are common in the first trimester.
  - Increasing number of leukocytes in pregnancy.
  - ALP produced by placenta is increased in pregnancy.

Management

- Observation for asymptomatic gallstone.
- Surgical intervention is indicated in the case that medical intervention was failed.
- Laparoscopic surgery could be safely performed.

GENITAL BLEEDING IN PREGNANCY

First Trimester in Pregnancy

Abortion, hydatidiform mole, ectopic pregnancy.

Second to Third Trimester in Pregnancy

Labor onset, placental previa, abruption placenta, vasa previa.

Postpartum

Uterine atonic bleeding, cervical/vaginal laceration, uterine inversion, placental retention

Placenta Previa

Etiology

- Frequency is 0.4-0.5 percent of all pregnancies.
- Risk factors: Previous cesarean section, instrumental abortion.

Diagnosis

- Painless vaginal bleeding.

Management

- Bed rest with possible tocolytics if bleeding ceased.
- Betamethasone to promote fetal lung maturity: c-section once maturity is confirmed.
- Delivery with c-secion in full term.

Uterine Atonic Bleeding

Etiology

- More than 500 ml of blood loss in the first 24 hours after delivery.
- Risk factors: Multiparity, macrosomia, use of $MgSO_4$, rapid or prolonged labor.

Management

- Vaginal exam to rule out other causes of bleeding.
- Bimanual massage, oxytocin drip is initial management.
- Hysterectomy or embolization of uterine artery is performed to refractory cases.

DEEP VENOUS THROMBOSIS AND PULMONARY EMBOLISM

Etiology

- Frequency while in pregnancy is increased 5-10 times compared to nonpregnant women.
- Frequency of DVT in pregnancy is 0.5-1/1,000 deliveries.
- Frequency of PE in pregnancy varies from 1/2,500 to 1/10,000.
- PE in pregnancy is the most common cause of maternal death.
- Factors for increased risks: Increased concentration of coagulators including fibrinogen—increased concentration of fibrinolysis inhibitors—venous obstruction by gravid uterus.

Diagnosis

Pulmonary Embolism

- Taking clinical presentation including prolonged immobilization after c-section.
- Important physical examination includes tachycardia (90%), dyspnea, and chest pain.
- SaO_2, chest X-ray, ECG, and ABG are indispensable for ruling out other conditions.

- Initial laboratory workup includes CBC, PT, aPTT, FBG, FDP, and AT-III.
- V/Q scan comes first for making diagnosis.
- Pulmonary angiogram comes for the inconclusive or moderate risk in V/Q scan.
- Pulmonary angiogram is golden standard of diagnosis.

Deep Vein Thrombosis

- Calf swelling with erythema or pain for symptoms.
- Homan's sign with physical examination.
- Diagnosis is made by duplex ultrasonography.

Management

Pulmonary Embolism

- O_2, IV fluid support during workup.
- IV heparin or LMWH for the initial treatment: Bolus for 60 U/kg following maintain does with continuous IV.
- aPTT is monitored for IV heparin (PTT 2.0-3.0).
- IV heparin is gradually shifted to oral warfarin with monitoring PT.

Deep Vein Thrombosis

- IV heparin or LMWH while pregnancy.

OBSTETRICAL EMERGENCY

Following conditions are highly known as the cause of maternal or fetal death, and need prompt management:

- Obstetrical hemorrhage due to either atonic bleeding, placenta previa, abruption placenta, and severe cervical laceration
- Uterine rupture complicated in VBAC (A-8)
- Eclampsia (A-7)
- Fetal prolonged deceleration due to umbilical cord prolapse
- Pulmonary embolism
- Sepsis due to pyelonephritis
- Amniotic embolism.

NAUSEA AND VOMITING IN PREGNANCY

- 70-80 percent of patients are affected.
- Hyperemesis gravidarum (HG) is severe form of N&V in pregnancy, affecting less than 1 percent of pregnancy.
- HG is defined as poor oral intake, severe N&V, body weight loss >=5 percent, ketonuria, etc.

- Need to rule out various differential diagnoses; gastroenteritis, appendicitis, diabetic ketoacidosis, hyperthyroidism, pseudotumor cerebri, cerebral tumor, pre-eclampsia, etc.

PRE–ECLAMPSIA AND ECLAMPSIA

Etiology

- 6-7 percent of incidence for pre-eclampsia. Eclampsia is rare in developed country.
- Primigravida, previous history, multiple pregnancy, pre-existing hypertension, hyperthyroidism, lupus erythematosus, and diabetes mellitus are known as high risks.
- Intrauterine growth retardation, eclampsia, preterm delivery, placenta previa, HELLP syndrome, hepatic rupture, and cerebral vascular hemorrhage are possible complications.

Diagnosis and Classification

- Pregnancy induced hypertension (PIH): BP>140/90 mm Hg without proteinuria and edema.
- Chronic hypertension: BP > 140/90 mm Hg prior to 20 weeks of gestation.
- Mild pre-eclampsia: BP > 140/90 mm Hg, proteinurea > 300 mg/24 hrs, and mild edema.
- Severe pre-eclampsia: BP>160/110 mm Hg, proteinurea > 5.0 g/24 hrs, and systemic edema.
- HEELP syndrome: Hemolysis, elevated liver enzyme, and low platelet.

Management

Periodical monitoring for symptoms, blood pressure, CBC, liver enzyme, uric acid, urine protein, and fetal nonstress test is mandatory.

Mild Pre-eclampsia

- Delivery if gestational age (GA) >=37 weeks.
- Expectant management with bed rest if GA <37 weeks.
- IV MgSO$_4$ if labor is in active phase (4 g for half hour as loading dose, 1-2 g/hr as maintain dose).

Severe Pre-eclampsia

- Delivery if GA>=34 weeks.
- Careful expectant management if GA<34 weeks (IV dexamethazon is optional).

- Delivery if the condition worsens.
- IV MgSO$_4$ once diagnosed as severe type.

Eclampsia

- Secure airway, and stabilization of maternal circulation.
- IV valium for antiseizure drug.
- MgSO$_4$ for prevention of further seizure.
- Work-up including head CT to rule out other condition is necessary.
- As long as fetal shows no distress, trial of vaginal delivery is recommended.

HELLP Syndrome

- Immediate delivery.

Antihypertensive Drug in Pregnancy

- Indicated if BP>160/105 mm Hg.
- Hydralazine, labetalol, and sodium nitroprusside are used while in pregnancy.

VAGINAL BIRTH AFTER CESAREAN (VBAC)

- Rate of cesarean section (c-section) at 2002 was 26 percent.
- Rate of VBAC at 2002 was 12.7 percent.
- Previous c-section with the indication of malpresentation is favorable factor for success.
- Uterine rupture is serious complication causing fetal demise (0.6%).

BIBLIOGRAPHY

1. ACOG Technical Bulletin Series
2. Creasy RK, Resnik R, Iams J, et al. Maternal-Fetal Medicine, 5th edn. Philadelphia, Saunders, 2003.
3. Cunningham G, Gant NF, Leveno KJ, et al. Williams Obstetrics, 21st edn. New York: McGraw-Hill Professional, 2001.
4. Iyengar SS. Pre-eclampsia. Lancet 2000;356(9237):1260-5.
5. Landon MB, Hauth JC, Leveno KJ, Spong CY, Leindecker S, Varner MW, et al. National Institute of Child Health and Human Development, Maternal-Fetal Medicine Units Network. Maternal and perinatal outcomes associated with a trial of labor after prior cesarean delivery. N Engl J Med 2004;351(25):2581-9.
6. Lipscomb GH, Stovall TG, Ling FW. Nonsurgical treatment of ectopic pregnancy. N Engl J Med 2000;343(18):1325-9.
7. Niebyl JR, Gabbe JR, Jennifer RN, Joe LS, et al. Obstetrics: normal and problem pregnancies, 4th edition. New York, NY: Churchill Livingstone, 2001.

Gynecological Problems for Surgeons

Koji Matsuo, Norichika Ushioda

DIFFERENTIAL DIAGNOSIS OF PELVIC MASS

Various lesions could be the cause of pelvic mass formation. MRI and ultrasound is useful for the diagnosis.

Benign Tumor

- *Ovarian cyst*: Teratoma, serous cyst adenoma, mucinous cyst adenoma, endometrial cyst, Meigs' syndrome (characteristic pleural effusion).
- Uterine myoma, uterine adenomyosis, pyometra.
- *Others*: Abscess in tube, hematoma, ectopic pregnancy, luteal cyst, polycystic ovary.

Benign to Borderline Malignancy

- Granulosa cell tumor, thecoma, Sertoli-Leydig cell tumor.
- Gastrointestinal stromal tumor.

Malignant Tumor

- *Ovarian cancer*: Cystadenocarcinoma, mucinous cystadenocarcinoma, dysgerminoma, metastatic tumor (Metastasis from gastric cancer called Krukenberg's tumor).
- *Uterine cancer*: Cervical cancer, endometrial cancer, uterine sarcoma, choriocarcinoma.
- *Others*: Retroperitoneal malignancy, e.g. angiosarcoma.

PAP SMEAR, CERVICAL INTRAEPITHERIAL NEOPLASIA, CERVICAL CANCER

Pap Smear

- Contributed to the decreasing number of cervical cancer.
- Recommended over the age of 18, or time of first sexual intercourse.
- Annual checkup is desired.

- Not necessary for the age >65 if result is normal (but not clearly defined).
- Every 5 years of cuff smear after hysterectomy due to benign reason.
- Endocervical cells must be obtained.

Cervical Intraepitherial Neoplasia (CIN)

Classification

- CIN I: Mild dysplasia that involves lower 1/3 of epithelium.
- CIN II: Moderate dysplasia that involves lower 2/3 of epithelium.
- CIN III: Severe dysplasia to carcinoma *in situ* that is full thickness dysplasia.

Management

- Abnormal pap smear findings (class IIb or more) required further evaluation with colposcopy or cone biopsy.
- Low-grade squamous intraepithelial lesion: 15-30 percent of chance of CIN II or more with biopsy—colposcopy is required.
- High-grade squamous intraepithelial lesion: 70-75 percent of chance of CIN II or more with biopsy—colposcopy and endocervical curettage are required.
- Atypical squamous cells of undetermined significance (ASCUS): 5-17 percent of chance of CIN II or more with biopsy—colposcopy, HPV test, and repeat cytology are required.
- Colposcopy: Transformation zone needs to be visualized by acetic acid.
- Cone biopsy: Loop electroexcision procedure, laser, and cold knife are used.

Cervical Cancer

Etiology and Classification

- Squamous cell carcinoma (most common), adeno-carcinoma, squamoadenocarcinoma.
- HPV 16 and 18, smoking, and immunosuppression are known causes.
- Stage IIIb is complicated with hydronephrosis due to the ureter involvement.
- 5-year survival rate is more than 80 percent in stage I, >60 percent in stage II, >30 percent in stage III, 10 percent in stage IV.

Management

- Modified radical hysterectomy for microinvasion (stages Ia1 and Ia2).
- Stages Ib1/IIa is indication of radical hysterectomy with pelvic lymph node dissection. Adjuvant chemotherapy with cisplatin-based regimen for positive lymph node.
- Stages Ib2 to IVa: Radiation therapy (external/brachytherapy) with cisplatin-based chemotherapy.
- Stage IVb: Palliative therapy with radiation.

ENDOMETRIAL HYPERPLASIA AND ENDOMETRIAL CANCER

Endometrial Hyperplasia

Etiology

- Premalignant lesion of endometrial cancer.
- Risk factors: Obesity, anovulatory cycle, tamoxifen.
- History of vaginal bleeding mostly postmenopause (however, many cases are asymptomatic).

Diagnosis and Classification

- Endometrial biopsy with following dilation and curettage is the mainstay of making diagnosis.
- Simple hyperplasia: Progression to cancer 1 percent.
- Complex hyperplasia: Progression to cancer 3 percent.
- Atypcial hyperplasia: Progression to cancer 9 percent.
- Complex hyperplasia with atypia: Progression to cancer 27 percent.

Management

- Diagnostic dilation and curettage for atypical hyperplasia in cytology.
- Medical curettage: Progesterone agent is treatment of choice.

- Repeat endometrial biopsy with 3-6 months of period.
- High-dose progesterone agent for persistent hyperplasia.
- Hysterectomy is indicated if medical curettage is failed.

Endometrial Cancer

Etiology

- Most common gynecologic cancer with best prognosis.
- Most cases are diagnosed >60 years old.
- Postmenopausal vaginal bleeding is the most common symptom.
- Hereditary nonpolyposis syndrome. DNA repair gene defect. Colorectal cancer and endometrial cancer are involved.
- 5-year survivor: 81-91 percent in stage I, 67-77 percent in stage II, 32-60 percent in stage III, 5-20 percent in stage IV.

Diagnosis, Histology and Classification

- Transvaginal ultrasound shows endometrial thickness.
- Endometrial biopsy with following dilation and curettage is golden standard.
- Pathology: Endometrioid, papillary serous, mucinous, clear cell type.
- Classification: Limited in endometrium (Ia), endocervical involvement (IIa), positive peritoneal cytology (IIIa), lymph nodes meta (IIIc), bladder or bowel invasion (IVa).

Management

- Surgical hysterectomy with salpingo-oophorectomy is treatment of choice.
- Additional lymph adnectomy dissection: >Ic, >IIa, grade 3, clear cell type, etc.
- Adjuvant chemotherapy or radiation therapy after hysterectomy.

ENDOMETRIOSIS AND ADENOMYOSIS

Endometriosis

- Endometrial gland or stroma outside the uterus, e.g. peritoneum, ovary, etc.
- Occur only in reproductive mense reserve female.
- Dysmenorrhea, pelvic pain is most common cause.
- Endometrial cyst (chocolate cyst) is complicated in the lesion of ovary.
- Infertility is complicated in the lesion of tube and ovary.
- Laparoscopy is used for both diagnosis and treatment.
- GnRH could be used as medical management.

Adenomyosis

- Endometrial gland or stroma is in myometrium.
- Enlarged myometrial thickness is typical finding.
- Dysmenorrhea and pelvic pain are most common symptom.

OVARIAN CYST AND OVARIAN CANCER

Ovarian Cyst

Etiology

- Follicular cyst is most common overall ovarian mass.
- Most ovarian tumors in women age of <45 years are benign.
- Serous cystadenoma is most common type.
- Teratoma causes torsion of steel.
- Ruptured mucinous cystadenoma could be the cause of pseudomyxoma peitonei.
- 1 percent of teratoma shows malignant transformation.
- Cystectomy for women desired pregnancy, salipingo-oophorectomy for nondesired.

Ovarian Cancer

Etiology

- Over 20,000 for annual incidence with over 13,000 deaths by ovarian cancer.
- 85 percent of epitherial type, 10 percent of germ cell type, and 5 percent of sex cord stromal type.
- Family history of breast or ovarian cancer has associated.
- Mutation of BACA 1 and 2 are associated with ovarian cancer development.
- OCPs reduce the risk of ovarian cancer.
- No useful screening tool for general population.
- Screening with CA125 is low specificity.

Findings and Diagnosis

- Pelvic mass and ascites are most common findings.
- Final diagnosis with staging is done by intraoperative histology.
- Paracentesis with cytology is indicated for ascites.

Management

- Postmenopausal ovarian mass is absolute indication of surgical exploration.
- Ovarian mass with < 8 cm in reproductive age: Careful observation.
- Ovarian mass with > 8 cm in reproductive age: Surgery is indicated.

- Surgical exploration is performed for all stage.
- Cytoreductive surgery (resection of as much tumor) is treatment concept.
- Optimal surgery (tumor <1 cm) is good prognostic indicator.
- Adjuvant chemotherapy with platinum and pacliitaxel-based regimen.
- Findings of second look surgery have important value of making prognosis.

UTERINE MYOMA

- Most common uterine tumor affecting 20-40 percent of reproductive female.
- Hypermenorrhea is seen in intramyometrial type.
- Could be the cause of infertility, preterm delivery.
- Symptomatic is indicated for the treatment with either myomectomy or hysterectomy.
- Recurrence after treatment is relatively common.

MENOPAUSE AND OSTEOPOROSIS

Menopause

- Menopause is defined as secondary amenorrhea more than 12 months.
- Average age is 50.6 years.
- Symptoms include vasomotor instability, e.g. hot flashes, sweating, palpitation.
- Postcoital vaginal bleeding as the sign of genital atrophy.
- HRT (E + P) as treatment of choice.

Osteoporosis

- Absolute decrease in amount of bone: Serum Ca, P, and PTH is normal.
- Bone mineral density >2.5 SDs below the mean (T score <-2.5).
- Diagnosis: Dual-energy X-ray absorptiometry (DEXA).
- Complications: Weightbearing bone fracture in supine, hip bone, etc.
- Management: Ca supplement with vitamin D, alendronate agent, raloxifene, calcitonin, HRT, exercise.

STD AND PID

Sexually Transmitted Disease

Chlamydia Trachomatis

- Most common cause of STD in both females and males.
- Symptoms appear after one week of sexual intercourse.
- Pap smear: Intracytoplasmic vacuoles, elementary body.

Neisseria Gonorrhoeae

- Characteristic purulent discharge half week after sexual intercourse.
- Pelvic inframatory disease including pelvic abscess is complicated.
- Gram-negative *Diplococcus* in white blood cell.
- Treatment with ceftriaxone.

Human Papilloma Virus

- Type 6 and 11 associated with condyloma acuminate.
- Koilocytic change in squamous epithelium.

Herpes Virus Type 2

- Tzanck preparation for diagnosis.
- Treatment with acyclovir.

Gardnerella Vaginalis

- Pathogen of bacterial vaginosis.
- Symptoms include fishy order, noninflammatory discharge.
- Test: pH more than 5.5, characteristic clue cells.
- Treatment with metronidazole.

Treponema Pallidum

- Pathogen of syphilis.
- Primary syphilis: Painless genital ulcer (usually solitary lesion), chancre.
- Secondary syphilis: Systemic maculopapular rash (mostly palm).
- Tertiary syphilis: Involved in central nervous system—neurosyphilis.
- Diagnosis: RPR, VDRL, and FTA-ABS. Dark field microscopy for primay syphilis.
- Treatment with penicillin G.

Trichomonas Vaginalis

- Motile protozoa in microscopy.
- Symptom includes greeny frothy discharge.
- Treatment with metronidazole.

PELVIC INFLAMMATORY DISEASE (PID)

Etiology

- Pathogens causing STD, mainly *Chlamydia trachomatis*, *Neisseria gonorrhoeae*.
- Ascending transmission through cervix.

- Major cause of infertility.
- Major cause of ectopic pregnancy.
- Chronic pelvic pain is long-term complication.

Symptoms and Findings

- Symptoms include pelvic pain, fever, and discharge.
- Physical findings: BT >38.5C, cervical motion tenderness, adnexal mass and tenderness, flamed cervix.

Management

- Indication of hospitalization: Abscess formation, teenager, pregnancy, necessity for surgery, symptoms of severe N/V, peritonitis, use of IUD, etc.
- IV antibiotics for hospitalized case.
- Counseling to prevent recurrent PID is important treatment process.

OCP AND HRT

Oral Contraceptive Pills

Introduction

- High success rate: 0.1 percent of failure rate with complete medication compliance (14% in condom use).
- Estrogen and progesterone are contained. Gonadotropin secretion is inhibited.
- Progesterone causes endometrial decidualization.
- Emergency contraceptive is effective if taken within 72 hours (75% of effectiveness).

Complications and Contraindications

- Increased risk of deep venous thrombosis and pulmonary embolism, stroke, myocardial infarction, hypertension, hepatic adenoma, cholelithiasis, and dyslipidemia (LDH increased, HDL decreased).
- Absolute contraindication: Smoke cigarette > = 15/day, smoker aged> = 35 years, h/o MI and stroke, h/o cardiovascular disease, h/o DVT/PE, breast cancer, and abnormal liver function.
- Relative contraindication: Long-term affected DM, hypertension, migraine headaches with aura, lupus erythematosus, hypertriglycemia, anticonvulsant drug, etc.
- OCPs are not allowed for following medication prescribed: Carbamazepine, phenobarbital, rifampin, phenytoin, topiramate, griseofulvin.
- Taking antibiotics increase the clearance of OCPs (hepatointestinal clearance).

Hormone Replacement Therapy

- Prescribed for symptomatic menopause or preventing osteoporosis.
- HRT increases the risk of coronary heart disease, stroke, breast cancer, and DVT/PE.
- Patient with intact uterus needs to take progesterone in addition to estrogen to reduce the risk of endometrial cancer.
- Periodical follow-up is necessary for: Liver function, lipid profile, breast exam, pap smear, etc.

URINARY INCONTINENCE

Diagnosis

- Urinary analysis with cytology and culture is necessary to rule out urinary infection.
- Pelvic examination for evaluate possible pelvic organ prolapse.
- Postvoid residual exam.
- Urodynamics is used to distinguish stress urinary incontinence from detrusor overactivity.

Classification and Management

Mixed type of incontinence could happen:

Stress Urinary Incontinence

- Occurs when intravesical pressure > urethral closure pressure.
- Pathophysiology: Intrinsic sphincter deficiency.
- Pelvic muscle exercise, surgical treatment, e.g. tension-vaginal taping.

Detrusor Overactivity

- Detrusor unintentionally contracts and results in incontinence.
- Detrusor hyperreflexia in neurological disorder, while detrusor instability in non-neurological disorder.
- Management: Timed voiding, pharmacotherapy.

BIBLIOGRAPHY

1. ACOG Practice Bulletin series.
2. Berek JS, Hacker NF. Practical gynecologic oncology, 3rd edn. Philadelphia: Lippincott Williams & Wilkins, 2000.
3. Hillard PA, Berek JS, Novak E, et al. Novak's Gynecology, 13th edn. Philadelphia, Lippincott Williams & Wilkins, 2002.
4. Philip J, Md Disaia, William T, Md Creasman. Clinical Gynecologic Oncology. CV Mosby; 6th edn (January 15, 2002).

Role of Interventional Radiology in Surgery

Preet Singh Kang

INTRODUCTION

Interventional radiology is a specialty devoted to advancing patient care through the integration of clinical and imaging-based diagnosis with minimally invasive therapy. Since the advent of interventional radiology in the late 1960s this field has evolved into a specialized branch with ever expanding role in current day medicine and surgery.

Interventional radiology uses X-rays, fluoroscopy, ultrasound, CT or MRI for diagnoses and to treat diseases with minimally invasive techniques. Presently, many conditions that once required surgery can be treated using intervention radiology based treatments which offer less risk, less pain and shorter recovery time. In many disease conditions interventional radiology can be complimentary to surgical management to improve patient care and outcomes. This is applicable to patients with multiple co-morbidities or high-risk situations where intervention radiology procedure can help stabilize or prepare the patient for a definitive surgical management at a later time. Advances in procedural techniques and addition of newer devices have greatly expanded the role of interventional radiology.

PRINCIPLES

There are broadly 2 types of intervention radiology techniques. The first is a direct percutaneous puncture using a needle and/or a catheter introduced via Seldinger technique under fluoroscopic, ultrasound, CT or MR guidance to reach the target which could be within any visceral cavity or solid organ in order to treat the underlying disease process. Seldinger technique is a multistep procedure whereby a thin needle is introduced in a tubular structure such as artery or hollow viscera or cavity through which a

guidewire can be placed. The needle is removed while holding in the guidewire to be followed by placement of long diagnostic or drainage catheters or variety of ostomy tubes based on the indication.

Using direct needle technique, aspiration or biopsy of a solid lesion could be performed with image guidance (Figs 20.1A and B). Alternatively, a needle or a catheter could be placed within a fluid collection for drainage or removal of pus (Figs 20.2A to C). In addition, a special needle such as a thermal ablation needle can be placed percutaneously into neoplasm of the liver, kidney or lung for radiofrequency ablation or cryoablation (Figure 20.3). All these procedures can be performed with imaging guidance to avoid vital structures with minimal risk to the patient.

The second technique is percutaneous access into tubular channels such as the arterial system, venous system, urinary system, gastrointestinal system or the biliary system in order to treat specific disease processes. The catheter is introduced via Seldinger technique and guidewires are used for navigation under fluoroscopic guidance into specific locations for providing therapy. Once the catheter is able to reach a specific site, therapeutic devices can be introduced over a guidewire to open blockage using angioplasty balloons, deliver stent or stent graft (Figs 20.4A and B). In case of bleeding or leakage of urine or bile, catheter based procedures can be used to seal or exclude the disease process. The catheter can deliver therapeutic medications such as thrombolytic or chemotherapy to specific sites, thereby avoiding risk of exposure to remote organs. Embolotherapy via percutaneous catheters is another major advance in technique especially with addition of microcatheters to treat bleeding from remote sites (Figure 20.5).

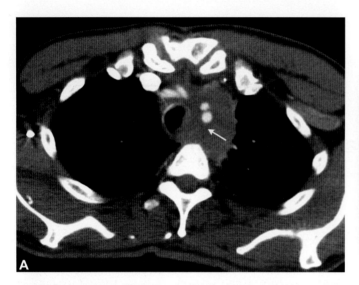

FIGURE 20.1A: Axial CT scan with iodine contrast showing a left upper lobe and mediastinal mass encasing the aortic arch vessels (arrow)

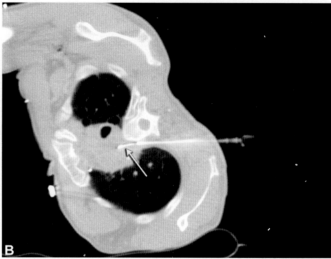

FIGURE 20.1B: Axial CT image of the same patient in prone oblique position with a trucut biopsy needle (arrow) introduced in the mass via left paravertebral posterior approach using iodine contrast enhanced CT guidance

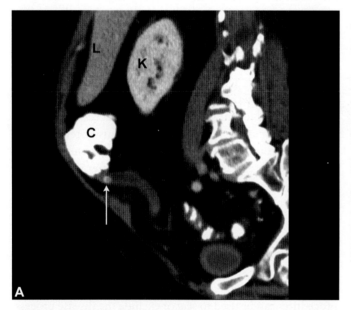

FIGURE 20.2A: CT scan reconstructed sagittal oblique image, obtained with oral and intravenous contrast, showing an enlarged inflamed appendix with an appendicolith at its junction with the cecum (C). The patient underwent laparoscopic appendectomy. (L–liver, K–right kidney)

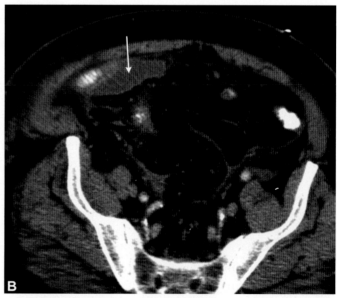

FIGURE 20.2B: Postappendectomy CT scan 2 weeks later shows fluid collection with peripheral enhancement (arrow) in this patient with lower abdominal pain and increased white blood cell count

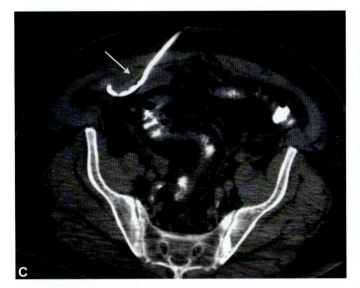

FIGURE 20.2C: CT scan demonstrating drainage of postoperative abscess with 8 Fr pigtail catheter (arrow) placed under CT guidance

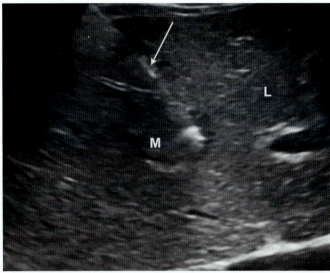

FIGURE 20.3: Axial ultrasound image of the liver (L), showing a radiofrequency ablation needle (arrow) guided into a hepatocellular carcinoma mass lesion (M) for treatment. The mass (M) had previously been biopsied using percutaneous needle

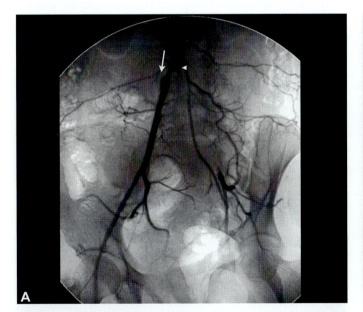

FIGURE 20.4A: Pelvic angiogram showing occluded left iliac artery at aortic bifurcation (arrowhead) and significant stenosis of proximal right common iliac artery. Percutaneous catheter placed via right common femoral artery (arrow)

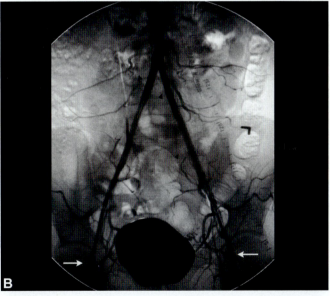

FIGURE 20.4B: Postintervention pelvic angiogram following revascularization of the left iliac artery with balloon expandable stent and placement of "kissing" aortic bifurcation stents (arrowheads) using bilateral femoral artery access (arrows)

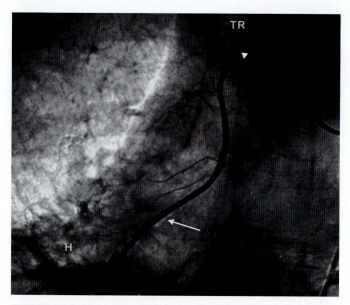

FIGURE 20.5: Right bronchial artery (arrowhead) angiogram, with microcatheter tip (arrow) is a distal location prior to embolization of hemoptysis (H) with polyvinyl alcohol particles. (TR–trachea)

PATIENT EVALUATION AND PRE-PROCEDURE REQUISITES

The evaluation of patient requires understanding of the patient's clinical condition, checking appropriate lab tests such as complete blood cell count including platelets, coagulation profile, basic electrolytes including renal function. Assessment of patient allergy and current medication is necessary. Since most of the interventional radiology procedures involve the use of iodine based contrast media, history and risk of contrast reactions should be addressed. In a patient with prior history of contrast reaction, premedication with steroids and antihistamines is performed. Most of the procedures are done under conscious sedation using short acting intravenous benzodiazepines and opioid medications in combination with local anesthetic. General anesthesia is rarely necessary. In any case, optimal patient outcome depends on close communication and consultation between the surgeon and the interventional radiologist. This is paramount in postoperative cases when a specific interventional procedure may avoid a second immediate surgery. Example of this situation is basket retrieval of retained common bile duct stone postcholecystectomy via the T-tube tract.

SCOPE OF INTERVENTION RADIOLOGY IN SURGERY

Interventional radiology procedures are used in the management of diseases affecting majority of the body organs and systems, such as gastrointestinal, hepatobiliary, cardiovascular, thoracic, obstetrics and gynecology, urinary and surgical infectious diseases, trauma, oncologic and transplant medicine. To illustrate the various IR procedures, case examples are presented as they are discussed in the following sections. These will be discussed in 2 broad groups, nonvascular interventions and vascular interventions.

Nonvascular Interventions

Percutaneous sampling and/or drainage of fluid collections, abscess within solid organs, pleural or peritoneal cavity is commonly performed for initial diagnosis or for post-operative patients. Percutaneous sampling could be performed using needle aspiration most commonly under ultrasound or CT scan guidance (Figure 20.6). Based on the gross and lab assessment of the fluid removed further treatment can be planned.

If the diagnosis of abscess is suspected or already established, percutaneous catheter placement ranging from

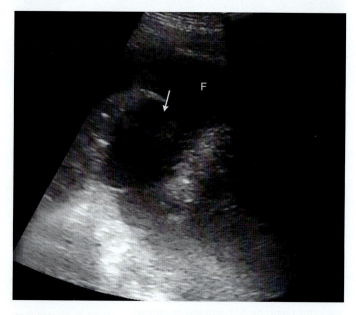

FIGURE 20.6: Ultrasound image of pleural effusion (F), showing the edge of the atelectatic lung (arrow) to be avoided, during guided thoracentesis of the fluid

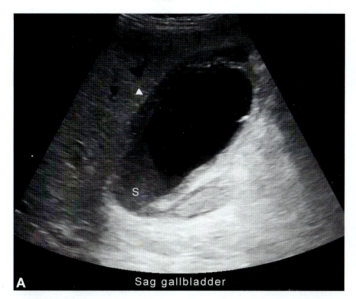

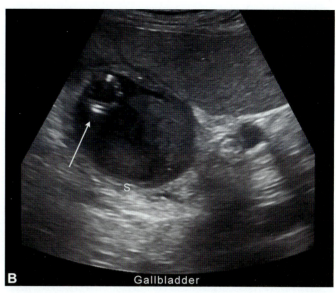

FIGURE 20.7A: Longitudinal ultrasound image of a distended gallbladder with wall thickening (arrowhead) and dependent sludge/pus (S), consistent with acute acalculous cholecystitis

FIGURE 20.7B: Ultrasound guided percutaneous transhepatic pigtail 8 Fr drainage catheter (arrow) placed within the gallbladder with removal of infected bile

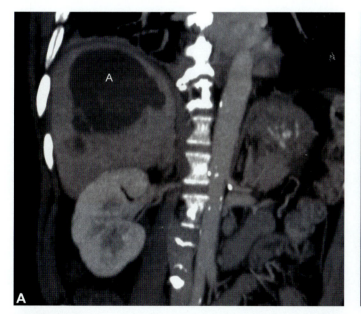

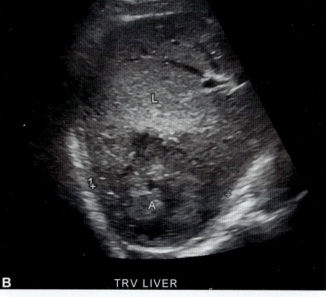

FIGURE 20.8A: Coronal CT scan image showing a large irregular abscess (A) in the right lobe of liver in a patient with fever, abnormal liver function tests and increased white cell count

FIGURE 20.8B: Ultrasound image of the liver (L), obtained during guided placement of a percutaneous 10 Fr pigtail drainage catheter to remove thick pyogenic material from the abscess (A)

6-18 French size could be performed within intra-abdominal abscess cavities, acute cholecystitis (Figs 20.7A and B), liver abscess (Figs 20.8 A to C), lung abscess, pyothorax, pneumothorax, hydronephrosis, tubo-ovarian abscess, etc.

Noninfected fluid collection such as pleural effusion, pericardial effusion or ascites can also be drained by simple aspiration. These can be easily repeated without significant risk in case of recurrent ascites in cirrhotic patients.

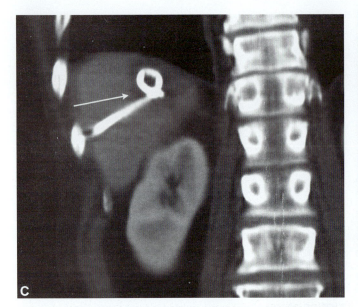

FIGURE 20.8C: Coronal CT scan image at 2-week follow-up showing near complete resolution of the abscess with the pigtail catheter (arrow) in position. The catheter was removed due to negligible output at this point

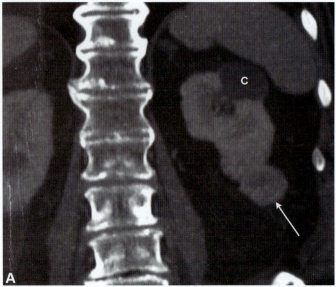

FIGURE 20.9A: Coronal CT scan image of the left kidney demonstrating a solid 3 cm enhancing mass lesion (arrow) at the lower pole. Incidental note made of a cortical renal cyst (C) at the upper pole

Malignant recurring pleural effusion can be managed by placement of implanted tunneled pleural cuffed catheters to facilitate fluid removal as necessary. This can significantly improve patient quality of life. In addition, sclerosing agents can be introduced via the pleural catheter to cause pleurodesis and prevent recurrent fluid accumulation.

Percutaneous biopsy is commonly performed for pulmonary nodule or masses, mediastinal lymph nodes, and abdominal or retroperitoneal masses or lymph nodes as well as viscera of the abdomen and pelvis. These are typically performed using ultrasound or CT scan for guidance. Alternatively fluoroscopy guidance can be used for large pulmonary lesion or rarely MRI if available. Various biopsy techniques include aspiration for cytology or histology as well as core biopsy to obtain larger samples. In patients with high risk of bleeding due to low platelets or elevated prothrombin time, transjugular biopsy of liver or kidney can be obtained. This can help with essential diagnosis as well as staging of neoplasm for preoperative planning.

Recent innovations in thermal ablation techniques have advanced the application of interventional radiology procedures for the management of renal cell carcinoma, nonsurgical hepatocellular carcinoma and nonsurgical lung neoplasm. One of the methods available is heat ablation using radiofrequency or microwave technology (Figs 20.9A to C). The other method of tumor treatment is cryoablation,

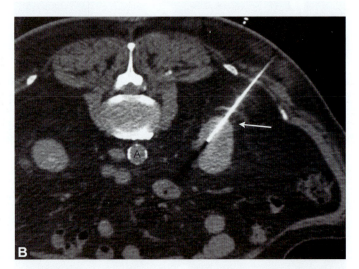

FIGURE 20.9B: Axial prone CT scan during image guided percutaneous biopsy and radiofrequency ablation of the lower pole mass (arrow) in this patient with high surgical risk. Biopsy revealed clear cell renal carcinoma. (A–aorta)

which essentially causes tissue death by freezing. These techniques consist of specialized needles which are introduced percutaneously under imaging guidance and placed accurately within the tumors for thermal ablation. Chemical ablation of hepatocellular carcinoma with absolute

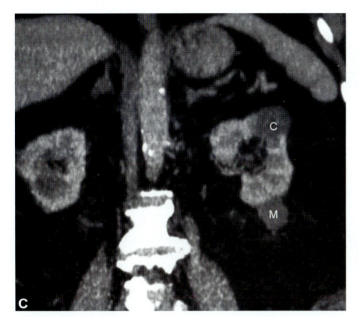

FIGURE 20.9C: Coronal CT image at 6-month follow-up post-radiofrequency ablation shows shrinking left renal lower pole mass (M) without significant enhancement consistent with successful treatment (C–cortical renal cyst)

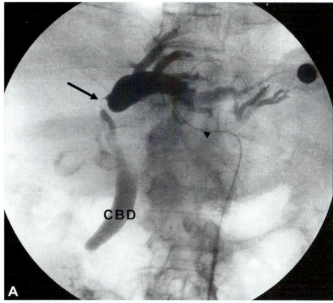

FIGURE 20.10A: Percutaneous transhepatic cholangiogram from a left ductal approach (arrowhead) showing Klatskin lesion causing severe stenosis at the confluence of intrahepatic ducts (arrow) with slow flow into the common bile duct (CBD). No communication with right ductal system seen

alcohol injection is a viable option in select cases. These nonsurgical ablative techniques are usually performed in patients who are not surgical candidates or need to be down graded in terms of tumor burden to become eligible for surgical treatment.

In the gastrointestinal tract, esophageal dilatation of benign strictures can be performed under fluoroscopic guidance. In case of malignant obstruction, esophageal, gastric or colonic stenting can be performed for palliative management of symptoms. Percutaneous gastrostomy tube placement is also feasible. In case the patient has risk of aspiration, the gastrostomy tube can be combined with an additional coaxial jejunostomy tube for safely feeding the patient.

Percutaneous transhepatic biliary access is useful in the management of postoperative bile leak or obstruction. Dual percutaneous biliary access and catheter drainage is performed for Klatskin type of neoplasm (Figs 20.10A and B). In case of malignant biliary obstruction, percutaneous biliary catheter drainage and/or biliary stenting can be performed for palliative therapy of neoplasms such as unresectable pancreatic carcinoma or cholangiocarcinoma

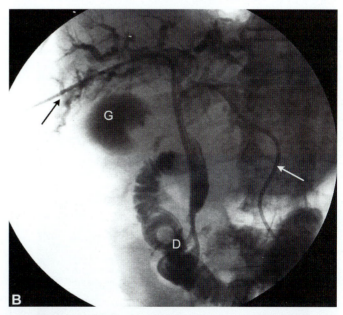

FIGURE 20.10B: Cholangiogram image showing bilateral transhepatic biliary access (arrows) with placement of internal/external drainage catheters ending in the duodenum (D). Small amount of retained contrast in the gallbladder (G)

(Figs 20.11A and B). The frequency of biliary interventions has decreased with advances in endoscopic biliary interventions. However, if the ERCP is unsuccessful or

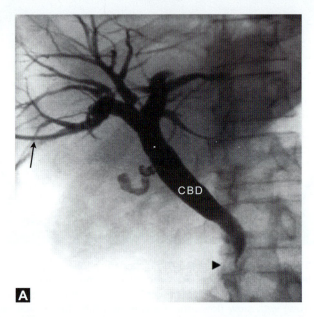

FIGURE 20.11A: Percutaneous transhepatic cholangiogram from right sided access (arrow), shows severe stricture (arrowhead) of the common bile duct (CBD), caused by nonresectable pancreatic carcinoma

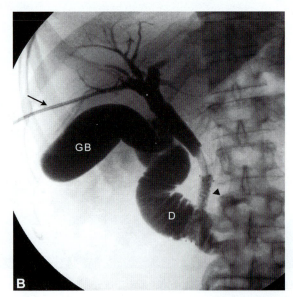

FIGURE 20.11B: Cholangiogram image via right sided access (arrow), showing internal metal stent (arrowhead) across the mass lesion with contrast flow into the duodenum (D)(GB–gallbladder)

difficult to perform due to prior surgery, percutaneous transhepatic biliary access is a viable option in such cases. This allows for bile sampling as well as brush or forceps biopsy of obstructing mass.

Benign biliary strictures can be treated with balloon angioplasty and long-term external biliary catheters. Percutaneous biliary access can sometimes be combined with endoscopic intervention using rendezvous guidewire snare technique for optimal patient care by collaboration.

Percutaneous cholecystomy catheter drainage for acute cholecystitis is useful in otherwise sick or unstable patients who are unable to undergo cholecystectomy. Patients with retained common bile duct stones following cholecystectomy and T-tube can undergo stone extraction using a basket catheter placed via an established T-tube tract, thereby avoiding a second exploration.

Celiac plexus block using absolute alcohol in widespread pancreatic or upper abdominal malignancy causing intractable pain deserves special mention as it can be accurately performed under CT guidance, using minimal contrast media for confirming location (Figure 20.12). Total of 30-50 ml absolute alcohol can be injected with a local anesthetic for a good response.

In the urinary system a simple procedure as percutaneous nephrostomy can be the initial access to a variety of interventions (Figs 20.13A to C). Some of the indications

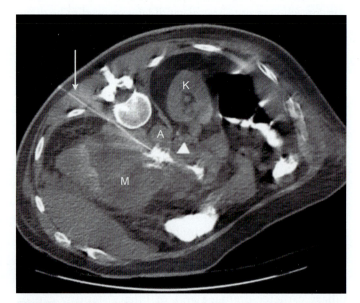

FIGURE 20.12: Celiac plexus block using CT guidance. Percutaneous needle (arrow) placed via paravertebral trajectory into the mass (M) encasing the celiac plexus region as confirmed with small amount of contrast (arrowhead), prior to injection of absolute alcohol (K- left kidney, A–aorta)

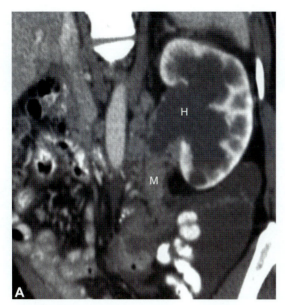

FIGURE 20.13A: Coronal CT image showing severe left hydronephrosis (H), caused by malignant retroperitoneal mass (M)

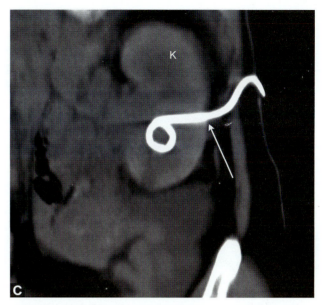

FIGURE 20.13C: Coronal CT scan obtained in follow-up during treatment shows relief of left kidney (K) hydronephrosis with nephrostomy catheter in position (arrow)

nephrolithotomy, double J ureteral or nephroureteral stent, ureteral stricture dilatation. In case of nonoperable malignant urinary obstruction, long-term bilateral nephrostomy drainage provides palliative relief. Some of the nonoperable urinary fistulas may be managed by bilateral ureteral occlusion using coils and gelfoam combined with bilateral nephrostomy drainage catheters (Figs 20.14A and B).

Vascular Interventions

Within the arterial system most diagnostic information can be obtained by high resolution CT or MR angiography. Most of the invasive arterial procedures are now combined with interventions. Peripheral arterial diseases such as arterial stenosis, occlusions or aneurysms can be treated using angioplasty, stent and/or stent graft placement. This is applicable in wide variety of anatomical sites such as aorto-iliac, femoro-popliteal, aortic arch vessels, carotid, renal, etc. Thrombolysis using percutaneous methods can significantly decrease the morbidity and mortality in peripheral arterial disease (Figs 20.15A to D). In the pulmonary arterial system, thrombolysis can be performed for massive pulmonary embolism using either mechanical thrombectomy tools or pharmacological thrombolytics. In several cases where open surgery has high morbidity and mortality, endograft can achieve comparable results as in the repair of abdominal aortic aneurysm or thoracic aortic

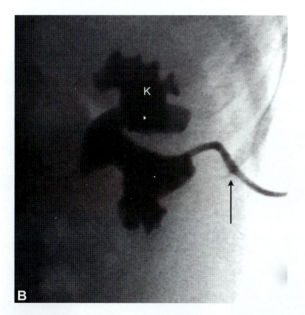

FIGURE 20.13B: Nephrostogram obtained during placed of percutaneous 8 Fr pigtail catheter (arrow) into the collecting system of the left kidney (K), via lower pole calyx, using ultrasound for access guidance

are relief of infection, stone disease, urinary diversion for distal obstruction, fistula or injury. Percutaneous nephrostomy also provides access for percutaneous

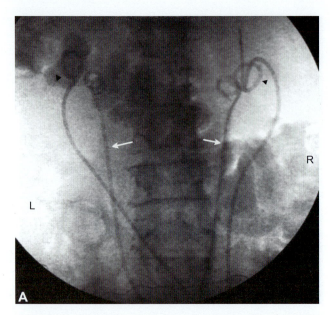

FIGURE 20.14A: Fluoroscopic spot image of patient with malignant recto-vesicular fistula, initially managed with placement of bilateral diverting percutaneous nephrostomy catheters (arrowheads) and double J stents (arrows)

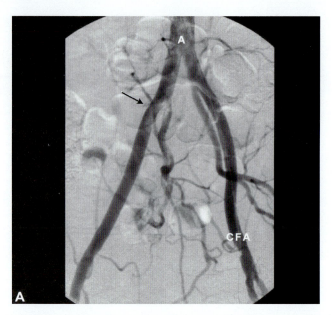

FIGURE 20.15A: Pelvic arteriogram showing significant stenotic lesion in the right iliac artery (arrow) causing distal thrombo-embolism as seen on next image (15B). Percutaneous access obtained via the left common femoral artery (CFA) (A–aorta)

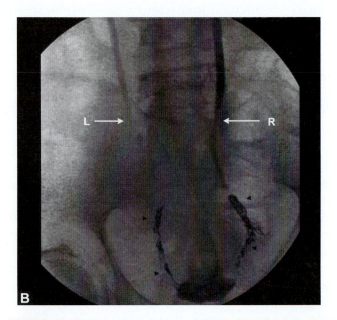

FIGURE 20.14B: Following unsuccessful resection of rectal cancer and persistence of the urinary fistula, both double J stents were removed from the ureters (arrows) via nephrostomy access using snare technique. Both distal ureters were occluded using embolization coils with permanent diverting bilateral nephrostomy catheters

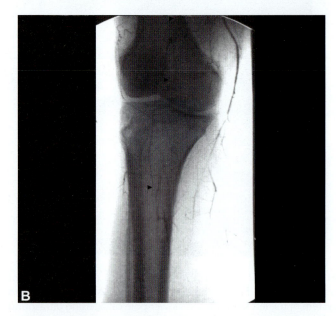

FIGURE 20.15B: Arteriogram of the right leg below the knee demonstrating absence of flow in the right popliteal artery and tibial branches (arrowheads) consistent with thromboembolism in this patient with cold ischemic right foot

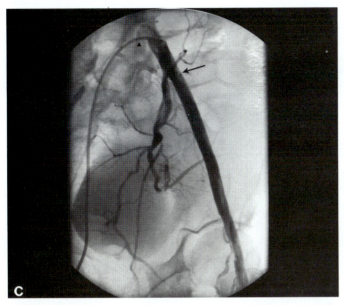

FIGURE 20.15C: Postintervention arteriogram shows patent right iliac artery after stenting (arrow), performed via sheath over the aortic bifurcation (arrowhead)

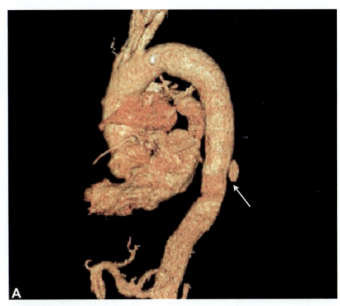

FIGURE 20.16A: CT scan 3-D image of the thoracic aorta showing a leaking thoracic aneurysm (arrow) presenting with chest pain and left hemothorax

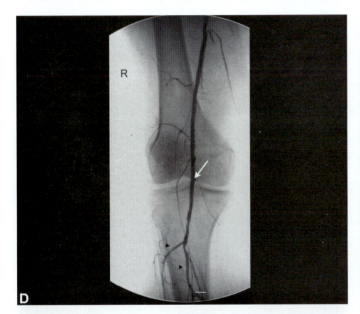

FIGURE 20.15D: Right leg arteriogram following 24 hours thrombolysis using infusion catheter showing patent right popliteal artery (arrow) and tibial arteries (arrowheads). Foot amputation was averted in this patient

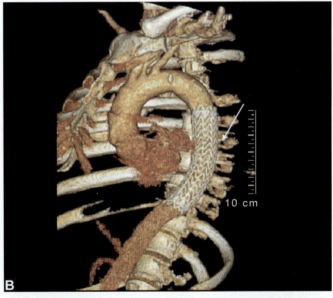

FIGURE 20.16B: CT scan 3-D image following thoracic aortic endograft (arrow) showing successful exclusion of the aneurysm

aneurysm (Figs 20.16A and B) with minimally invasive techniques. Intracranial aneurysms can now be successfully treated via percutaneuos embolization methods by neurointerventionalists.

Treatment of various types of bleeding with the use of percutaneous transcatheter embolotherapy is a highly developed field especially with the advancement of microcatheter techniques and development of embolic material such as polyvinyl alcohol particles, microcoils and glue.

Hemoptysis from chronic condition such as bronchiectasis, tuberculosis or less commonly lung malignancies can be managed using bronchial artery embolization. In cases of pulmonary artery malformations, aneurysm or injury selective branch embolization can be performed.

Symptomatic fibroids are now commonly treated with uterine artery embolization, thereby avoiding a hysterectomy for treating a benign disease (Figs 20.17A and B). Similar embolization procedure can be used in the treatment of postpartum hemorrhage.

Treatment of gastrointestinal bleeding requires the detection of source and possible intervention for its management. Examples include embolization of the gastroduodenal artery for bleeding duodenal ulcers, detection and embolization of bleeding from diverticular disease, vascular malformation or complication following colonoscopic procedures. Some of these are managed entirely using interventional radiology procedures, in other cases a critical patient can be stabilized for definitive surgical management later (Figs 20.18A and B). Vascular complication of pancreatitis can lead to pseudoaneurysm formation, which is best treated using percutaneous embolization if accessible (Figs 20.19A to C).

Portal hypertension from liver disease can cause complications of gastrointestinal bleeding commonly from varices or result in severe ascites and abdominal distension. Creation of transjugular intrahepatic portosystemic shunt by IR techniques can significantly relieve the portal hypertension and control the recurrence of bleeding and ascites (Figure 20.20).

Life-threatening hematuria from renal cell carcinoma can be effectively managed with percutaneous embolization (Figs 20.21A to C). Some surgeons routinely prefer to have the renal tumor embolized preoperatively for facilitating surgical excision and decreasing blood loss during surgery. Postoperative complications resulting in hemorrhage and pseudoaneurysm can at times be successfully treated with percutaneous catheter embolization as shown in this case of partial nephrectomy (Figs 20.22A to C).

There has been significant development in the management of liver neoplasms especially hepatocellular carcinoma. Nonsurgical patients with HCC can undergo transarterial chemoembolization (TACE) with improvement in survival and outcome. Selective patient can be downgraded following TACE and/or selective portal vein embolization to eventually undergo definitive surgical

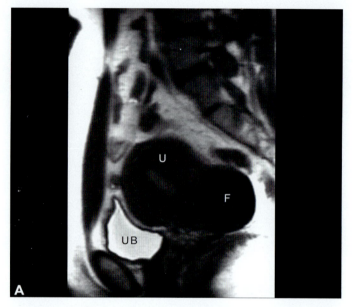

FIGURE 20.17A: Sagittal MRI image of the pelvis demonstrating an enlarged uterus (U), with an additional large posterior fibroid (F) in this patient with lower abdominal pain, excessive vaginal bleeding, urinary frequency and anemia (UB–urinary bladder)

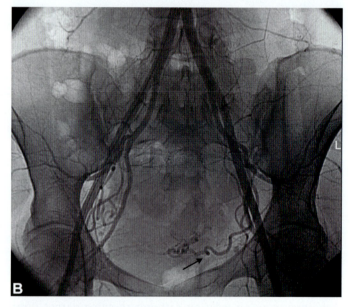

FIGURE 20.17B: Pelvic arteriogram image obtained during uterine artery (arrow) embolization using polyvinyl alcohol particles with successful relief of symptoms in 2-3 months

therapy such as liver transplant or resection (Figs 20.23A to D). Recurrence of hepatocellular carcinoma in post-resection cases can be treated with TACE. Hepatic metastases from

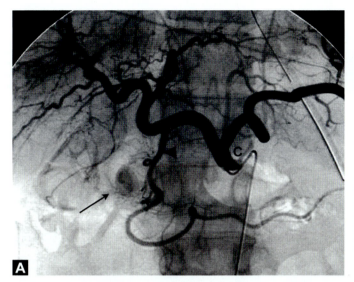

FIGURE 20.18A: Celiac axis arteriogram (C) in a patient with recurrent hemetemesis following unsuccessful endoscopic treatment of a bleeding duodenal ulcer. Contrast extravasation (arrow) seen arising from a gastroduodenal artery (arrowhead) branch

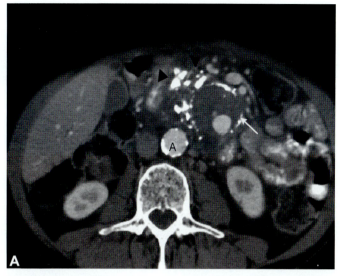

FIGURE 20.19A: Axial CT scan of the abdomen demonstrating a pseudocyst of the pancreas with pseudoaneurysm (arrow), in this patient presenting with hemetemesis. Multiple pancreatic calcifications (arrowheads) are seen. Endoscopy revealed bleeding from the ampulla (A–aorta)

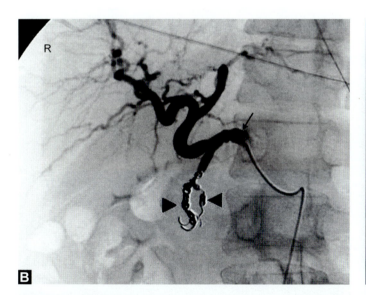

FIGURE 20.18B: Hepatic arteriogram (arrow) after successful coil occlusion of the gastroduodenal artery bleeders (arrowheads). This allowed for the critical patient to recover for a subsequent definitive surgical management

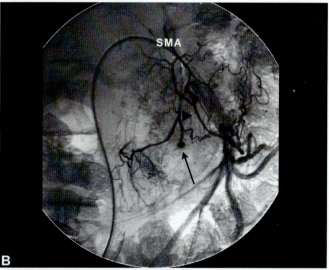

FIGURE 20.19B: Arteriogram of the superior mesenteric artery (SMA) showing the branch (arrowhead) feeding the pseudo-aneurysm (arrow)

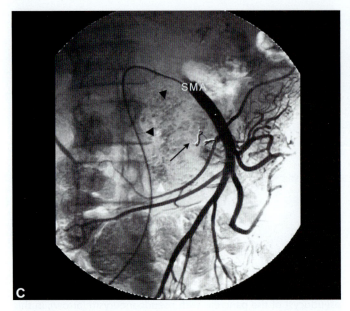

FIGURE 20.19C: Superior mesenteric arteriogram (SMA), following successful coil embolization of the pseudoaneurysm (arrow), thereby avoiding a high risk open surgery. Scattered pancreatic calcifications are seen (arrowheads)

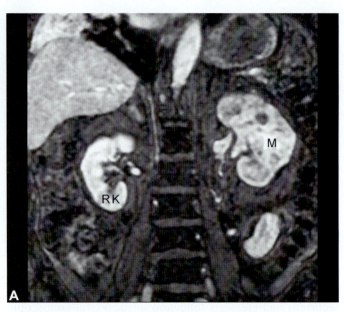

FIGURE 20.21A: Coronal MRI scan with gadolinium contrast showing large enhancing mass (M) in the left kidney in this patient with hematuria. Normal right kidney (RK) is seen

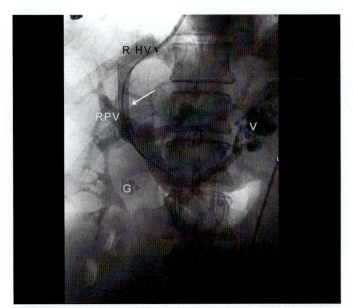

FIGURE 20.20: Angiogram obtained during creation of a transjugular intrahepatic portosystemic shunt (TIPS), from the right hepatic vein (R HV) to the right portal vein (R PV) using a metal stent (arrow). Also noted are gastroesophageal varices (V) and gallstones (G)

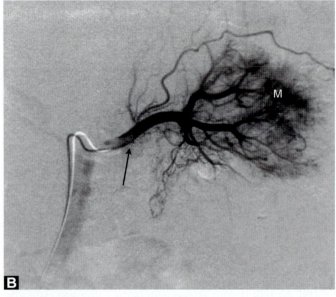

FIGURE 20.21B: Arteriogram of the left kidney (arrow), obtained when the hematuria exacerbated to become life-threatening. Large enhancing mass (M) seen consistent with renal cell carcinoma

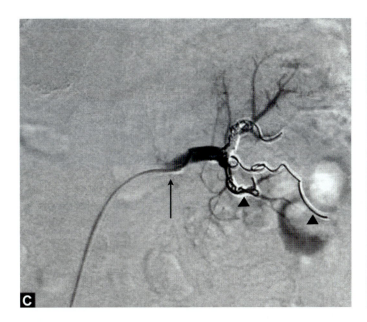

FIGURE 20.21C: Postembolization arteriogram of the left kidney (arrow) following occlusion of the left renal artery with polyvinyl alcohol particles and coils (arrowheads). The hematuria was emergently controlled and the patient subsequently has a nephrectomy

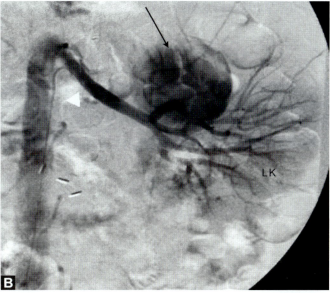

FIGURE 20.22B: Arteriogram image with catheter in the left renal artery (arrowhead) showing a large pseudoaneurysm in the partial nephrectomy site and preserved lower half of the left kidney (LK)

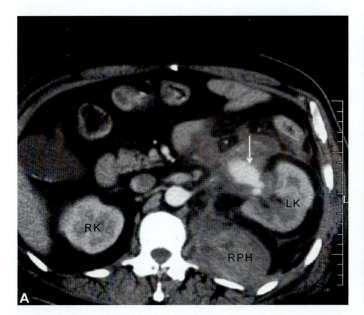

FIGURE 20.22A: Axial CT scan image with IV contrast showing left sided retroperitoneal hemorrhage (RPH) in a patient with recent partial nephrectomy of the left kidney (LK) for a upper pole neoplasm. Also seen is a large pseudoaneurysm (arrow) of the left renal artery (arrowhead) branch

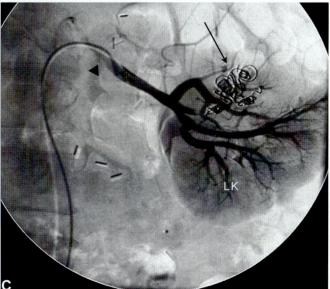

FIGURE 20.22C: Arteriogram of the left renal artery (arrowhead) following successful coil embolization of the pseudoaneurysm (arrow) and its feeding branches. The lower half of the left kidney (LK) was preserved

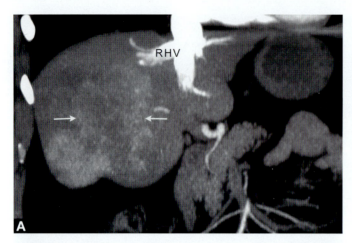

FIGURE 20.23A: Coronal CT image of the liver showing a large enhancing mass (arrows) occupying most of the right lobe. Percutaneous biopsy proved a diagnosis of hepatocellular carcinoma (RHV–right hepatic vein)

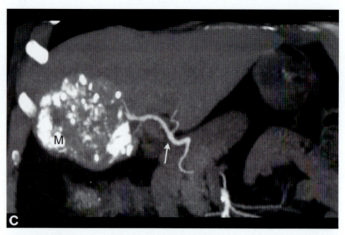

FIGURE 20.23C: Coronal CT image 1 month following TACE shows significant reduction in the ethiodol stained mass (M) with compensatory hypertrophy of the unaffected left lobe. Note preserved main hepatic arterial supply (arrow)

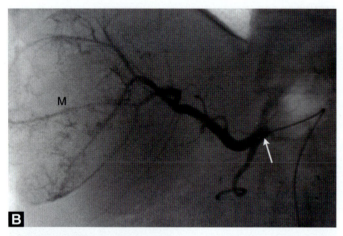

FIGURE 20.23B: Hepatic arteriogram (arrow) image performed during transarterial chemoembolization (TACE) shows the large mass (M) in the right lobe with tumor blush and displaced hepatic arterial branches. Cisplatin, mitomycin and doxorubicin admixed with ethiodol was injected followed by polyvinyl alcohol particles

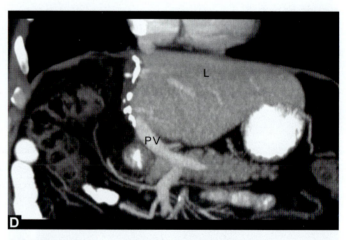

FIGURE 20.23D: Coronal CT image post right hepatectomy showing normal appearing hypertrophied left lobe liver (L) and patent main and left portal venous system (PV)

carcinoid or intestinal adenocarcinoma in selected cases are sometimes a candidate for TACE or other transarterial embolization procedures. Close cooperation between liver physicians and surgeons can significantly impact on patient survival.

Venous procedures and interventions performed by IR have come to play a dominant role in patient care. These consist of central venous access such as placement of non-tunneled or tunneled catheters and implanted ports. Hemodialysis access maintenance involving angioplasty, declot and management of arteriovenous fistulas or grafts are routinely performed. Superior vena cava syndrome can result from mediastinal involvement from inflammation or neoplasm resulting in SVC and/or brachiocephalic vein obstruction with and without thrombosis. Stenting and/ or thrombolysis of central venous occlusions due to benign or malignant etiology can be performed (Figs 20.24A to C). Placement of vena cava filters as well as retrieval of filters no longer indicated has a significant role in management of venous thromboembolic disease (Figure 20.25).

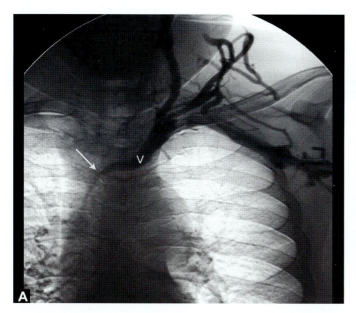

FIGURE 20.24A: Central venogram of the chest from left brachial vein percutaneous access in a patient with left arm and facial swelling due to superior vena cava (SVC) syndrome. Occlusion at the upper SVC (arrow) and medial left brachiocephalic vein (V) seen with multiple venous collaterals in the left upper chest and neck

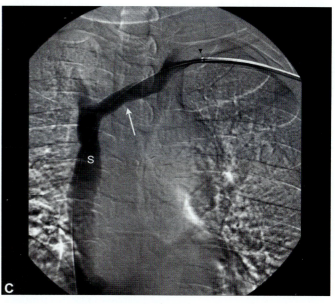

FIGURE 20.24C: Postintervention venogram via sheath (arrowhead) injection shows patent left brachiocephalic vein with stent (arrow) and patent superior vena cava (S)

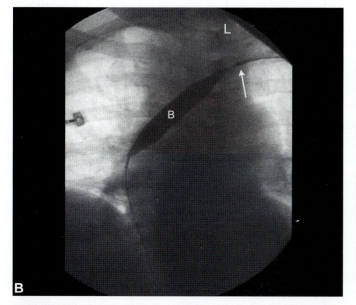

FIGURE 20.24B: Fluoroscopic image during large diameter (12-16 mm) percutaneous transluminal balloon (B) angioplasty of the occlusion following guidewire crossing via a vascular sheath (arrow)

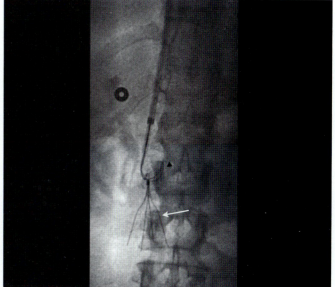

FIGURE 20.25: Fluoroscopic image of an inferior vena cava filter (arrow) in a patient with lower extremity deep venous thrombosis and a short term indication to stop anticoagulation to undergo major sugery for gynecological malignancy. The filter was retrieved via percutaneous snare (arrowhead) following successful recovery from surgery and resuming anticoagulation

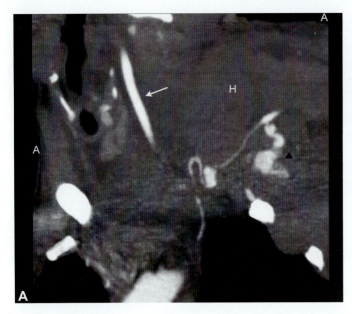

FIGURE 20.26A: Coronal CT angiogram reconstructed image of the left upper chest and neck in a stab injury showing large displacing hematoma (H) arising from laceration of the left subclavian artery branches (arrowhead). Patent left common carotid artery (arrow)

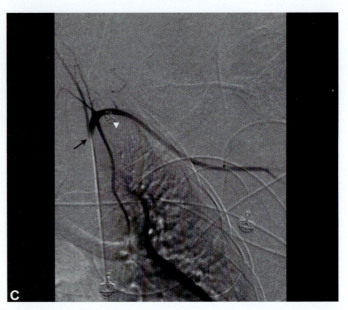

FIGURE 20.26C: Postcoil embolization (arrowhead) arteriogram of the left subclavian artery (arrow) following successful treatment of the bleeder

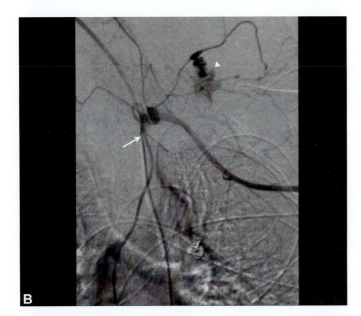

FIGURE 20.26B: Emergent arteriogram of the left subclavian artery (arrow) showing patent left vertebral and left internal mammary artery. Active bleeding (arrowhead) with extravasating contrast seen from costocervical branch

Retrievable vena cava filters placed for high thromboembolic risk surgical patients can be later removed once the patient can either be anticoagulated or no longer needs caval filtration. Common conditions such as symptomatic varicose veins in the lower extremity can be sclerosed with percutaneous endovenous laser or radiofrequency technique. Varicocele causing infertility or scrotal pain can be embolized via percutaneous transvenous access with sclerosing agents or coils.

Role of IR in trauma deserves special mention as clinical and radiological assessment of injured patients can help triage them into appropriate management pathway. Significant injury to solid viscera such as liver, spleen or kidney can now be treated with IR embolic techniques and avoid the need of a laparotomy. There is an emerging role of endograft for thoracic aortic injuries. Other specific sites such as bleeding from pelvic fracture, intercostal or epigastric arterial bleed, etc. can be selectively or subselectively embolized using percutaneous transarterial catheters with embolic material such as gelfoam, coils or polyvinyl alcohol particles. Bleeding from high risk areas such as epistaxis or neck injuries can be effectively treated with percutaneous transcatheter embolization (Figs 20.26A to C).

Role of Imaging in Trauma

Some examples of ideal images are illustrated in Figures 20.27A to C.

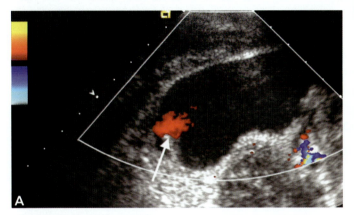

FIGURE 20.27A: Ultrasound image right lower quadrant with color Droppler in a patient with history of blunt trauma showing free fluid with some internal echoes, and slow ooze from a vascular structure (arrow)

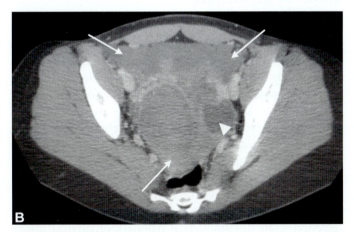

FIGURE 20.27B: CT pelvis axial image in a 25-year-old female with history of blunt trauma, showing high density free fluid (arrows) consistent with hemorrhage. Low density ovarian cyst (arrowhead) noted on the left side

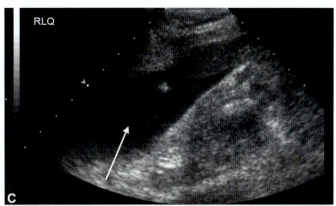

FIGURE 20.27C: Ultrasound right lower quadrant in a patient with blunt trauma showing free fluid in the peritoneal cavity (arrow)

CONCLUSION

Interventional radiology offers a wide variety of procedures based on innovation and development of minimally invasive techniques over the past 35 years. Currently many disease conditions have the option of benefiting from IR interventions. There is role for interventional radiology in both presurgical and postsurgical management of patients. The best patient outcome needs close cooperation between the interventional radiologist and the surgeon in order to select the most appropriate form of treatment. Current data, availability and best evidence should factor in the decision making of optimizing patient care.

BIBLIOGRAPHY

1. Kandarpa, Krishna, Aruny, John E. Handbook of interventional radiologic procedures, 2002.
2. Kaufman, John A, Lee, Michael J. Vascular and interventional radiology: The Requisites, 2004.

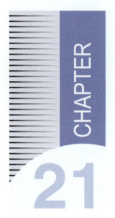

CHAPTER

21

Surgical Infections

Puja Van Epps, Gopala K Yadavalli

SURGICAL INFECTIONS

Joseph Lister revolutionized the surgical landscape and gave birth to the modern surgical era with his use of carbolic acid to reduce germs and subsequently refining the use of aseptic principles in surgery. Over 140 years later, despite the widespread use of antisepsis and modern antimicrobials, surgeons cannot escape the need to not only be aware of surgical infections but also how to treat them and continue their efforts to reduce these infections.

Surgical infections can be categorized into two main groups: infections that occur postoperatively in a surgical site and infections that require a surgical treatment. Of these, surgical site infections (SSIs) are a major cause of morbidity and mortality around the world.[1] In 1999, the Center for Disease Control and Prevention (CDC) reported that between 14-16 percent of all nosocomial infections were related to surgical sites, making SSI the third most common type of nosocomial infections.[2] Similarly, most studies report a comparable impact on Indian healthcare system. Reported rates of SSI in Indian hospitals have varied from 3 percent to around 40 percent.[3,4]

Staphylococcus aureus remains the most common isolate from surgical wounds in India and around the world. A growing proportion of these isolates are methicillin-resistant (MRSA), which is of concern due to its impact on morbidity and mortality.[5] Surgical patients are not immune to the emergence of virulent and resistant strains of bacteria, viruses and fungi. With the ubiquitous use of antibiotics and increasing complexity of patients (including immuno-suppressed patients), the surgeon must become familiar with both the basic knowledge as well as new challenges arising in the practice of infectious diseases in surgical patients. This chapter will include a discussion on the setting of infection including its immune basis as well as host factors, common infections and pathogens encountered in surgical patients, their management as well as the role of infection control.

INFLAMMATION AND THE IMMUNE BASIS OF INFECTION

Surgical intervention is associated with disruption of barrier defenses as well as with acquired lesions in innate and adaptive immunity.[6] Incisions, placement of indwelling catheters, and implantation of hardware can facilitate entry of microorganisms and allow establishment of infection in the early postoperative period. Extensive study of patients undergoing accidental trauma, thermal burns, and significant surgical intervention has demonstrated that immunodepression is a common feature in these individuals.[7-9] Deactivation of monocytes and depletion of circulating dendritic cells has been observed in cardiac and noncardiac surgery settings.[10] Impairment of cytokine secretion is an immunological hallmark of surgical injury and can involve both innate (NK cell) and adaptive (T cell) pathways. The use of extracorporeal circulation (cardiopulmonary bypass) and corticosteroids intra- and perioperatively can further exacerbate these immune defects.[11]

HOST FACTORS

Microorganisms contaminate virtually all surgical wound, but only a minority of them causes disease. The development of infection depends on the interplay between the immune system of the host, procedure related risk factors as well as the microbe and its ability to adhere to and invade the host tissue. A number of host factors can increase the patient's risk of developing an infection, including diabetes, malnutrition, malignancy, hypoxemia, immunosuppression due to transplantation, and hypothermia. In surgical patients with the above risk factors or other states of immunodeficiency, care must be taken to correct or control the underlying condition to prevent wound infection.

Diabetes is a known risk factor for impaired wound healing and increased infections. It is thought to be a result of both long-term effect of diabetes on macro and microvasculature as well as impaired functioning of complement and antibodies due to hyperglycemia in the acute setting. Hyperglycemia in postsurgical patients has been shown to be associated with increased rate of SSI. Recent evidence suggests that tight glucose control in the preoperative period, even in nondiabetics, is associated with reduced frequency of infections.[12] Optimizing nutritional status in the perioperative period may also reduce the risk of infection. Low serum albumin levels have been associated with increased rates of infections. In a 2006 meta-analysis looking at 17 trials studying the use of specialized nutritional support with immune-modulating nutrients in the pre-, peri- and postoperative setting, it was found that improving the nutritional status was associated with a 39-61 percent reduction in infectious complications.[13]

Although it is presumed that increased oxygen availability is a positive host factor in terms of reduction of infections, studies on the use of supplemental oxygen in surgical patients have been conflicting. While the initial studies done in patients undergoing colon surgery indicated a 50 percent reduction in SSI in patients receiving 80 percent supplemental oxygen compared to 30 percent,[14] recent data by Pryor and colleagues suggests much higher rates of infections in patients receiving high FiO_2 in the perioperative setting.[15] Currently the use of supplemental oxygen is recommended with the goal to maintain adequate oxygenation and not to provide hyperoxia.

MICROBIOLOGY

Surgical Site Infections

SSI by definition is infection that occurs at any site related to and after a surgical procedure. As discussed above the impact of SSI on healthcare in both the resource-limited and well-resourced nations is far reaching. An Indian study looking at 1125 surgeries showed that not only was there almost a two-fold increase in expenditure associated with SSI, but the rate of mortality was also higher at 12.8 percent in patients who developed surgical site infections compared to 3.8 percent in those who did not.[16] Surgical site infections are categorized based on the anatomic level of infection (Table 21.1).

The risk of wound infection is in part determined by the degree of contamination present in a wound. Surgical wounds are classically divided into: (1) clean (2) clean-contaminated (3) contaminated and (4) dirty. Risk of infection, as predicted by the National Nosocomial Infection Surveillance (NNIS) score is directly related to, but not limited to, the degree of contamination.[2] The ranges of infection rates are around 3-5 percent for clean wounds to upward of 27 percent for dirty wounds.[4] The risk factors for developing a surgical site infection are listed in Table 21.2.

Table 21.1: Surgical site infections—categorized based on the anatomic level of infection
Incisional
Superficial—infection of the skin or the subcutaneous tissue
Deep—deeper infection involving the tissue beneath the superficial layer, fascia and muscles.
Organ/space
Infection involving any part of the body manipulated during a surgical procedure other than the body wall.

Table 21.2: Risk factors for surgical site infection	
Patient factors	*Procedure related*
Diabetes/hyperglycemia	Recent/prolonged hospitalization
Age	Wound class
Malnutrition	Preoperative shaving
Malignancy	Contamination of operating room/personnel
Steroid or other immunosuppressive use	Prolonged hypotension
Prior contamination/colonization or infection	Improper antimicrobial prophylaxis
Cigarette smoking	Poor postoperative wound care

Surgical wound infections typically present within the first or second week of surgery. Patients may complain of pain at the surgical site or may simply present with postoperative fever. The key is to thoroughly inspect the wound for signs of inflammation including edema, erythema as well as signs of abscess formation. Presence of fluctuance, tenderness or purulence may indicate subcutaneous tissue infection. Deep space infections in the absence of superficial signs can be more challenging to diagnose. In such cases imaging such as CT scan, if available, may be necessary. The definitive treatment of an established surgical site infection is drainage and wound debridement. Culture of the site should be performed to identify the etiology and aid in the proper antibiotic selection.

The microbiology of surgical infections is typically polymicrobial and isolates are increasingly resistant to commonly used antibiotics. In a study of one hundred and seventeen surgical infections, between 67-80 percent of non-abscess related infections were polymicrobial.[17] According to much of the published data, S. aureus is the most commonly isolated microorganism in the Indian setting. Rates of MRSA range from 20 - 40 percent in various studies done in India looking at SSI.[3,5] Other gram-positive bacteria of clinical importance are coagulase-negative staphylococci, Enterococcus spp and Streptococcus spp. The most common gram-negative isolates are Pseudomonas aeruginosa, E. coli and Klebsiella spp, Bacteroides fragilis, Peptostreptococcus and Clostridium spp are important anaerobes that cause disease in surgical patients. The antibiotic management of these infections will be discussed later in this chapter.

Community Acquired Infections

Infections requiring surgical treatment are also an important category of infections of which the surgeon needs to be aware. These include skin and soft tissue infections (SSTIs), cutaneous abscesses and intrabdominal infections. Brief discussion on tetanus will also be done in this section.

SSTIs range from cellulitis to diffuse necrotizing infections, including fasciitis, and myositis. Most superficial skin infections are easily treated with wound care and antibiotics. However, infections involving deeper layers of tissue including muscle and fascia can cause systemic illness and prove to be rapidly fatal. These infections generally require aggressive surgical debridement along with antimicrobials. Cellulitis is easily diagnosed based on clinical findings, which include localized erythema, tenderness and edema. Risk factors for developing cellulitis include diabetic neuropathy, peripheral vascular disease, and alcoholism

among others. Staphylococcus and Streptococcus species are most commonly implicated, with gram-negative bacilli playing an important role in immuncompromised or hospitalized patients. In a large study done at the All India Medical Institute of Medicine Sciences looking at over 5,000 samples from SSTIs, S. aureus was found to be the most common isolate.[18] Methicillin resistance in S. aureus was found to be over 38 percent. Additionally, over 66 percent of gram negative isolates were extended-spectrum beta-lactamase producers. On the other hand necrotizing infections can be difficult to diagnose and spread rapidly. Clinical findings can include presence of cellulitis, open wounds, necrotic tissue, intense pain, crepitus, and signs of systemic illness including fever, tachycardia, or hypotension. Plain film may reveal presence of gas in an extremity. Clostridium perfringens causes necrotizing cellulitis as well as myositis or myonecrosis, often termed gas gangrene. The organism usually enters open wounds through contaminated soil. As soon as this diagnosis is suspected radical tissue-saving debridement should be performed. Nonclostridial infections include necrotizing fasciitis and can be either due to mixed, synergistic flora from the peritoneum or perineum, or caused by Group A streptococci. Although both gangrene and fasciitis require surgical treatment, an important distinction between the two is that the latter often only requires removal of dead skin and fascia and generally not amputation. In terms of antimicrobial therapy, broad-spectrum antibiotics are usually clinically indicated. Coverage should include activity against gram-negatives, positives and anaerobes.

Mainstay of treatment for subcutaneous abscesses is drainage of infected area. An infectious process resulting in necrotic tissue composed of dead or dying cell components and bacteria characterizes abscess formation. Clinically this presents as localized tenderness, and signs of inflammation and the treatment requires drainage of pus. Furuncles usually begin in infected hair follicles or skin glands. These are the most common type of surgical infection and typically only require incision and drainage. Carbuncles occur when an infection in a number of furuncles spreads through the subcutaneous tissue resulting in multiple connecting tunnels. This gives the appearance of multiple small openings in the skin, usually draining pus. These not only require adequate drainage and often excision of sinus tracts but also require antibiotics with coverage against Staphylococcus and Streptococcus species. Hidradenitis suppurativa is abscess formation within apocrine sweat glands. Treatment varies depending on the extent of infection. It can involve drainage of individual abscess to excision and grafting of large affected areas. Perirectal abscesses result from infection of the crypts of the anorectal canal. These can extend into the pelvis as well as the genitourinary tract and can cause significant morbidity in immune-compromised patients. These require adequate drainage and antibiotic coverage against gram-negative and gram-positive organisms. Lastly, diabetic foot ulcers or abscesses typically result from repetitive injury to compromised tissue. These are also typically mixed flora infections and often not only require debridement but may also necessitate excision of dead tissue including bones. Osteomyelitis is a common complication of foot infections and should be evaluated for in any patient presenting with a diabetic foot ulcer.

Tetanus

Despite being a largely vaccine-preventable illness, tetanus continues to cause havoc in the developing world. There are 1,000,000 cases of tetanus per year worldwide and about 300,000 deaths as a result.[17] *Clostridium tetani* gains entry through contaminated wounds to infect the nervous system. Tetanus is a clinical diagnosis, as confirmatory tests are not usually available. Although the mean incubation period is 7 days, tetanus can occur with 1 day to several months post-exposure. Once the diagnosis is suspected, mainstay of therapy is neutralization of toxin with tetanus immune globulin, proper wound management, as well as IV antibiotics. Immunization recommendation for tetanus is listed in Table 21.3.

Intra-abdominal/retroperitoneal abscesses can carry with them significant amount of morbidity and mortality. Aside from some specific exceptions most of these infections usually require percutaneous drainage. Patients with these infections typically present with systemic signs of illness including fever, abdominal pain, and sepsis or frank shock.

Diagnosis often requires imaging such as a CT scan or abdominal ultrasound. Infections not typically requiring surgical intervention are spontaneous bacterial peritonitis, salpingitis, diverticulitis (first 2-3 episodes) and amebic liver abscesses. Majority of the remainder of intra-abdominal infection not only require empiric antibiotic coverage against gram negatives and anaerobes but also need surgical debridement or drainage. The key to the treatment of these infections is source control that can only be effectively achieved in the operative setting. Etiology of these infections can often be polymicrobial and fluid or tissue obtained in the operation theatre must be sent for culture to determine the exact organism for targeted therapy.

Postoperative Fever

Hospital acquired infections in surgical patients are an important component of this discussion. Although fever is a common occurrence in the postoperative setting, neither are all fevers infectious in nature, nor will all infections result in a fever. It is helpful to think of the 5 "W"s when trying to determine the cause of a postoperative fever (Table 21.4).

The most frequent nonsurgical infections in this setting are urinary tract infection, pneumonia, and invasive catheter related infection. The diagnosis is usually straightforward using physical exam, culture and laboratory data or plain film of the chest. Empiric antibiotic coverage should be based upon the suspected site of infection, common pathogens and **drug resistance data at each individual institution**. If the initial investigation is negative further imaging with a CT or MRI, if available, of the operative site maybe indicated. Abdominal ultrasound is a less costly alternative to CT when abscess is suspected. The likelihood of SSI increases the longer postoperative fever remains undiagnosed. Key is to promptly determine the need for surgical intervention, including debridement, drainage and/or removal of hardware. In the era of frequent antibiotic use,

Table 21.3: Tetanus immunization—quick review	
Indication	*Immunization/Prophylaxis*
Routine adult immunization	Td 0.5 ml every 10 years
Clean minor wounds	
Unknown or incomplete immunization	Td 0.5 ml, no TIG needed
Complete immunization	No Td or TIG needed
Tetanus prone wounds	
Unknown or incomplete immunization	Td 0.5 ml and 250 units TIG given IM
Complete immunization	Td 0.5 ml (unless last dose <5 years ago)

Td = Adult tetanus-diptheria vaccine; TIG = Tetanus immune globulin

Table 21.4: 5 "W"s—determine the cause of a postoperative fever				
Wind	*Water*	*Wound*	*Walk*	*Wonder drugs*
Pneumonia, pulmonary embolus, atelectasis	Urinary tract infection	Surgical site infection Infected hardware/catheter	Deep venous thrombosis	Drug fever Transfusion related fever

C. difficile colitis is an important emerging infection in both surgical and medical patients. A surgical patient presenting with diarrhea, abdominal pain, fever or leukocytosis should be started on empiric coverage against *C. difficile* with metronidazole and, where available, stool sample should be sent for toxin or antigen testing.

MANAGEMENT OF SURGICAL INFECTIONS

The decision to initiate antimicrobial therapy in a patient depends on several factors, including the clinical condition of the patient, the (often presumed) identity of the pathogen, and the site of suspected infection. The goal of therapy is to achieve control of the infection so that host defenses are able to clear it. Achieving this goal not only depends on the choice of antimicrobial but also on the ability to exceed minimum inhibitory concentration of the antibiotic at the site of infection against suspected or proven pathogens. Table 21.5 lists some common infections encountered in surgical patients and suspected pathogens. Once empiric antibiotics have been initiated the key is to observe for a therapeutic response in the patient and follow the appropriate cultures for identification and sensitivity patterns. Failure to respond to therapy could be due to a variety of reasons, including inappropriate initial choice or inadequate levels of antibiotics, presence of a secondary infection, failure to adequately drain a pocket of infection or development of drug resistance. Antimicrobial drug resistance is a major concern for medical and surgical patients alike. Antimicrobial drug resistance in Indian healthcare settings is rising steadily, including the spread of extended spectrum beta-lactamase and carbepenemase-producing organisms.[18] In a study looking at surgical infections in northern India, between 22-53 percent of gram negative isolates were multidrug-resistant.[17] Overuse of antimicrobial therapy has repeatedly been implicated in the spread of these drug resistant bacteria. Judicious use of antibiotics not only involves the appropriate choice of agent but also the duration of treatment. Infection control strategies such as strict hand washing between patient interactions and contact precautions also play a critical role in minimizing the development of multidrug-resistant organisms.

Fungal infections are an increasing cause of morbidity in surgical patients. *Candida* species, especially *C. albicans*, are the most commonly identified fungal pathogens. While the recovery of *Candida* species from open wounds or sputum usually reflect colonization rather than true infection, fungemia or intrabdominal fungal abscesses almost always represent an invasive infection and warrant therapy. Amphotericin B is the most commonly used antifungal; however, due to its toxicity careful dosing is required. Lipid-complex or liposomal preparations of amphotericin B are generally better tolerated than conventional (deoxycholate) preparations, but are considerably more costly, limiting their utility for many patients. Fluconazole is the appropriate antibiotic choice for *C. albicans* infections, however non-albicans species such as *C. glabrata*, *C. krusei* and others exhibit increasing levels of resistance to fluconazole and require therapy with an alternate antifungal such as voriconazole or caspofungin. Selection of appropriate antimicrobial therapy for resistant pathogens, both bacterial and fungal is best done in close consultation with a clinical microbiologist, and if available, a clinical infectious disease specialist.

Infection Control

While most risk factors for the development of infection can not be eliminated there is abundant data to suggest that perioperative antisepsis practices as well as antimicrobial prophylaxis reduces the risk of surgical infections. Although various sources of potential bacterial contamination of a surgical wound exist, including operating room staff and poor air quality, patient's endogenous flora is believed to be the major source of infection. For instance, nasal colonization of patient's with *S. aureus* is believed to be a risk factor for development of postoperative infection. The data on the routine use of topical mupirocin to reduce this risk however has been conflicting. There have been several studies showing reduction in *S. aureus* with the use of mupirocin, however, a randomized controlled trial involving around four thousand

Table 21.5: Common pathogens for various sites	
Site of infection	*Suspected pathogen*
Skin/soft tissue	*Staphylococcus, Streptococcus*
Gas gangrene	*Clostridium*
Billiary tract infections	*E. coli, Klebsiella, Enterococcus*
Peritonitis/intrabdominal abscess	*E. coli, Pseudomonas*, anaerobes
Hospital acquired colitis	*Clostridium difficile*
Urinary tract infection	*E. coli, Klebsiella*
Hospital acquired pneumonia	*Staphylococcus* (suspect MRSA), *Pseudomonas, Klebsiella, Acinetobactor*
Catheter related infection infection control	*Staphylococcus, Enterobacteriaceae*

patients failed to show a significant decrease in staphylococcal surgical site infections.[19] Additionally, there has been concern regarding the development of mupirocin resistance in S. *aureus* when used routinely.

The preparation of operative site using antiseptic agents is not a matter of debate, however. Antibiotics are given depending on the organ involved and the common pathogen for that particular operating area (Table 21.5). The site should be prepped with a thorough wash to remove any visible contaminants followed by application of an antiseptic agent for disinfection. These agents have evolved since Lister's carbolic acid, with alcohol or iodine containing products being among the most inexpensive and readily available. Chlorhexidine gluconate has greater antimicrobial activity when compared to these products but may not be readily available in resource limited settings. There have been numerous studies showing increased risk of SSI with preoperative shaving. And despite the CDC recommending against shaving with a razor, this practice remains ubiquitous. It is believed that the nicks and cuts caused by a razor mobilize the patient's endogenous flora and can result in infection. If hair needs to be removed, recommendation is to use electric hair clippers immediately before the operation. In a large 10-year study, the risk of infections was the highest when hair was removed using a razor (2.5%), as compared to electric clipper (1.4%) or no hair removal (0.9%).[20]

Preoperative antisepsis of the surgical team members is also a key component in reducing surgical infections. Surgical hand scrub is a well-established practice across the world. Alcohol based products are the most commonly used germicidal agents in Europe and the developing world. Effective hand scrub should be about 2-3 minutes long, and does not have to involve scrubbing with a brush.[21] Nails should be kept short to avoid colonization and achieve proper bacterial load reduction during scrubbing. Aside from

these, universal precautions to maintain sterility should be maintained throughout the operation. The operating room should be a controlled environment with proper ventilation, sterilized instruments as well as proper surgical attire that reduces bacterial shedding during a procedure.

Antimicrobial Prophylaxis

Antimicrobial prophylaxis refers to a short course of antibiotics given in the pre- (one hour before incision) and perioperative setting (24 hours after surgery), to reduce the risk of surgical site infection. The principle behind the use of prophylaxis is to eliminate or at least reduce the bacterial load that may be inoculated into the surgical wound at the time of the surgery. Despite the presence of evidence and proper guidelines for the use of antimicrobial prophylaxis, numerous studies have shown improper timing and choice of antibiotics usage in India.[22] A 2006 study looking at challenges in adherence to guidelines of antimicrobial prophylaxis identified lack of familiarity as the number one barrier to proper antimicrobial use in this setting.[23] As the study discusses, there are several areas of improvement when it comes to this issue in the Indian setting.

Cephalosporins are the mainstay of prophylaxis when it comes to surgical procedures. This also means that there is increasing prevalence of resistant organisms, the most concerning of which is S. *aureus*. As mentioned previously, this is the most commonly isolated organism in surgical infections, and the incidence of MRSA (including cephalosporin-resistant staphylococci) has increased between 30-40 percent in the Indian setting.[5] Additionally, the incidence of multidrug-resistant gram-negative bacilli, as well resistant fungal pathogens is also on the rise. There is an urgency to realize the prevalence of fungal infection in Indian setting. The timing of antibiotic administration is also important. Generally, the initial dose of antibiotics should be at the onset of procedure. For long surgical procedures antibiotics may have to be redosed to achieve adequate levels during the procedure. The issue of duration of prophylaxis remains up for debate. There have been studies leaning both ways when it comes to short versus long courses of antibiotics. Currently, a first-generation cephalosporin such as cefazolin is recommended for most procedures. In abdominal surgeries where there is a risk of ruptured viscous, addition of an aminoglycoside such as gentamicin or clindamycin is often warranted. Metronidazole in combination with cephalosporin is also occasionally used. In surgeries where there is a high risk of MRSA infection, vancomycin may be considered. **It should be noted that because of the aforementioned issues these recommendations will not remains static.**

REFERENCES

1. Kirkland KB, Briggs JP, Trivette SL, Wilkinson WE, Sexton DJ. The impact of surgical-site infections in the 1990s: attributable mortality, excess length of hospitalization, and extra costs. Infect Control Hosp Epidemiol 1999;20:725-30.
2. National Nosocomial Infections Surveillance (NNIS) System report, data summary from January 1990-May 1999, issued June 1999. Am J Infect Control 1999;27:520-32.
3. Kamat U, Ferreira A, Savio R, Motghare D. Antimicrobial resistance among nosocomial isolates in a teaching hospital in Goa. Indian J Community Med 2008;33:89-92.
4. Lilani SP, Jangale N, Chowdhary A, Daver GB. Surgical site infection in clean and clean-contaminated cases. Indian J Med Microbiol 2005;23:249-52.
5. Kownhar H, Shankar EM, Vignesh R, Sekar R, Velu V, Rao UA. High isolation rate of *Staphylococcus aureus* from surgical site infections in an Indian hospital. J Antimicrob Chemother 2008;61:758-60.
6. Yadavalli GK, Auletta JJ, Gould MP, Salata RA, Lee JH, Heinzel FP. Deactivation of the innate cellular immune response following endotoxic and surgical injury. Exp Mol Pathol 2001;71:209-21.
7. Hershman MJ, Cheadle WG, Appel SH, et al. Comparison of antibody response with delayed hypersensitivity in severely injured patients. Arch Surg 1989;124:339-41.
8. Livingston DH, Appel SH, Wellhausen SR, Sonnenfeld G, Polk HC Jr. Depressed interferon gamma production and monocyte HLA-DR expression after severe injury. Arch Surg 1988;123:1309-12.
9. Polk HC Jr, George CD, Wellhausen SR, et al. A systematic study of host defense processes in badly injured patients. Ann Surg 1986;204:282-99.
10. Yadavalli GK, Chien JW, Wener KM, et al. Interleukin 12 and interferon-gamma synthetic deficiency is associated with dendritic cell cytopenia after cardiac surgery. Shock 2005;24:26-33.
11. Butler J, Rocker GM, Westaby S. Inflammatory response to cardiopulmonary bypass. Ann Thorac Surg 1993;55:552-9.
12. Van den Berghe G. Insulin therapy for the critically ill patient. Clin Cornerstone 2003;5:56-63.
13. Waitzberg DL, Saito H, Plank LD, et al. Postsurgical infections are reduced with specialized nutrition support. World J Surg 2006;30:1592-604.
14. Greif R, Akca O, Horn EP, Kurz A, Sessler DI. Supplemental perioperative oxygen to reduce the incidence of surgical-wound infection. Outcomes Research Group. N Engl J Med 2000;342:161-7.
15. Pryor KO, Fahey TJ, 3rd, Lien CA, Goldstein PA. Surgical site infection and the routine use of perioperative hyperoxia in a general surgical population: a randomized controlled trial. Jama 2004;291:79-87.
16. Suchitra JB, Lakshmidevi N. Surgical site infections: Assessing risk factors, outcomes and antimicrobial sensitivity patterns. African J Microb Res 2009;3:175-179.
17. Saini S, Gupta N, Aparna, Lokveer, Griwan MS. Surgical infections: a microbiological study. Braz J Infect Dis 2004;8:118-25.
18. Mohanty S, Kapil A, Dhawan B, Das BK. Bacteriological and antimicrobial susceptibility profile of soft tissue infections from Northern India. Indian J Med Sci 2004;58:10-5.
19. Kalmeijer MD, Coertjens H, van Nieuwland-Bollen PM, et al. Surgical site infections in orthopedic surgery: the effect of mupirocin nasal ointment in a double-blind, randomized, placebo-controlled study. Clin Infect Dis 2002;35:353-8.
20. Tanner J, Woodings D, Moncaster K. Preoperative hair removal to reduce surgical site infection. Cochrane Database Syst Rev 2006;3:CD004122.
21. Loeb MB, Wilcox L, Smaill F, Walter S, Duff Z. A randomized trial of surgical scrubbing with a brush compared to antiseptic soap alone. Am J Infect Control 1997;25:11-5.
22. Srishyla MV, Rani MA, Damodar S, Venkataraman BV, Jairam N. A preliminary audit of practice—antibacterial prophylaxis in general surgery in an Indian hospital setting. Indian J Physiol Pharmacol 1994;38:207-10.
23. Khan SA, Rodrigues G, Kumar P, Rao PG. Current challenges in adherence to clinical guidelines for antibiotic prophylaxis in surgery. J Coll Physicians Surg Pak 2006;16:435-7.

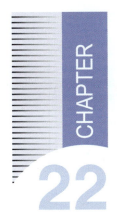

Perioperative Acute Kidney Injury

Abhishek Swami, Harish Reddy

INTRODUCTION

Perioperative kidney injury is a significant problem that is associated with considerable mortality, morbidity and increased length of hospital stay. Often there is incomplete recovery regardless of the baseline renal function. Only about 15 percent of patients who develop acute renal failure perioperatively fully recover. About half of patients who develop acute renal failure postoperatively, die.[1] Presently our ability to detect early kidney injury is limited and with the present means we are only able to detect renal dysfunction once the damage has been done. Therefore, a detailed evaluation in the perioperative period should include a thorough assessment of the risk for renal injury and measures should be instituted to prevent renal damage where possible.

DEFINITION AND INCIDENCE

The risk of kidney injury varies with different studies, because of variations in study population and definition of renal failure. Traditionally the term acute renal failure (ARF) covers many different meanings and several definitions are in use, ranging from 25 percent increase of serum creatinine to the need for renal replacement therapy. It has been realized that small changes in renal function have an impact on outcomes and this knowledge has led to the introduction of the terminology acute kidney injury (AKI). Recognizing the need for uniform definition of ARF, the Acute Dialysis Quality initiative (ADQI) group in 2004 proposed a consensus graded definition, called the RIFLE criteria (Fig. 22.1). These criteria emphasize the importance of less severe kidney injury in addition to renal failure and categorize the range of AKI into 3 severity categories and 2 outcome classes. This classification system has been validated in numerous

settings.[2,3] RIFLE stands for risk of renal dysfunction; Injury to kidney; Failure of kidney function; Loss of kidney function; and End-stage kidney disease. It relies on measurement of serum creatinine and urine output to classify the severity of ARF.

The reported incidence of postoperative AKI has ranged between 5-25 percent. Studies using RIFLE criteria have reported the postoperative AKI incidence to be about 20-25 percent.[4,5] Few studies have also looked at the risk of mortality in patients with postoperative AKI. In patients undergoing cardiac surgery, the risk of 90 day mortality has been reported to be as high as 32 percent in the more severe category RIFLE-F (failure) compared with 8 percent for those in RIFLE-R (risk) and 21 percent for RIFLE-I (injury). The

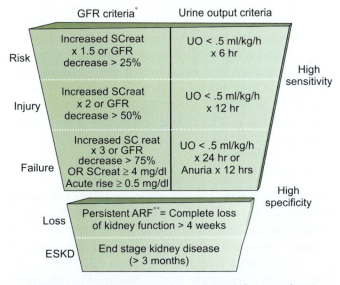

FIGURE 22.1: RIFLE criteria for uniform definition of ARF

RIFLE classification was found to be independent risk factor for mortality in these studies.[4]

In 2007, Acute Kidney Injury Network (AKIN) proposed an interim definition and staging system for AKI. Table 22.1 the diagnostic criteria for AKI are: an abrupt (within 48 hours) decrease in kidney function defined as an absolute increase in serum creatinine (SCr) of either > 0.3 mg/dl or increase of 1.5 fold from baseline or a reduction in urine output to < 0.5 ml/kg/hr for 6 hours (Table 22.1).[6]

Table 22.1: AKIN criteria		
Stage	S Cr criteria (48 hrs)	Urine output criteria
1	1.5–2 times baseline or >0.3 mg/dl rise	<0.5 ml/kg/hr for 6 hours
2	2-3 times baseline	<0.5 ml/kg/hr for 12 hours
3	>3 times baseline or S Cr > 4 + 0.3 mg/dl rise or Renal replacement therapy (RRT)	<0.3 ml/kg/hr for 24 hours or anuria for 12 hours.

AKI stages 1, 2 and 3 correspond to RIFLE Risk, Injury and Failure respectively. RIFLE loss and End stage were removed as they were felt to represent outcomes rather than stages of AKI. Patients who require RRT are considered to be in stage 3. This criteria is more sensitive as it includes patients with smaller increase in SCr (>0.3 mg/dl). AKI is not defined by GFR in AKIN criteria as estimated GFR is not reliable for acute changes in SCr.

Etiology

The etiology of acute kidney injury in the perioperative period is multifactorial and can be divided into prerenal, intrinsic renal, or postrenal causes. The most common pathophysiology is acute tubular necrosis (ATN). Prerenal AKI is reversible and is due to absolute or relative hypoperfusion. If the hypoperfusion is not corrected then ischemic ATN will result. Other intrinsic renal causes can be broadly categorized as glomerular, tubular, vascular or interstitial. Postrenal causes of AKI include obstruction of the bladder or ureters.

Risk Factors

There are no specific guidelines for identifying risk factors for AKI and preoperative renal risk stratification; furthermore the data about risk factors in literature is not uniform. The reason is lack of standardized definition and paucity of accurate biomarkers to detect AKI. There have been a variety of predictive models developed to risk stratify

Table 22.2: Preoperative and intraoperative renal failure risk	
Preoperative risk factors	Intraoperative risk factors
• Advanced age • Female gender • Obesity • Elevated preoperative S Cr and BUN • History of renal dysfunction • Left ventricular dysfunction • Hemodynamic instability • Peripheral vascular disease (PVD)/ Coronary artery disease • Septicemia • Comorbidities Diabetes, COPD, uncontrolled HTN, Liver disease • Severity of illness • Medications: Diuretic, vasopressors, NSAIDs, antibiotics, IV contrast. • Genetic	• Emergency surgery • Cardiac surgery: CABG, CPB • Vascular surgery • Liver transplantation • Hemodilution/Anemia • Medications: Diuretics, vasopressors, NSAIDs, antibiotics, aprotinin • General anesthesia

patients undergoing cardiac surgery but only a few studies have looked at noncardiac surgery population.

The risk factors can be broadly divided into those that can be identified preoperatively and those that occur intraoperatively (Table 22.2).

Preoperative Risk Factors

There are several preoperative factors that are predictive of postoperative renal dysfunction. The most important correctable risk factors are dehydration and hemodynamic instability. Elevated creatinine and chronic kidney disease are also substantial risk factors. Studies have shown that elevated creatinine is associated with exponential increases in postoperative ARF. Other diseases like COPD requiring bronchodilators, chronic liver disease, uncontrolled hypertension, PVD, CAD, CHF have been reported to confer kidney injury in those undergoing surgery.[7] Recent literature demonstrates an association between obesity and ARF after cardiac and noncardiac surgery. This association is independent of comorbidities such as diabetes and hypertension. **Women have been found to have a higher risk of developing acute renal failure than men at every level of baseline serum creatinine.**

There are some evidences for a genetic basis for renal risk. Patients who have inherited the epsilon-4 allele of apolipoprotein have decreased AKI compared to those who have other alleles.[8]

The use of diuretics and vasopressors can decrease renal perfusion and potentiate AKI. There is no evidence with the limited available data that angiotensin converting enzyme inhibitors (ACE-I) increase the risk of AKI, however several clinicians choose to withhold ACE-I prior to surgery as these can impair renal autoregulation and can compromise GFR in the face of other insults. There are several other medications administered commonly in the perioperative period, such as antibiotics, nonsteroidal anti-inflammatory drugs and contrast dyes that can be nephrotoxic. There is widespread use of herbal medications and alternative forms of medicines in the developing world which are potentially nephrotoxic and one should always inquire about their use, since such information is not always forthcoming.

Intraoperative Risk Factors

Surgery itself leads to reduction in GFR. Surgery causes a release of catecholamines, rennin, angiotensin, and arginine vasopressin. These lead to a redistribution of renal blood flow and a decrease in GFR.[9] Additionally, general anesthesia results in some degree of hypotension and depresses cardiac output, which further reduces renal perfusion and affects renal function.

Emergency surgeries confer greater risk as these patients are usually more ill and hemodynamically compromised. Furthermore, there is no opportunity to stabilize their volume status and optimize medical treatment preoperatively.

Certain types of surgery such as those undergoing cardiac surgery, vascular surgery or liver transplantation are much more likely to compromise renal blood flow. The risk of AKI after liver transplant has been reported to be greater than 50 percent. Low serum albumin and intravascular volume depletion are predisposing factors. The risk of AKI appears to be increased by prolonged duration of cardiopulmonary bypass (CPB) and aortic cross clamping time.[10] Patients who undergo more complex procedures such as combined CABG and valve surgery have a greater risk. Hemodilution or anemia on CPB also increases risk of AKI significantly. The mechanism is not clear. Contact activation plus release of vasoconstrictor hormones (epinephrine, angiotensin) and inflammatory cytokines may be responsible. Cardiac and vascular surgeries can also induce AKI from atheroembolism.

Diuretics and vasopressors are commonly used during surgeries and cause a reduction in GFR. Aprotinin is a protease inhibitor that has been used to reduce perioperative bleeding in CABG, orthopedic and liver transplant surgeries. There have been numerous reports of an association between aprotinin administration and elevation in postoperative creatinine. It affects kinin pathways that alter intrarenal hemodynamics. FDA suspended marketing of aprotinin in November 2007.

PREOPERATIVE RISK PREDICTION SCORES

Noncardiac Surgery

There is a lack of validated risk predictor scores for patients undergoing noncardiac surgery whereas there have been a variety of predictive models described for patients undergoing cardiac surgery. Kheterpal et al recently studied about 15,000 patients with normal preoperative renal function undergoing noncardiac surgery in a prospective observational study in an attempt to identify risk profiles for ARF (defined as GFR of 50 ml/min or less within the first seven postoperative days) in general surgical population. They identified seven independent preoperative predictors and developed propensity scores related to specific preoperative risk factors (See Table below).[7] This score might help to predict the risk of developing ARF after surgery. The model needs further validation but may prove useful in allowing timely interventions to prevent kidney injury and as a guide for preoperative discussions with patients.

Preoperative predictors of postoperative ARF
• Age, year (59 yrs or greater)
• Emergent surgery
• Liver disease
• Body mass index, kg/m^2 (32 kg/m^2 or greater)
• High risk surgery (intrathoracic, intraperitoneal, suprainguinal, vascular, surgeries involving large blood loss or fluid shifts)
• Peripheral vascular occlusive disease
• Chronic obstructive pulmonary disease necessitating bronchodilator therapy

Frequency and hazard ratio of ARF based on number of preoperative risk factors.

Preoperative risk class	*Acute renal failure %*	*Hazard ratio*
Class I (0 risk factors)	0.3	
Class II (1 risk factor)	0.5	2
Class III (2 risk factors)	1.3	4.7
Class IV (3 or more risk factors)	4.3	16

Cardiac Surgery

One of the useful risk prediction scoring models was developed by Thakar et al based on their study of about 33,000 patients undergoing open heart surgery regardless of preoperative renal function. The scoring model was developed on a randomly selected test set (n = 15,838) and was validated on remaining patients. In this system points are awarded based on risk factors, (see Table below) and patients can be assigned to one of four risk categories of increasing severity. The risk of ARF requiring dialysis in these risk categories ranged between 0.5 to 22 percent.[11]

Table 22.3: ARF score[a]

Risk factor	Points
Female gender	1
Congestive heart failure	1
Left ventricular ejection fraction <35 percent	1
Preoperative use of IABP	2
COPD	1
Insulin-requiring diabetes	1
Previous cardiac surgery	1
Emergency surgery	2
Valve surgery only (reference to CABG)	1
CABG + valve (reference to CABG)	2
Other cardiac surgeries	2
Preoperative creatinine 1.2 to <2.1 mg/dl (reference to 1.2)	2
Preoperative creatinine 2.1 (reference to 1.2)	5

[a] Minimum score, 0; Maximum score, 17.

Risk categories based on score	Frequency of ARF requiring dialysis
0–2	0.4 percent
3–5	1.8 percent
6–8	7.8 percent
9–13	21.5 percent

MEASURES TO PREVENT KIDNEY INJURY

1. Assess the risk: Using the tools described above (Table 22.3), the degree of overall risk should be assessed based on patient's individual risk and the characteristics of the procedure. This will help identify the high-risk patients. These tools can be used in limited resource settings easily as the parameters are mostly clinical and incorporate simple diagnostic tests.
2. Calculate estimated GFR, based on the modification of diet in renal disease (MDRD) equation. This will help in establishing preoperative renal dysfunction (GFR < 60 ml/min) patients with GFR equal to or less than 60 ml/min should be considered high-risk regardless of other risk factors.
3. Adjust medications: Based on the renal function (eGFR using MDRD equation) ascertain which medications need dose adjustment. Avoid medications such as ACE-I, angiotensin receptor blockers, NSAIDs, aminoglyco-

sides, aprotinin or excessive diuretic use, especially in patients with pre-existing renal dysfunction.

4. Assess and optimize volume status: A thorough clinical assessment should always be done to look for signs of dehydration or decreased volume status such as orthostatic hypotension, tachycardia, decreased skin turger, collapsed peripheral veins or low urine output. Physical exam may be useful but is not very sensitive in detecting volume status. High BUN or uric acid, metabolic alkalosis, dysnatremias may provide further clues. Central venous pressure measurements can be reliably used to assess and monitor volume status. If there is evidence of hypovolemia, it should be corrected prior to surgery. Uncorrected hypovolemia may lead to renal medullary hypoxia and ischemic ATN. The ideal fluid for correcting hypovolemia and hypotension is controversial. There is no evidence that colloids are better than crystalloids. Colloids are expensive and hence their use is not justified. The amount of crystalloids administered should be directed according to hemodynamic parameters, urine output (UO) and invasive monitors such as CVP. Mean arterial pressure (MAP) should be maintained > 65-70 mm Hg, UO > 0.5 cc/kg/hr, and CVP 10-15 mm Hg.[12] Excessive fluid resuscitation may be harmful and patients should be monitored closely for volume overload.

5. Preserve renal perfusion: Hypotension should be prevented. Renal injury can occur with any antihypertensive medication due to lowered blood pressure. In patients with long-standing hypertension, acute lowering of blood pressure to values even in the normal range should be avoided. ACE-I and angiotensin receptor blockers can decrease renal perfusion due to efferent arteriolar vasodilatation. These medications can affect renal autoregulation and should be held until fluid volume is restored. Hypotensive anesthesia should also be avoided for patients at risk of AKI. Abdominal insufflation for laparoscopic procedures may compromise renal perfusion. Lower pressures (< 15 mm Hg) or gasless laparoscopy should be considered for patients at risk of AKI.

6. Limit use of contrast agents: Risk factors for development of contrast induced nephropathy (CIN) include chronic renal insufficiency, dehydration, diabetes mellitus, congestive heart failure, high contrast volume and high osmolar contrast. If contrast is needed a low osmolar nonionic agent is preferred. Intravenous fluids such as normal saline should be used before and after procedures to increase urine flow. Adequate intravenous volume

expansion with isotonic crystalloid (1.0 to 1.5 ml/kg per hr) for 3 to 12 hr before the procedure and continued for 6 to 24 hr afterward can lessen the probability of CIN in patients who are at risk. The data on oral fluids as opposed to intravenous volume expansion as a CIN prevention measure are insufficient. Sodium bicarbonate infusion may also reduce the risk of CIN and can be used. The role of acetylcysteine is controversial and there have been both positive and negative studies. The benefit may be undefined but it is certainly harmless and should be used in high-risk patients. Prophylactic hemodialysis and hemofiltration have not been validated as effective strategies. In all high-risk patients, a follow-up serum creatinine should be obtained at no less than 24 hours or no more than 72 hours after contrast exposure.[13,14]

7. Optimize hematocrit levels: There is some evidence that low hematocrit levels are associated with increased mortality in dialysis patients. Furthermore, cardio-pulmonary bypass hemodilution is associated with increased likelihood of AKI. Hematocrit should be maintained at >24%.

8. Identify acute kidney injury: RIFLE criteria are a reasonable tool to assess kidney injury. Timely identification of AKI is very important as early intervention may reverse injury. Urine output and creatinine should be monitored closely in the perioperative period.

There has been enormous research aimed at finding pharmacotherapeutic options for prevention or treatment of AKI. Many promising treatments in experimental models or initial studies have failed to translate into successful clinical therapies. Renal dose dopamine has not shown any benefit. Fenoldopam (dopamine 1 receptor antagonist), loop diuretics, anaritide (recombinant atrial natriuretic peptide), and calcium channel blockers have been tried and not shown consistent benefit. Further studies are needed and some of these agents may show promise in future.

SUMMARY

Acute kidney injury (AKI) is the term to describe abrupt reduction in kidney dysfunction and it replaces previous terms such as ARF. The new definition is more sensitive in detecting AKI but needs to be validated further. Mortality secondary to perioperative AKI often exceeds 50 percent and small changes in SCr correlate to significant increases in mortality. Major risk factors include prior history of renal dysfunction, elevated SCr, hemodynamic insult, dehydration, decreased cardiac function, and cardiac and vascular surgery. Perioperative interventions most importantly should focus on maintenance of euvolemia, preservation of renal perfusion and avoidance of nephrotoxins.

PERIOPERATIVE EVALUATION OF PATIENTS WITH KIDNEY DISEASE

Chronic kidney disease (CKD), refers to a decline in the glomerular filtration rate (GFR) caused by a variety of diseases. Chronic kidney disease (CKD) is defined as either a glomerular filtration rate (GFR) of <60 ml min-1/1.73 m^2 for 3 months or more, irrespective of cause, or kidney damage leading to a decrease in GFR, present for 3 months or more. The damage may manifest as abnormalities in the composition of blood or urine, on radiological imaging, or in histology. Among patients with chronic kidney disease, the stage of disease should be assigned based on the level of kidney function, irrespective of diagnosis, according to the KDOQI CKD classification.

Stage	Description	GFR (mL/min/1.73m^2)
1.	Kidney damage with normal or ↑ GFR	> 90
2.	Mild ↓GFR	60-89
3.	Moderate ↓GFR	30-59
4.	Severe ↓GFR	15-29
5.	Kidney failure	< 15 or dialysis

KDOQI recommends the modification in diet in renal disease (MDRD) equation to estimate GFR. The MDRD equation has been validated in patients with CKD but it is not precise at high values of GFR, and in patients with a grossly abnormal muscle mass, patients with a very low BMI, pregnant patients, and where renal function is changing rapidly.

PREOPERATIVE ASSESSMENT

CKD is a risk factor for postoperative cardiovascular complications. Patients with a creatinine level greater than or equal to 2 are considered to have a clinical predictor of at least intermediate pretest probability of increased perioperative cardiovascular risk in the updated American College of Cardiology/American Heart Association (ACC/AHA) guidelines on perioperative cardiovascular evaluation of noncardiac surgery.

In addition patients with advanced kidney disease have electrolyte and acid base abnormalities which can be further aggravated by the effects of surgery and anesthesia. It is probably safe to avoid general anesthesia in patients with chronic kidney disease who have a serum potassium level above 5.5 mEq per L.

Patients with advanced CKD are predisposed to anemia and are at increased risk of worsening anemia with blood loss. They are also at increased risk for excessive bleeding during surgery from defect in platelet aggregation. Optimization of hemoglobin prior to surgery is helpful. To decrease the bleeding risk DDAVP can be administered prior to surgery in select patients who have advanced renal failure with high blood urea nitrogen levels. Patients who are adequately dialyzed donot warrant any therapy.

Preoperative diagnostic testing in patients with chronic kidney disease should include serum electrolytes, blood urea nitrogen, creatinine, calcium, complete blood count and chest radiograph. Patients who are on dialysis are advised to undergo dialysis a day before surgery to avoid any electrolyte disturbances.

Preoperative and intraoperative hypertension is common in patients with chronic kidney disease. With few exceptions, patients who have kidney disease and hypertension should continue antihypertensive drug therapy throughout the surgical period.

Noninvasive cardiac diagnostic testing is recommended on patients who are about to receive intermediate-risk or high-risk procedures and have a poor functional capacity.

POSTOPERATIVE ASSESSMENT

Chronic kidney disease is an independent risk factor for postoperative death and cardiovascular events after elective, noncardiac surgery.[15] CKD is a risk factor for multiple postoperative complications, including acuter renal failure, hyperkalemia, acid-base disturbances, volume overload, infections, drug toxicity, etc. All these impact surgical morbidity and affect postoperative outcomes.

Fluid, Electrolytes and Acid-base Disturbances

Patients with advanced CKD have an impaired ability to concentrate and dilute urine. The decrease in ability to excrete a sodium load predisposes patients with CKD stage 4 and 5 to volume overload and hyperchloremic metabolic acidosis, when large volumes of saline solutions are administered. Hyponatremia may occur from hypotonic fluids or inappropriate secretion of antidiuretic hormone.

Patients with advanced CKDSTAGE 5 and patient with diabetic nephropathy (Type 4 RTA) cannot excrete a potassium load. A reduction in ammonia synthesis and the ability to excrete hydrogen ions leads to metabolic acidosis in patients. It is important to avoid potassium load unless significant hypokalemia exists. Hyperkalemia may be precipitated by tissue breakdown, transfusions, acidosis, ACE inhibitors, beta-blockers, heparin, rhabdomyolysis, and the use of Ringer lactate solution as a replacement fluid.

Acute Renal Failure

Patients with CKD are at an increase risk of acute renal failure. Acute renal failure in is an independent risk factor for increased postoperative morbidity and mortality. Attention to fluid balance is paramount. Avoiding medications which can potentiate acute renal failure are best avoided. NSAIDs are contraindicated. ACE inhibitors are best avoided in the immediate postoperative setting unless there is a compelling reason. Radiocontrast agents should be avoided unless absolutely necessary. Antibiotics like aminoglycosides should not be used unless absolutely necessary.

Pharmacology

Chronic kidney disease (CKD) affects both the pharmacokinetics and the pharmacodynamics of large number of drugs. This effect will predispose these patients to adverse side effects. Adjusting medications is therefore an important aspect of medical management of the surgical patient with CKD. The effect of altered clearance must be addressed and dose adjustments should be done based on the estimated GFR to avoid unwarranted toxicity. Patients with acute renal failure estimated GFR is a poor predictor of true renal clearance and adjustments should be made based on the severity of renal failure.

Dialysis Access

Dialysis access care is important in patients with endstage renal disease. Vascular access may be either permanent or temporary. Permanent access include native arteriovenous fistulas and arteriovenous grafts and peritoneal dialysis catheters. Temporary vascular access includes tunneled and non tunneled catheters. Avoiding intravenous lines in the arm with fistulas and grafts is important. When new catheters are placed, the subclavian vein should be avoided as the risk of stenosis after catheterization is high. If a femoral vein is cannulated it is best to utilize it for short-term and catheter changed to internal jugular vein as the risk of infections is much higher with a femoral Quinton.

REFERENCES

1. Schreiber MJ. Minimizing perioperative complications in patients with renal insufficiency. Cleve Clin J Med. 2006;73 Suppl 1:S116-20.
2. Bellomo R, Ronco C, Kellum JA, Mehta RL, Palevsky P. Acute renal failure - definition, outcome measures, animal models, fluid therapy and information technology needs: the Second International Consensus Conference of the Acute Dialysis Quality Initiative (ADQI) Group. Crit Care. 2004;8(4):R204-212.
3. Hoste EAJ, Kellum JA. Acute kidney injury: epidemiology and diagnostic criteria. Curr Opin Crit Care. 2006;12(6):531-37.
4. Kuitunen A, Vento A, Suojaranta-Ylinen R, Pettilä V. Acute renal failure after cardiac surgery: evaluation of the RIFLE classification. Ann. Thorac. Surg. 2006;81(2):542-6.
5. Lombardi R, Ferreiro A. Risk factors profile for acute kidney injury after cardiac surgery is different according to the level of baseline renal function. Ren Fail. 2008;30(2):155-60.
6. Mehta RL, Kellum JA, Shah SV, et al. Acute Kidney Injury Network: report of an initiative to improve outcomes in acute kidney injury. Crit Care. 2007;11(2):R31.
7. Kheterpal S, Tremper KK, Englesbe MJ, et al. Predictors of postoperative acute renal failure after noncardiac surgery in patients with previously normal renal function. Anesthesiology 2007;107(6):892-902.
8. Chew ST, Newman MF, White WD, et al. Preliminary report on the association of apolipoprotein E polymorphisms, with postoperative peak serum creatinine concentrations in cardiac surgical patients. Anesthesiology 2000;93(2):325-31.
9. Wagener G, Brentjens TE. Renal disease: the anesthesiologist's perspective. Anesthesiol Clin 2006;24(3):523-47.
10. Rosner MH, Okusa MD. Acute kidney injury associated with cardiac surgery. Clin J Am Soc Nephrol 2006;1(1):19-32.
11. Thakar CV, Arrigain S, Worley S, Yared J, Paganini EP. A clinical score to predict acute renal failure after cardiac surgery. J Am Soc Nephrol 2005;16(1):162-8.
12. Vincent J, Gerlach H. Fluid resuscitation in severe sepsis and septic shock: an evidence-based review. Crit. Care Med 2004;32(11 Suppl): S451-54.
13. Solomon R, Deray G. How to prevent contrast-induced nephropathy and manage risk patients: practical recommendations. Kidney Int. Suppl. 2006;(100):S51-53.
14. McCullough PA, Stacul F, Becker CR, et al. Contrast-induced Nephropathy (CIN) Consensus Working Panel: executive summary. Rev Cardiovasc Med 2006;7(4):177-97.
15. Mathew, et al. Chronic kidney disease and postoperative mortality: A systematic review and meta-analysis International 2008;73: 1069–81.

CHAPTER

23

Surgical Education

Vijay Mittal, Subhas Gokul

INTRODUCTION

Learning is a complex process. The quality of surgical training and competence defines the quality of patient care.[1] Surgical residency programs aim at producing competent professionals in a safe and pedagogically efficient environment.[2] The training of surgeons has undergone remarkable evolution in the millennia that have passed since the inception of the art of surgery.[3] Our basic model of surgical training has remained unchanged for over a century. Much of this is being dramatically challenged by unprecedented changes to the training environment. Increasing intolerance of error, diminution in the degree of independence given to trainees, increasingly challenging technological changes and an appropriate focus on patient safety have fundamentally changed the complexion of surgical training.[2]

Attempts at improving surgical education began almost a millennium ago; the first tiny steps in a long process to advance training in the craft of surgery.[3] The modern surgeon, in addition to a lifelong commitment to learning and honing his craft, is also required to fulfill his role as a teacher and a manager.

The indian medical education system, one of the largest in the world, has produced many physicians, who have emigrated to the United States, United Kingdom and several other countries. The quality of these physicians, therefore, has had a broad global impact. Medical schools in India have rapidly proliferated in the past 25 years.[5] The qualities of the indian surgeon, include the tenacity to milk the most out of patient load, experience, improvisation and innovation. In addition, they have the desire and capacity to transfer these immeasurable and essential ingredients to both the surgical trainee and the poor patient.[1]

In the early part of the 20th century, the surgical residency program was introduced at Johns Hopkins University by William Halsted. At that time, surgeons did not officially subspecialize or differentiate, and they performed operations in several different anatomic areas and organ systems. As surgical knowledge expanded and the variety of possible operations increased, the tree of surgery began to grow branches. Nevertheless, they all maintained a connection to the trunk of the tree for a long time.[6]

SELECTION OF RESIDENTS/POSTGRADUATES

Traditionally in the western countries, surgical residency programs have selected individuals based on their academic achievements (USMLE scores, evaluation on clinical rotations) and a subjective impression from a 15–20 min interview. Consideration is also given to the previous research activities.

In India the residents are selected based on a competitive entrance examinations, which are held nationally as well as regionally. These exams consist of multiple choice questions that test the overall basic and clinical knowledge of applicants. Based on their performance, ranks are awarded and entrance into various specialities is by basis of merit, with the higher ranking applicants having the right of choice over their compatriots. No personal interviews are conducted for selecting the residents.

Academic achievements and competitive examinations reflect theoretical knowledge; however, they do not ensure that the candidate can apply this knowledge in practice. The development of new surgical approaches, such as minimally invasive techniques and endoluminal therapies, requires mastering unique psychomotor skills. The issue of psychomotor testing as a selection tool for procedural specialities is complex and controversial.[2]

National attrition rate in general surgery in the USA is 5.8 percent. Surgery is a team sport, and self-promoting behavior may compromise success. Assimilating a new resident to the culture of the department remains a significant challenge. Thus resident selection imposes significant challenges. Suboptimal test-takers may be excluded despite the paucity of data supporting an association of test performance with eventual performance as a practicing physician.[7]

SURGICAL TRAINING

Although technical proficiency is definitely an important prerequisite for a successful outcome, other qualities such as intellectual abilities, personality and communication skills, and a commitment to practice are important elements in the profile of a competent surgeon.[2] Optimizing educational experiences is of importance in many fields, not in the least due to constraints imposed by limited resources such as time and personnel. Medical school and residency education, in particular, is vulnerable to the stress imposed by the scarcity of resources juxtaposed with the sheer volume of information that students and residents must master, which must occur in a setting that also carries significant restrictions on time.[8]

There is a changing picture of general surgical training due to proliferation of fellowships in subspecialities of surgery, as well as the increasing desire of these subspecialities for recognition as independent specialities in their own right. The proliferation of advanced fellowships in gastrointestinal surgery, surgical oncology, endocrine surgery, breast surgery, and other core areas of general surgery has eroded the general surgery residency experience and has created a system, in which residents now realize that they need to take advanced training to gain additional experience in core areas of general surgery. This drives the proliferation of fellowships, which erodes core training. Laparoscopic fellows now perform procedures which used to be regularly performed by general surgeons, such as partial colectomy and fundoplication.[6]

TRAINING IN THE USA

There are approximately 250 hospitals that train residents in general surgery in the United States; approximately half of these are "university hospitals", meaning they are part of a medical university, and the rest are "community" or regional hospitals affiliated to a university. The maximum number of surgery residents that an individual hospital is allowed to train is set by a nongovernmental nonprofit entity called the Accreditation Council for Graduate Medical Education (ACGME). The ACGME is responsible for the quality of residency programs and accredits all surgery programs through a subentity called the Residency Review Committee for Surgery (RRC). The RRC performs on-site visits to residency programs once every 5 years, and more often if problems that require correction are noted. Each year, approximately 1,100 medical graduates choose to enter graduate education in general surgery. Ultimately, approximately 300 of these residents complete 5 years of general surgery training and then enter practice of surgery. The rest go beyond the basic general surgery training to enter various subspecialty fields that require general surgical training as a prerequisite.[6]

Surgical residency training programs face many challenges in producing competent surgeons. The Accreditation Council for Graduate Medical Education (ACGME) requires residents to receive training in 6 competencies (Table 23.1), and programs must document the achievement of those competencies with great precision. These are intended to ensure both quality patient care and competent trainees.[9] Teaching patterns in most of the residency programs across USA include weekly grand rounds, didactics covering core curriculum, and morbidity and mortality discussions held weekly (Table 23.2). The Surgical Council on Resident Education (SCORE) is a consortium formed in 2006 by the principal organizations involved in US surgical education. SCORE's mission is to improve the education of general surgery residents (trainees) in the United States through the development of a standard national curriculum for general surgery residency training.

Morbidity and mortality (M&M) meetings aim to improve the standards of surgical care, and are required in all hospitals responsible for training junior surgical staff. M&M meetings must be carefully planned and well organized. They are essentially peer reviews of mistakes occurring during the care of patients. The objectives of a well-run M&M conference are to learn from complications and errors, to modify behavior and judgment based on previous experiences, and to prevent repetition of errors leading to complications. Meetings should be nonpunitive and focus on the goal of improved patient care. They also highlight recent cases and identify areas of improvement for clinicians involved in the case. Meetings are also important for identifying systems issues (e.g. outdated policies, changes in patient identification procedures, arithmetic errors, etc.) which affect patient care.

Table 23.1: ACGME competencies

1. Patient care
Residents must be able to provide patient care that is compassionate, appropriate, and effective for the treatment of health problems and the promotion of health.
2. Medical knowledge
Residents must demonstrate knowledge of established and evolving biomedical, clinical, epidemiological and social-behavioral sciences, as well as the application of this knowledge to patient care.
3. Practice-based learning and improvement
Residents must demonstrate the ability to investigate and evaluate their care of patients, to appraise and assimilate scientific evidence, and to continuously improve patient care based on constant self-evaluation and life-long learning.
4. Interpersonal and communication skills
Residents must demonstrate interpersonal and communication skills that result in the effective exchange of information and collaboration with patients, their families, and health professionals.
5. Professionalism
Residents must demonstrate a commitment to carrying out professional responsibilities and an adherence to ethical principles. Residents are expected to demonstrate.
6. Systems-based practice
Residents must demonstrate an awareness of and responsiveness to the larger context and system of health care, as well as the ability to call effectively on other resources in the system to provide optimal health care.

Table 23.2: Typical teaching schedule in surgical residency in USA Community Teaching Hospital

Weekly

Tuesday	7 am - 8 am	Morbidity and mortality meeting
Wednesday	7 am - 8 am	Grand rounds with an expert speaker
Wednesday	8 am - 11 am	Core topics in surgery discussion
Thursday	7 am - 8 am	(Alternate) video conference teaching in core topics in surgery on consortium basis
Thursday	9 am - 10 am	Teaching rounds
Friday	7 am - 8 am	Multidisciplinary tumor board meeting
Friday	11 am - 12 pm	Meeting of program director with senior residents
Saturday	8 am - 10 am	(Not fixed) grand rounds with an expert speaker
Tuesday/Thursday	2 pm - 4 pm	Skills lab/gross anatomy dissection

Monthly

1st Monday	4 pm - 5 pm	Research update meeting
1st Monday	5 pm - 6 pm	Journal club meeting /Evidence based discussion
4th Wednesday	6 pm - 8 pm	Regional surgical association meeting
4th Friday	8 am - 10 am	Feedback and monthly evaluation by program directors

As the body of medical literature continues to expand, physicians must develop the necessary skills to keep up with the vast amount of information available. The journal club provides a forum to allow residents to remain current with the literature while also teaching them the methods to evaluate it critically. Periodic evaluation of this conference will allow the organizers to assess the concordance of the resident's goals with those of the faculty. Formal evaluation will also provide an objective assessment of the knowledge gained by the house-staff through participation in journal club. Journal clubs have become a forum to teach its members critical appraisal techniques thereby enriching their understanding of the medical literature. They also have emerged as a method to promote the practice of evidence-based medicine. It is important to design a format to make it both stimulating and educational for its members. The journal club requires audience participation to best educate its participants. It is the constant exchange of ideas and interactions amongst members that help optimize its teaching potential (Table 23.3).

Table 23.3: Journal club
Structure
- Structure journal club to conveniently fit into residency schedule
- Preselect one or two residents to lead the discussion
- Article selection should occur at least three weeks before scheduled presentation
- Assigned resident(s) should meet with faculty advisor before presentation to plan areas of emphasis and approach to moderating the discussion
- Distribute articles to participants two weeks before meeting
- Encourage participants to read the article in preparation for the discussion
Article
- Selecting articles emphasizing different aspects of experimental design
- Creating a controversy-utilizing debate format
- Selecting classic articles
- Meticulous analysis of a single article
- Problem-based learning method
Evaluation
- Use periodic written surveys to assess the goals and overall satisfaction of participants
- Survey residents if attendance is suboptimal to decide whether a change in meeting time and/or duration may improve attendance
- Evaluate knowledge gained by participants using either self evaluation surveys or by more objective measurements using a pretest/post-test format

Tumor boards are an integral part of cancer patient treatment. Tumor Board is a treatment planning approach includes discussions of current medical and surgical oncology cases. Imaging, pathology and modes of treatment are discussed. Residents are expected to post and present cases as they become available. The tumor board incorporates factors such as' assessing learning needs, interacting among provider-learners with opportunities to practice the skills learned, and sequenced and multifaceted educational activities.

A fundamental aspect of surgical residency training includes the teaching of basic principles of surgical science. This is accomplished with a formal, didactic core curriculum. The basic surgical curriculum is implemented in most programs as a weekly teaching conference with all resident levels in attendance at the same conference. Here residents do the presentation and in addition to core surgical principles, an increased emphasis is now being placed on areas such as professionalism, leadership and communication, and systems-based practice.

MEDICAL COUNCIL OF INDIA/NATIONAL BOARD OF EXAMINATION

The Medical Council of India (MCI) was established in 1934 under Medical Council Act of 1933, with the main function of establishing uniform standards of higher qualifications.[1] MCI is an autonomous organization to develop standards in postgraduate medical education, training, and examination for resident pursuing MS (General Surgery). Whereas the National Board of Examinations (NBE) looks over the Diplomate in National Board (DNB) training in surgery was established in 1974. The majority of the NBE trainees are in private sector nonteaching hospitals with excellent facilities for clinical and investigative evaluation, but with limited "hands on" experience compared with the MCI-recognized teaching hospitals, because most DNB seats in surgery are in private hospitals.[1] Association of surgeons of India (ASI) is a national level association of both the certified surgeons and surgeons in training. It has branches at state and district level. Activities are undertaken for promoting surgical education at different levels (Table 23.4).

Tougher implication of the guidelines and laws, with regards to surgical education by the MCI is needed.[10] More active participation is needed from ASI for governing surgical education.

ETHICS

Indian surgery has an incredibly high standard of overall efficiency, empathy, and recognition. Ancient India's

Table 23.4: Governing bodies in Indian surgical training		
Governing bodies	Medical Council of India (MCI)	National board of examination (NBE)
Degree/Diploma	MS (Gen surgery)	DNB (Gen surgery)
Established	1934	1974
Hospitals	Mostly government funded	Mostly private hospitals
Enrolment based on	National/State/Institutional level examinations	National level examinations
Examination	Conducted by several different universities	Conducted by one body at various centers

contributions to ethics and surgical training are remarkable. Now, almost 3,000 years later, they still continue to have great relevance, despite widespread concerns about the erosion of long-held value systems and cherished codes of medical practice.[11]

Many surgeons face profound ethical issues as part of their daily work. An ethics curriculum would certainly meet most components of professionalism. Residents are expected to demonstrate respect, compassion, and integrity; a responsiveness to the needs of patients and society that supersedes self-interest; accountability to patients, society, and the profession; and a commitment to excellence and on-going professional development. They should demonstrate a commitment to ethical principles pertaining to provision or withholding of clinical care, confidentiality of patient information, informed consent, and business practice. They should also demonstrate sensitivity and responsiveness to patients' culture, age, gender, and disabilities,[12] which are part of 6 competencies laid down by ACGME.

WORKING HOURS

Historically, extensive work hours have always been believed to be a necessary component of resident education and have become the public symbol of a profession that requires hard work and dedication. Long working hours for surgical residents is a time honored tradition of presumed merit, but is the one that has recently come under scrutiny and criticism.[13]

The universal pressure to reduce working hours for surgical trainees is driven by concerns for patient safety and quality of life of surgical residents. This is being implemented in the west. The European working hour directive limits the average work week to a maximum of 48 h, including overtime, and a minimum uninterrupted rest period of 24 h per week and 11 h per day.[2,14] The challenge will be to achieve the same educational goals of a surgical residency

in fewer hours. Newer training models like the "mentorship model," "case-based model," and "night float model" offer new ideas aimed at improving efficacy of surgical residency training to accommodate the 80-hour workweek in the USA. Care should be taken not to optimize resident training at the expense of patient care, while following these models.[15] However, there is a growing concern that this may lead to lengthening of the training programs, reduced volume and complexity of operative experience, and narrowing of surgical expertise. Ultimately, there is a growing body of opinion that graduating residents are less skilled than their teachers[2] (Table 23.5).

Unlike the western countries, the surgical resident in India has no limited work hours. He could be at work for indefinite hours every day and still find his patient care incomplete. As he progresses from the first to the third year of residency, his responsibilities for patient care and operative experience widen.[1] Furthermore, many programs maintain a fairly strict hierarchical approach to training, which often relegates junior residents to the completion of many mundane tasks resulting in an enormous amount of wasted educational time among this group of trainees.[2]

STRUCTURED CURRICULUM

Curricula in most Indian surgical training programs are haphazard. What residents learn often has more to do with available opportunity than predicated on structured educational objectives. Most programs have long lists of educational objectives, which often look like the 'index' of a textbook, but there is rarely an integral link between these objectives and a curricular plan to accomplish them.[2]

Operative elective, day surgery, dedicated supervised training lists and emergency lists with the keeping of a surgical logbook detailing experience, on-call duties, and outpatient clinics will of course continue.[4] We need to refocus on the service to education ratios for all our trainees, aiming where possible, to maximize educational

Table 23.5: Working hours			
System	*USA*	*United Kingdom*	*India*
Week	80 hrs	48 hrs	No limit
One shift	Up to 24 hrs	Up to 13 hrs	No limit
Minimum rest	24 hour/week	24 hour/week	None set

opportunities while minimizing those service elements that provide little value added to the overall training of a surgeon. We need a structured training program that allows for a quicker ascent to technical competence coupled with the safeguards of a rigorous assessment program to gauge a resident's progress with respect to their procedural knowledge and technical proficiency.[2,16,17]

Defining key modules for general surgery with clear educational objectives, clear expectations and assessment of competence has the potential to significantly improve the training process. This type of training would mandate rigorous competency benchmarks, which would need to be met prior to promotion to the next training level. This approach, which would be centered on objective assessment and structured feedback, has the potential to dramatically change the pace of skills acquisition. Each training module would need to be based on a comprehensive training and assessment curriculum using a systematic, stepwise approach.[2]

Evidence-based medicine is not something solely mentioned in lectures, but should be actively taught by faculty and observed and practiced by residents in the clinical setting. Residents directly benefit and acquire medical knowledge and experience from their teaching faculty. Surgical procedures can and have been studied systematically to evaluate almost all feasible aspects, from preoperative skin preparation and antibiotics to methods of performing incisions and techniques for dissection to complication rates and mortality. When new surgical procedures are introduced, they can be studied and evaluated first by the scientific community. In this way, a safe, effective, and validated operative procedure that has passed through the rigorous scrutiny of other physician-scientists can then be passed on to surgical trainees.[3]

The surgical trainee is expected to maintain a log book of his operative work during the 3-year period. Due to lack of supervision, this often is a minor formality.[1] Where as in the USA there is an online record of operative logbook which is monitored by the ACGME. There are 11 areas of expertise with a certain minimum number of required cases

in each; these needs to be achieved in order to graduate. The program must document that residents are performing a sufficient breadth of complex procedures to graduate qualified surgeons. Residents must enter their operative experience concurrently during each year of the residency in the ACGME case log system. A total of at least 750 major cases should be logged in by the resident at the time of graduation. This should include 150 Major cases logged in as a Chief resident (Table 23.6).

Timely and regular feedback is critical. There is a growing body of evidence that expert feedback, delivered in a pedagogically sound way, can shorten the learning curves associated with new procedures.[2] Resident-led teaching on surgical services is typically disorganized, which restricts the quantity and quality of such teaching. Responsibility for instruction is usually unassigned, so various team members intermittently teach students when convenient. Surgical residents' educational skill has traditionally not been a part of their evaluations, even for trainees planning on academic careers. Resident development as educator has received increasing attention in recent years, and various programs have been developed to encourage maturation of residents as teachers (Table 23.7).[18]

SKILLS LAB

During the past 2 decades, the practice of surgery has undergone rapid transformation. Extensive acceptance and utilization of minimally invasive surgical techniques has occurred, and more recently, robotic technologies have been

Table 23.6: Operative requirements in the USA	
Pancreas	3
Liver	4
Plastics	5
Endocrine	8
Trauma operative	10
Thoracic	15
Trauma nonoperative	20
Pediatric surgery	20
Head and neck	24
Laparoscopic advanced	25
Skin, soft tissues and breast	25
Vascular	44
Laparoscopic basic	60
Abdomen	65
Alimentary	72
Endoscopy	85
Total chief cases	150
Total	750 cases
Teaching assistant	50 (atleast)

Table 23.7: Evaluation

Resident evaluation

The faculty must evaluate and document resident performance in a timely manner.
The program should:
- Do objective assessments of ACGME competencies
- Document progressive resident performance improvement appropriate to educational level
- Provide each resident with documented semiannual evaluation of performance with feedback
- Monitor the resident's knowledge by use of a formal exam such as the American Board of Surgery in Training Examination (ABSITE) or other cognitive exams

Summative evaluation for each resident upon completion of the program, which then becomes part of the resident's permanent record maintained by the institution.

Faculty evaluation

- Should be done at least annually.
- Review of the faculty's clinical teaching abilities, commitment to the educational program, clinical knowledge, professionalism, and scholarly activities.
- Annual written confidential evaluations by the residents.

Program evaluation

- Done by the residents and faculty
- Must document formal, systematic evaluation of the curriculum at least annually
- Monitor graduate performance, including performance of program graduates on the certification examination

Rotation evaluation

- Done in a timely manner by the residents and faculty

360 Degrees evaluations

- Done by multiple evaluators (e.g. peers, patients, self, and other professional staff like nurses in floor and operating rooms)

developed. The use of surgical devices, such as mechanical staplers, electrosurgical dissection tools, and laser therapies enable surgeons to enhance the quality of the operative procedure, with subsequent benefits to patients.[19]

Training would start with simulated models and clinical situations in the skills lab until predefined proficiency criteria are met. Only then, would the trainee be able to progress to clinical situations on the ward and the operating room. There has been extensive evaluation of teaching and testing methods for surgical skills. Research has demonstrated that an hour spent in a virtual reality simulator translates to 2 h in the operating room. Furthermore, randomized trials have demonstrated that skills acquired in a virtual environment can be transferred to the operating room. Equally important is the pace of skills laboratory sessions. Studies have shown that when compared with single sessions in the skills laboratory, multiple distributed sessions result in augmented learning.[2]

Same day laparoscopic cholecystectomy is now the accepted standard of care. With these advances in care and with a greater awareness of the science of patient safety, we as healthcare professionals need to develop and hone our skills to meet patient demand. In the past, the "learning curve" for acquisition of skill was based on repeated, albeit supervised, "practice" on patients. By definition, the early part of the learning curve led to longer operating times and may have led to an increased likelihood of complications. This approach is no longer an ethically or economically viable option. Nonetheless, the inexperienced surgeon must acquire the knowledge, skills, and attitudes necessary to deliver their trade. This concept is not only true for junior trainees but also for established surgeons who must learn new techniques. The delivery of a surgery-training curriculum, with the bulk of the learning curve endured on simulators rather than on patients, is now becoming a reality.[19]

The organization of the tools, space, learners, and faculty is a substantive challenge that is tempered only by the greater challenge of keeping up with the constant evolution of new technologies such as telerobotics and natural orifice transendoscopic surgery into daily practice.[19] As our knowledge in this field expands, the use of well designed local and national simulation-based curricula will likely become increasingly widespread.[20]

RESEARCH

Scholarly activities include journal clubs, case reports, case series, basic science and research projects. Development of the next generation of surgical scientists begins by attracting the best students into surgery and by providing a structured research curriculum with appropriate oversight. The future of academic surgery depends on the continuous influx of young people with creative and inquisitive minds that are nurtured and trained to investigate novel frontiers dedicated to the advancement of knowledge and science.[21]

Before being accepted as a candidate for the examination, a thesis/dissertation is required on one specific researched surgical topic. This also is perfunctionally examined in most centers and loses its value as a research training tool.[1]

The research and innovation of surgeons throughout the centuries has contributed significantly to scientific knowledge and has helped develop the best patient care. The future of surgery as an academic and professional discipline that will continue to contribute to the discovery and clinical translation of new knowledge, technology, and surgical therapeutic innovation might depend on how high research is on the priority scale of surgical education and practice.

Institutions must be committed to maintaining the highest standards of research training, such that following completion successful trainees will be able to function independently as scientific investigators. This implies that the institution must provide the facilities, resources, dedicated course work and curriculum, and an environment conducive to the production of high quality work. Mentoring is critical for the trainee but this requires substantial time and commitment from the mentor.[21] Appointment of basic scientist (PhD holder) as director of research helps in providing guidance and assistance to residents with their research activities.[22]

Following completion of their training, trainees should be able to formulate meaningful hypotheses independently, design and conduct experiments to test their hypotheses, critically analyze their results, and understand the significance and potential application of their research findings. The development of presentation skills is likewise important in the form of oral and written communications. During and after their research training it is imperative that trainees be taught to uphold the highest ethical standards in regards to all aspects of research and patient care.[21]

CERTIFICATION

There is a yearly in-training examination conducted nationally by the American Board of Surgeons. The scores of this examination are used for assessment of the program, residents and for fellowships selection.[23] Most of the programs conduct annual mock oral examination either on a free standing in-house, or on a consortium basis. Both these examinations help the residents and program by providing an insight in the deficiencies and their remedies.

In India, on the other hand, there is only a one-time assessment at the end of the 3 years of residency. This is a theory examination is essay type consisting of four papers each with long questions and short notes. The practical examination comprises clinical evaluation on a long case for detailed discussion and a few short cases to assess clinical skills and quick responses. There are two vivas covering radiology, pathology, anatomy, and operative discussion.[1] The MS examination of the MCI suffers from gross disparity in standards, evaluation, even transparency, as it is conducted by several disparate universities, each with its own agenda and standards of competence. The NBE diploma of the National Board of Examination by contrast has one uniform standard of evaluation and competence because it is conducted by one body all over the country at various centers. Furthermore, there is greater transparency and less bias in the clinical evaluation because candidates have to appear in centers and cities away from their own hospitals.[1]

In the current era of surgical education, a training program must examine a resident's performance under individual core competencies, objectifying and documenting against a set of criteria, to develop a measure of the "soundness" of training of each resident.[24] Effective communication with patients is an essential skill for surgical trainees in the diagnosis and management of clinical problems. This is an area that may be suboptimally tested.[4]

FURTHER TRAINING

Based on a survey done in the USA, there is an increasing orientation of surgical trainees toward fellowship training.

Indeed, nearly 75 percent of current trainees plan to pursue fellowships after general surgery training.[25] Fellowships available postgeneral surgery residency in USA include: bariatric, breast, burns, colorectal, endoscopy, hepato-pancreatobilliary, minimally invasive, plastic, surgical critical care, surgical oncology, transplant, trauma, and vascular surgery. To help residents decide on future career and fellowships, specialty rotations are provided in the general surgery residency curriculum (Table 23.8).

Majority of the institutions training surgical residents in India lack a setting for critical care, vascular surgery, plastics, thoracic surgery and trauma. As these training in these specialities are integral part of general surgery training, residents should be sent on outside rotations to nearby institutions with such facilities. There is an ever-increasing role of imaging and interventional radiology in surgical management. Residents should have posting in radiology as a completion of their training.

In India, super specialization is available in the form of MCh and DNB. They are available in the following fields—cardiothoracic surgery, neurosurgery, plastic, surgical gastroenterology, surgical oncology, and vascular surgery.

CHANGES NEEDED IN THE SYSTEM

The traditional time-based approach to surgical education relies on the assumption that all surgical trainees learn at the same rate. There is emerging evidence that this is not the case. The current time-based model needs to be replaced by an outcome-based system, which would lead to certification after demonstration of competence rather than based on length of training. All the competencies should be objectively evaluated and successfully met by each resident before graduation.[2]

Table 23.8: Specialty rotations
Apart from general surgery residents rotate in the following specialty:
• Anesthesiology
• Burn care
• Cardiac surgery
• Gastroenterology
• Gynecology
• Neurosurgery
• Orthopedic surgery
• Pediatric surgery
• Radiology
• Thoracic surgery
• Transplant surgery
• Urology

To have the entire surgical training program under the aegis of one body with one uniform strictly implemented training program, syllabus, standards, and one examination conducted by this one regulatory body fairly and transparently all over the country would tone up and improve the entire training program even without any further embellishment or expenses.[1] Changes are needed in the admission system of surgical residents while maintaining transparency. Also the regulatory body MCI should be more vigilant that the standards in individual programs are met.

Surgeons of future will have to meet higher expectations and deal increasingly with complex, demanding procedures in patients who may have a number of challenging health-care issues. A constellation of recent pressures would seem to indicate that we will not be able to meet these challenges with traditional methods. We need to change the training system, else we may be at risk of graduating residents who may be less skilled than the previous generation. We need to deploy bold new methods of training, experiment with new paradigms and above all, study our new approaches to ensure that we are on track for producing better surgeons; surgeons who will deliver superlative care that focuses on quality and patient safety.[2]

Reforms should be based on sound educational research, with government agencies being held accountable for evidence based regulations. If these reforms are successful, the impact of improving indian surgical education will be felt around the world.[5]

REFERENCES

1. Udwadia TE, Sen G. Surgical training in India. World J Surg 2008;32(10):2150-5. PMID: 18679746.
2. Grantcharov TP, Reznick RK. Training tomorrow's surgeons: what are we looking for and how can we achieve it? ANZ J Surg 2009;79(3):104-7. PMID: 19317771.
3. Franzese CB, Stringer SP. The evolution of surgical training: perspectives on educational models from the past to the future. Otolaryngol Clin North Am. 2007;40(6):1227-35, vii. PMID: 18021837.
4. West H. Training of general surgical residents: What model is appropriate? Am J Surg 2008;195(1):136-8. PMID: 18070737.
5. Supe A, Burdick WP. Challenges and issues in medical education in India. Acad Med 2006;81(12):1076-80. PMID: 17122473.
6. Bell RH Jr. Graduate education in general surgery and its related specialities and subspecialities in the United States. World J Surg 2008;32(10):2178-84. PMID: 18581168.
7. Longo WE, Seashore J, Duffy A, Udelsman R. Attrition of categoric general surgery residents: results of a 20-year audit. Am J Surg 2009; PMID: 19178898.
8. Mammen JM, Fischer DR, Anderson A, James LE, Nussbaum MS, Bower RH, Pritts TA. Learning styles vary among general surgery

residents: analysis of 12 years of data. J Surg Educ 2007;64(6):386-9. PMID: 18063274.

9. Webb TP, Weigelt JA, Redlich PN, Anderson RC, Brasel KJ, Simpson D. Protected block curriculum enhances learning during general surgery residency training. Arch Surg 2009;144(2):160-6. PMID: 19221328.

10. Srivastava SK. Surgical training in India. Natl Med J India 2003;16(1):48-9. PMID: 12715961.

11. Singh B, Saradananda S. Ethics and surgical training in ancient India—a cue for current practice. S Afr Med J 2008;98(3):218-21. PMID: 18350226.

12. Helft PR, Eckles RE, Torbeck L. Ethics education in surgical residency programs: a review of the literature. J Surg Educ 2009;66(1):35-42. PMID: 19215896.

13. Mittal V, Salem M, Tyburski J, Brocato J, Lloyd L, Silva Y, Silbergleit A, Shanley C, Remine S. Residents' working hours in a consortium-wide surgical education program. Am Surg 2004;70(2):127-31; PMID: 15011914.

14. Council directive 93/104/EC. Official J Eur Commun 1993; L307:18–24.

15. Mittal VK, Portenier D. Continuity of care in the 80-hour workweek era. Curr Surg 2006;63(1):31-4. PMID: 16373157.

16. Grantcharov TP, Reznick RK. Teaching procedural skills. Br Med J 2008;336:1129–31.

17. Aggarwal R, Grantcharov TP, Darzi A. Framework for systematic training and assessment of technical skills. J Am Coll Surg 2007; 204:697–705.

18. Jamshidi R. Formalizing teaching responsibilities for junior surgical housestaff encourages educator development. J Surg Educ 2008;65(6):514-7. PMID: 19059187.

19. Aggarwal R, Darzi A. From scalpel to simulator: a surgical journey. Surgery 2009;145(1):1-4. PMID: 19081469.

20. Scott DJ, Cendan JC, Pugh CM, Minter RM, Dunnington GL, Kozar RA. The changing face of surgical education: simulation as the new paradigm. J Surg Res 2008;147(2):189-93. PMID: 18498868.

21. Suliburk JW, Kao LS, Kozar RA, Mercer DW. Training future surgical scientists: realities and recommendations. Ann Surg 2008;247(5):741-9. PMID: 18438110.

22. Sabir M, Penney DG, ReMine SG, Mittal VK. Scholarly activities—essential to surgical education. Curr Surg 2003;60(4):459-62. PMID: 14972241.

23. Schneider JR, Coyle JJ, Ryan ER, Bell RH Jr, DaRosa DA. Implementation and evaluation of a new surgical residency model. J Am Coll Surg 2007;205(3):393-404. PMID: 17765154.

24. Chung R. Evaluating surgical residents the old school way: clues to how surgical training works and why. J Surg Educ 2008;65(6):512-3. PMID: 19059186.

25. Foley PJ, Roses RE, Kelz RR, Resnick AS, Williams NN, Mullen JL, Kaiser LR, Morris JB. The state of general surgery training: a different perspective. J Surg Educ 2008;65(6):494-8. PMID: 19059183.

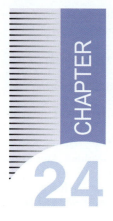

24

Cancer: An Epidemiology

BB Yeole

HISTORICAL CONTEXT

Epidemiology has its origins in the idea, first expressed over 2000 years ago by Hippocrates and others, that environmental factor can influence the occurrence of disease. However, it was not until the nineteenth century that the distribution of disease in specific human population groups was measured by any great extent. This work marked not only the formal beginnings of epidemiology but also some of its spectacular achievements; for example, the finding by John Snow that the risk of cholera in London was related, among other thing, drinking of water supplied by a particular company. Snow's epidemiological studies were one aspect of a wide-ranging series of investigations that involved an examination of physical, chemical, biological, sociological and political processes into.

The epidemiological approach of comparing rates of disease in subgroups of human population became increasingly huge in the late nineteenth and early twentieth centuries. The main application was to communicable diseases. This method proved to be a powerful tool for showing associations between environmental conditions or agents and specific diseases.

Today, communicable disease epidemiology remains of vital importance in developing countries where malaria, schistosomiasis, leprosy, poliomyelitis and other diseases remain common. This branch of epidemiology has again become important in developed countries with the emergence of new communicable diseases such as Legionnaire's disease and the acquired immunodeficiency syndrome (AIDS).

DEFINITION AND SCOPE OF EPIDEMIOLOGY

Epidemiology has been defined as "the study of the distribution and determinants of health-related states or events in specified populations, and the application of the study to control of health problems". This emphasizes that epidemiologists are concerned not only with death, illness and disability, but also with more positive health states and with an objective to improve health.

The target of a study in epidemiology is a human population. Population can be defined in geographical or others terms, for example, a specific group of hospital patients or factory workers could be the unit of study. The most common population used in epidemiology is in a given area of a country at a given time. This forms the base for defining of subgroups with respect to sex, age group, and ethnicity and so on. The structures of populations vary between geographical areas and time periods. Epidemiological analysis has to take such a variation into account.

In the broad field of public health, epidemiology is used in a number of ways, earlier studies in epidemiology were concerned with the causes (etiology). In this sense, epidemiology is a basic medical science with a goal of improving the health of populations.

The causation of some diseases can be linked exclusively to genetic factors, as with phenylketonuria, but is more commonly the result of an interaction between genetic and environmental factors. In this context, environment is defined broadly to include any biological, chemical, physical, psychological or other factors that can affect health.

Epidemiology is also concerned with the causes and outcome (natural history) of diseases in individuals and groups. The application of epidemiological principles and methods to problems encountered in the practice of medicine with individual patients has led to the development of clinical epidemiology. **Epidemiology lends strong support to both preventive and clinical medicine.**

Epidemiology is often used to describe the health status of population groups. Knowledge of disease burden in populations is essential for health authorities, and help optimize use limited resources to the best possible effect by identifying priority health programs for prevention and care. In some specialist areas such as environmental and occupational epidemiology, the emphasis is on studies of population with particular types of environmental exposure.

Recently, epidemiologists have become involved in evaluating the effectiveness and efficiency of health services, by determining the appropriate length of stay in hospital for specific condition, the value of treating high blood pressure, efficiency of sanitation measures to control diarrhea diseases, efficiency of sanitation measures to control diarrhea, the impact on public health of reducing lead additives in petrol, and others.

MEASURES OF DISEASE FREQUENCY

Population at Risk

Several measures of disease frequency are based on the fundamental concept of prevalence and incidence. It is important to note that the calculation of measures of disease frequency depends on correct estimates of the number of people under consideration. Ideally these figures should include only people who are potentially susceptible to the disease studied. Clearly, men should not be included in calculations of the frequency of carcinoma of the cervix. That part of population that is susceptible to a disease is called the population at risk.

Prevalence and Incidence

The prevalence of disease is the number of cases in a defined population at a specified point in time, while its incidence is the number of new cases arising in a given period in a specified population. Measuring prevalence and incidence basically involves the counting of cases in the defined population at risk. Data on prevalence and incidence become much more useful if converted into rates. A rate is calculated by dividing the number of cases by the corresponding number of people in the population at risk, and is expressed as cases per 10^n people.

The prevalence rate (P) for a disease is calculated as follows:

$$P = \frac{\text{Number of people with the disease or condition at a specified time}}{\text{Number of people in the population at risk at the specified time}} \times (10^n)$$

In the calculation of incidence rates the numerator is number of new events that occur in a defined time period and the denominator is the population at risk of experiencing the event during this period.

Incidence rate (I) is calculated as follows:

$$I = \frac{\text{Number of people who get a disease in a specified time}}{\text{Sum of the length of time during which each person in the population is at risk}} \times (10^n)$$

The numerator strictly refers only to first events of disease. The units of incidence must always include a dimension of time.

Cumulative Incidence Rate of Risk

Cumulative incidence rate is a simpler measure of the occurrence of a disease. Cumulative incidence rate (CI) can be calculated as follows:

$$CI = \frac{\text{Number of people who get a disease during a specified period}}{\text{Number of people free of the disease in the population at risk at the beginning of the period}} \times (10^n)$$

Cumulative incidence rate is after presented as cases per thousand populations.

Comparing Disease Occurrence

Measuring the occurrence of disease or other health states is only beginning of the epidemiological process. The next essential step is the comparison of occurrence in two or more groups of people whose exposures have differed in a qualitative sense and individual can either be exposed or unexposed to a factor under study. An unexposed group is used as a reference group. In a quantitative sense, exposed people can have different levels and duration of exposure. The total amount of a factor that has been exposed to an individual is called the dose.

The process of comparing occurrence can be used to calculate the risk that a health effect will result from an exposure. Both absolute and relative comparisons can be made; the measures describe the strength of an association between exposure and outcome.

ABSOLUTE COMPARISON

The risk difference, also called attributable risk (exposed), excess risk or absolute risk, is the difference in the difference in the rates of occurrence between exposed and unexposed groups. It is useful measure of the extent of the public health problem cased by the exposure.

Attributable Fraction (Exposed)

The attributable fraction or etiological fraction is determined by dividing the risk difference by the rate of occurrence among the exposed population when an exposure is believed to be a cause of given disease, the attributable fraction is the proportion of the disease in specific population that could be eliminated in the absence of exposure. Attributable fraction is a useful tool for assessing priorities for public health action.

Population Attributable Risk

The population attributable risk is a measure of the excess rate of disease in a total study population which is attributable to an exposure. This measure is useful for determining the relative importance of exposures for the entire population and is the proportion by which the incidence rate of the outcome of the entire population would be reduced, if exposure would be eliminated. It may be estimated by the formula:

$$Afp = \frac{Ip\text{-}Iu}{Ip}$$

where **Ip** is the incidence rate of the disease in the total population. **Iu** is the incidence rate of the unexposed group.

Relative Comparison

The risk ratio or relative risk is the ratio of the risk of occurrence of a disease among exposed people to that among the unexposed. The risk ratio is better indicator of an association that the risk difference, because it is expressed relative to a baseline level of occurrence. It is thus related to the magnitude of baseline incidence rate unlike the risk difference, population with similar risk differences can have differing risk ratios; depending on the magnitude of the baseline risk. The risk ratio is used in assessing the likelihood that an association represents a casual relationship.

Types of Epidemiological Studies

Epidemiological studies can be classified as either observational or experimental. The most commonly used type of study is stated in following Table 24.1 together with the units of study and their alternative names.

Observational studies allow nature to take its course; the investigator measures but does not intervene. They include studies that can be called descriptive or analytical.

Table 24.1: Types of epidemiological studies

Type of study	Alternative name	Unit of study
Observational studies		
Descriptive studies		
Analytical studies		
Ecological	Correlational	Populations
Cross-sectional	Prevalence	Individuals
Case-control	Case-reference	Individuals
Cohort	Follow-up	Individuals
Experimental studies	Intervention studies	
Randomized controlled Trials	Clinical trials	Patients
Field trials		Healthy people
Community trials	Community intervention studies	Communities

A descriptive study is limited to a description of the occurrence of a disease in a population and is often the first step in an epidemiological investigation. An analytical study goes further by analyzing relationship between health status and other variables. Apart from the simplest descriptive studies, epidemiological studies are analytical in character.

Limited descriptive information such as a case series, in which the characteristics of a number of patients with a specific disease are described but are not compared with those of a reference population, often stimulates the initiation of a more detailed epidemiological study.

Experimental or intervention studies involve an active attempt to change a disease determinant, e.g. an exposure or a behavior or the progress of a disease, through treatment and are similar in design in other sciences, However, they are subject to extra constraints, since the health of the people in the study group may be at stake. The major experimental study design is the randomized controlled trial using patients as subjects. Field trials and community trials are other experimental designs in which the participants are respectively healthy people and communities.

In all epidemiological studies it is a essential to have a clear definition of a case of the disease being investigated i.e. the symptoms, signs or other characteristics indicating that a person has the disease. Also necessary is clear definition of an exposed person, i.e. the characteristics that identify definitions of disease and exposure, great difficulties are likely to be experienced in interpreting the data from an epidemiological study.

Cancer Registries

Rates of the incidence of cancer can be derived only from population based cancer registries. The number of such registries in the world has increased steadily over a last 50 years but in comparison of availability of data of mortality, the population so covered remains relatively limited, Furthermore, the populations served by cancer registries are often not representatives of a country as a whole, comprising only the inhabitants of a major city, community or a province.

Cancer registration is a quite a complex undertaking and careful quality control is essential to ensure that the resulting data on incidence are valid and reliable. The major problem, however, is ensuring that every new case of cancer is identified. The case with which this can be done depends on the medical facilities available and the quality of the statistical and recording systems already in place. A further difficulty is identifying individuals and ascertaining that they do in fact, come from the population under study. These problems are more difficult to surmount in developing countries, which explains why relatively few registries have succeeded in surviving for long.

Incidence statistics from cancer registries around the world are published in the series of compilations—Cancer Incidence in five continents. So far nine volumes have been published. These volumes contain a description of the methods used to measure the validity of registry data.

International Comparison

Last forty years have seen a rapid growth in the development of cancer registration worldwide. International Agency for Research on Cancer and International Association of Cancer Registries recently published the "Cancer Incidence in Five Continents, Vol–IIX. In this volume, data on the incidence are presented for about 200 populations in 56 countries for the period of 1998-2002.[1]

Cancer Registration in India

The first population based cancer registry named Bombay Cancer Registry, was established by the Indian Cancer Society, in Mumbai (formerly Bombay) in 1964 covering the urban population of Greater Bombay. This was followed by the setting up three satellite registries of the Bombay Cancer Registry in the state of Maharashtra at Poona in 1972, at Aurangabad in 1978 and at Nagpur in 1980. In 1981, realizing cancer as a significant health problem and need to implement cancer control activity in the country, Indian Council of Medical Research of Government of India launched the National Cancer Registry Programme (NCRP). The main objectives of NCRP were: (i) to generate authentic data on the magnitude of the cancer problem (ii) to undertake epidemiological investigations and advice control measures and (iii) to promote human resource development in cancer epidemiology. By this way, two new population based cancer registries were founded in Chennai (formerly Madras) and Bangalore in 1981, besides augmentaining the Bombay Cancer Registry, with the systematic data collection starting from 1st January 1982. Subsequently new population based cancer registries were commissioned by NCRP in Bhopal in 1984, New Delhi in 1986 and rural registry in Barshi, Maharashtra in 1987. Ahmedabad population based cancer registry was functioning since 1980 at Gujarat Cancer Research Institute, Ahmedabad. The rural population based registry at Karunagappally was established in 1990 as a special purpose registry by the Regional Cancer Center, Trivandrum. Chittaranjan National Cancer Institute, Kolkata, established Kolkata Population Based Cancer Registry in 1991. Ambilikai Rural Cancer Registry in Tamil Nadu State was established in 1995 by International Agency for Research on Cancer, Lyon, France. A North-East Regional Cancer Registry (NERCR) project was started in January 2003 in four states. Regional Research Center for North-East (RMRC-NE), Dibrugarh, was designated as monitoring unit for these registries. The six population based cancer registries in the northern part of India covers the following areas: in Assam State, Dibrugarh District, Kamrup Urban District and Silchar Town; in Manipur State, Imphal West District, and other two covering entire states of Mizoram and Sikkim. Rural Cancer Registry at Ahmedabad was started from 1st January 2004 under the network project of National Cancer Registry Programme of Indian Council of Medical Research.[2]

At present there are sixteen urban population and four rural population based cancer registries are functioning in India covering about 20 percent urban population and 1.5 percent of rural population. From 1st January 2007, population based registries functioning[3-7] at Poona, Nagpur, Aurangabad, Karunagappally and Trivandrum are incorporated in the network of NCRP. The existence of the population-based registries in India to date is given Table 24.2 as well as in Figure 24.1.

The description of the basic registries of population based cancer registries functioning in India are given in Table 24.2. The area covered by urban registries varied from 142 sq km in Trivandrum and 685 sq km in Delhi. The population covered varied between 0.09 million in

Table 24.2: Area and population covered, number of cases, proportion of histologically verified and death certificate only cases and incidence rates in each registry[3-7]

Registry/Period	Area in kms	Sex	Population in million	Cases	CR	AAR	TR
Bangalore 2006	365.7	M	3.55	2655	74.7	108.5	161.4
		F	3.23	3282	101.6	133.5	276.4
Barshi 2006-07	3713.4	M	0.27	250	45.9	50.3	98.5
		F	0.25	247	49.5	51.8	125.0
Bhopal 2006-08	284.9	M	0.95	2054	71.8	106.4	179.7
		F	0.85	1987	77.1	106.8	227.8
Chennai 2006	170.0	M	2.35	2375	100.9	113.4	195.4
		F	2.28	2622	114.8	123.9	264.6
Delhi 2006	685.3	M	8.88	6805	76.6	125.1	209.9
		F	7.26	6118	84.2	119.7	261.6
Mumbai 2006	437.7	M	7.33	5356	73.0	103.1	161.6
		F	5.90	5685	96.3	111.4	214.7
Kolkata 2006		M	2.52	2134	84.4	80.1	142.6
		F	2.13	2061	96.4	90.0	209.6
Dibrugarh 2006-07		M	0.65	975	74.3	109.0	203.0
		F	0.62	689	55.4	78.6	181.8
Kamrup Urban 2006-08		M	0.59	1912	106.8	156.7	247.4
		F	0.52	1279	81.8	120.0	239.1
Cachar 2007-08		M	0.83	1555	93.4	130.9	264.1
		F	0.52	940	59.2	77.3	180.9
Mizoram 2006-07		M	0.53	1150	108.5	167.5	306.1
		F	0.50	969	96.9	144.9	283.9
Sikkim 2006-08		M	0.34	601	57.8	88.5	132.3
		F	0.30	556	61.3	101.1	184.8
Manipur 2006-07		M	1.21	1235	50.9	69.4	127.6
		F	1.20	1301	54.2	70.1	141.3
Ahmedabad-R 2006-07		M	0.86	911	52.9	70.0	136.5
		F	7.77	682	43.8	49.9	111.4
Ahmedabad-U 2006-07		M	2.46	3069	62.3	82.7	154.7
		F	2.17	2508	57.8	67.3	141.6
Aurangabad 2006	50.5	M	0.57	232	40.5	66.3	112.9
		F	0.52	224	42.9	64.0	160.8
Nagpur 2006	236.9	M	1.19	845	70.9	87.9	159.8
		F	1.12	902	79.9	90.6	211.9
Pune 2006	344.8	M	2.35	1320	56.0	80.5	120.0
		F	2.11	1423	67.2	84.3	163.7
Thi'puram 2006	142	M	0.57	703	123.2	119.5	201.1
		F	0.60	701	116.8	104.7	218.5
Kollam 2006	212	M	1.28	1504	116.9	111.5	197.7
		F	1.39	1365	97.6	85.7	176.8

Aurangabad Registry and 12.15 million in Mumbai. The Barshi rural registry covers the maximum area of 3713.4 sq km and the least population about 0.5 million.

Regional Variation within India

The number of cases registered per year during 2001-2004 ranged between 145 in Silchar town and 9022 in Mumbai.

The age-adjusted incidence rate standardized to the world population ranged between 43.8 in Barshi and 194.5 in Mizoram among males and 39.8 in Ahmedabad and 157.4 in Mizoram among females.[2]

The first five leading sites of cancer based on age-adjusted incidence rates by sex are presented in Figure 24.2 for males and in Figure 24.3 for females. Among males, in Mumbai the lung is the most frequent cancer followed by larynx, mouth and esophagus; in Poona, larynx was a leading cancer followed by mouth, prostate and lung; in Aurangabad, esophagus is the most frequent cancer followed by hypopharynx and mouth; in Nagpur, larynx is the most frequent cancer followed by esophagus and lung; in Bangalore and Chennai, stomach is the most prominent cancer followed by lung and esophagus; in Bhopal, Delhi, and Imphal, lung is the most frequent cancer while in Dibrugarh and Kamrup, esophagus is the leading site; in Mizoram and Sikkim state, stomach is the most common cancer followed by lung and esophagus. In females except Barshi, Kamrup, and Imphal registries breast is the leading cancer followed by cervix and ovary. In Barshi and Mizoram, cervix is the leading site and in Imphal, lung is the most predominant site.

National Estimates

The International Agency for Research on Cancer has played a primary role in the establishment of cancer registries, the

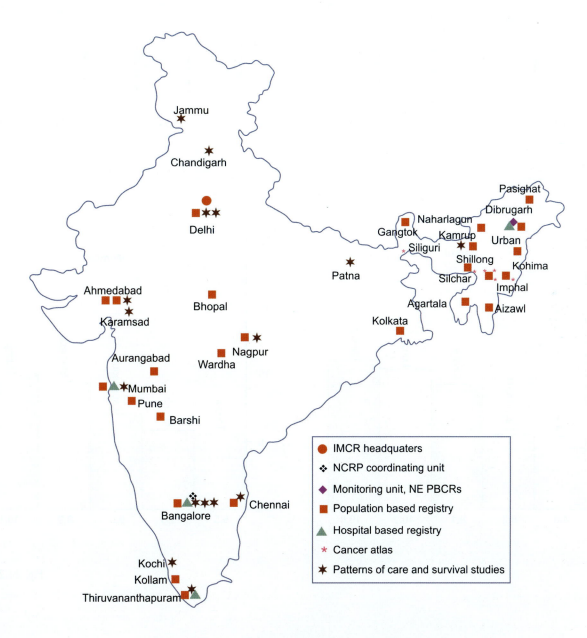

FIGURE 24.1: Map of India showing cancer registries in India

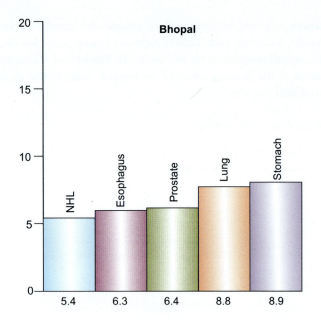

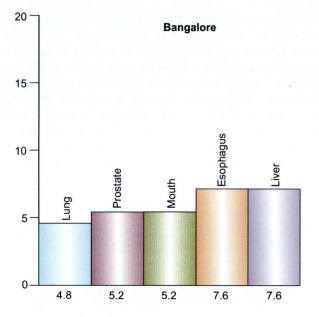

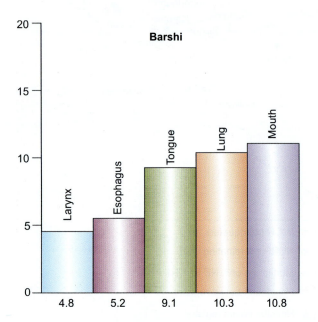

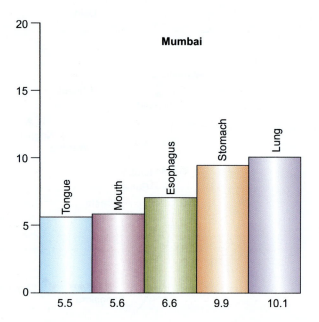

Fig. 24.2 contd...

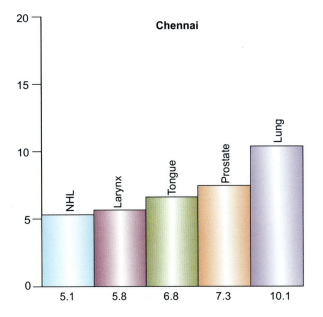

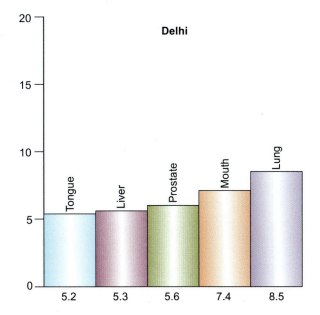

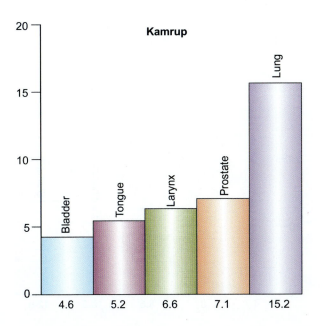

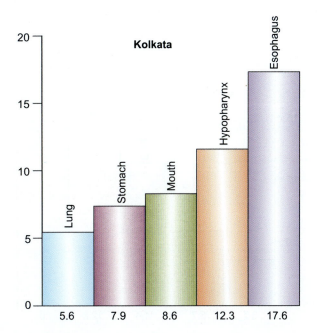

Fig. 24.2 contd...

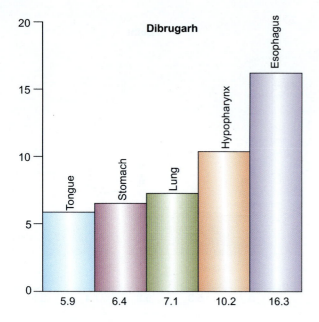

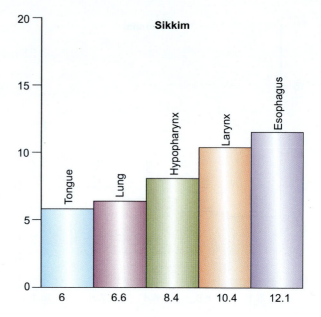

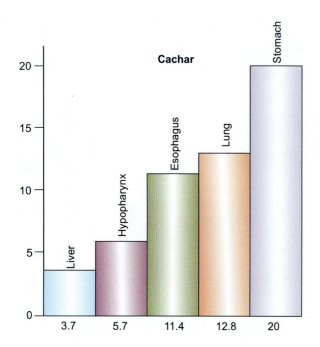

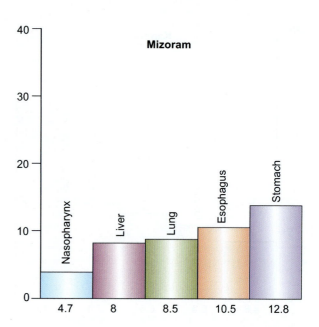

Fig. 24.2 contd...

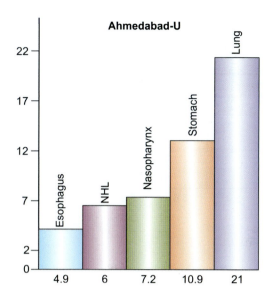

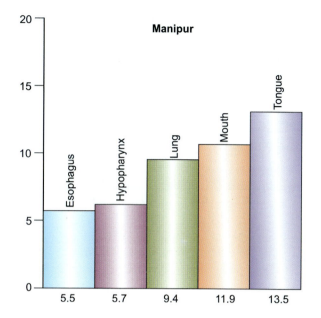

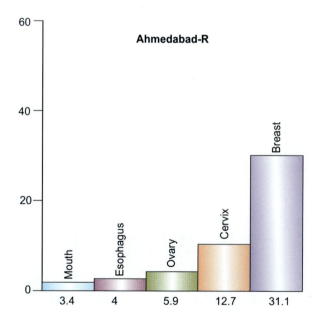

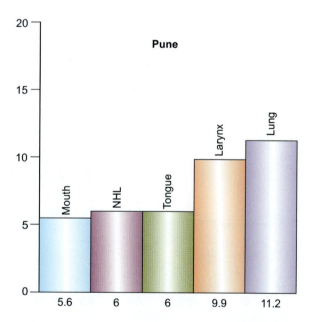

Fig. 24.2 contd...

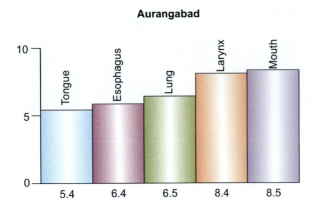

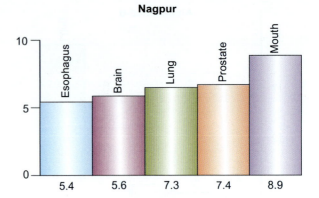

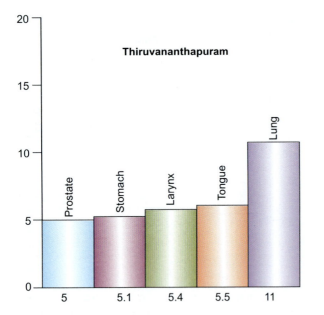

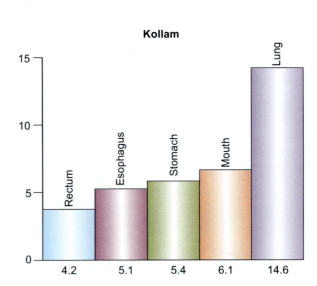

FIGURE 24.2: Most predominant cancers, males

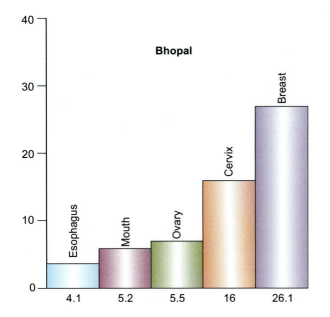

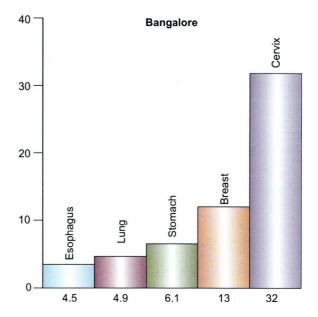

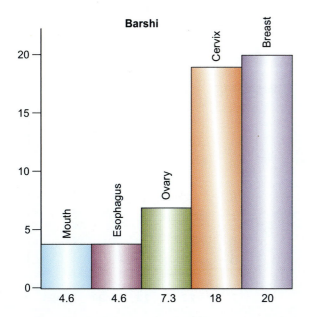

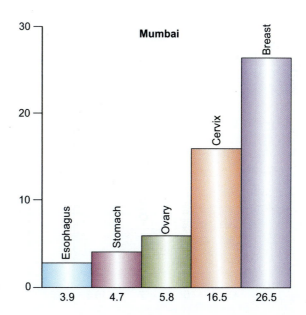

Fig. 24.3 contd...

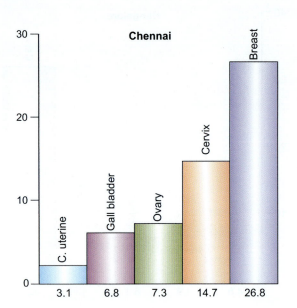

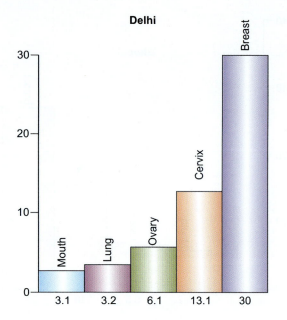

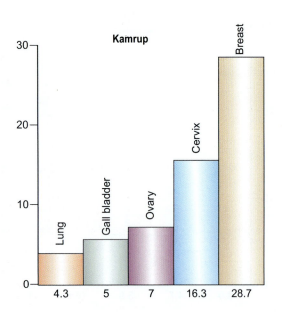

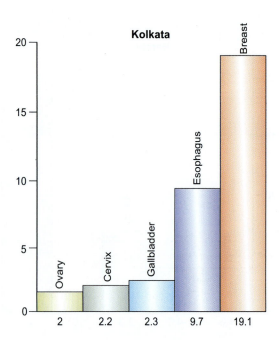

Fig. 24.3 contd...

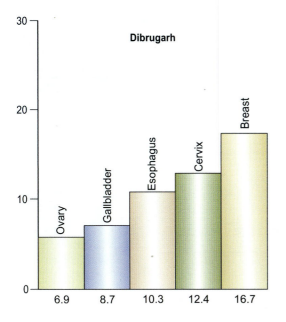

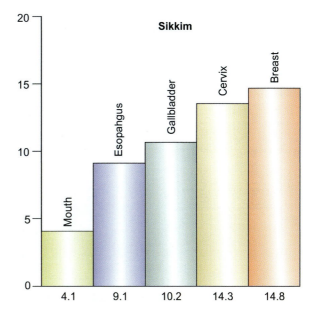

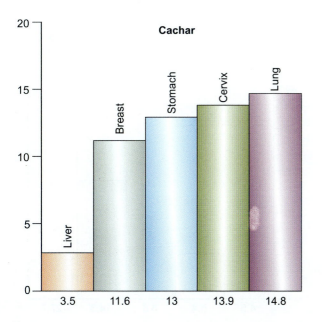

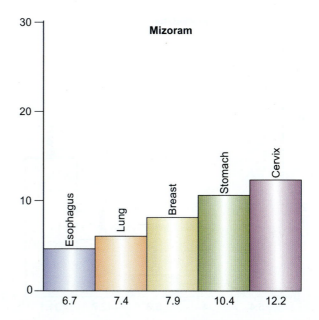

Fig. 24.3 contd...

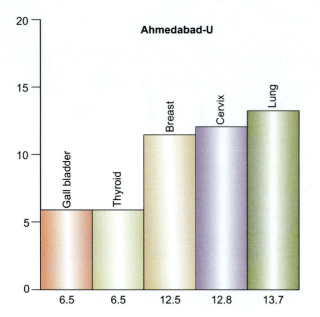

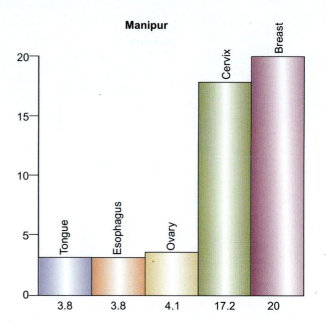

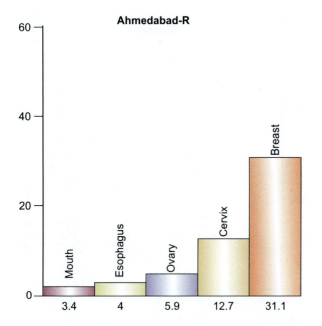

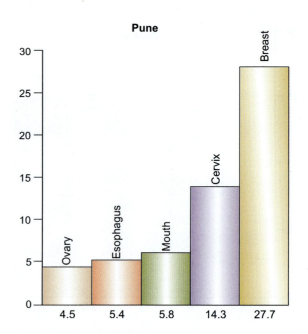

Fig. 24.3 contd...

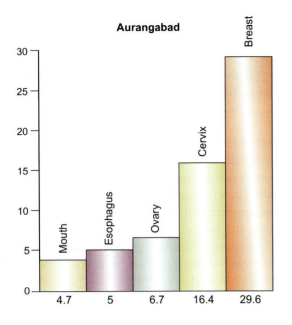

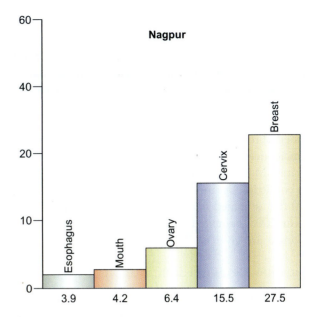

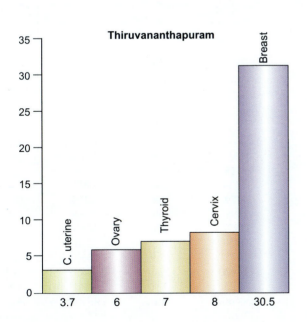

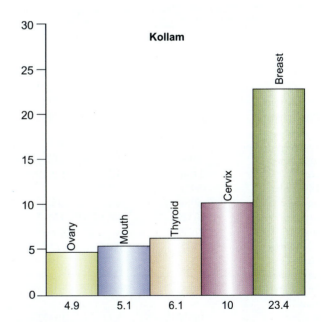

FIGURE 24.3: Most predominant cancers—females

accreditation of data collection procedures and the integration and reporting findings.[8]

International Agency for Research on Cancer has prepared national estimates of cancer incidence and mortality for the year 2008 for many countries. For estimations incidence data has been used reported in Cancer Incidence in Five Continents Vol. IX. Many registries provided statistics on cancer survival. With this survival and incidence data, the prevalence of cancer cases has been estimated. Mortality data by cause of death are available for many countries. Because of registration of vital events (birth/death) the estimated figures for incidence and mortality for the year 2008 estimated by International Agency Research on Cancer are given in Table 24.3.

Worldwide Regional Distribution

Worldwide, 12 million people are diagnosed with cancer annually and more than 7 millions die of the disease every year, currently, over 25 million people in the world are cancer patients. All communities are burdened with cancer, but there are marked regional differences. The total cancer burden is highest in affluent societies, mainly due to high incidence of tumors associated with smoking and Western life-style, e.g. tumors of the lung, colorectal, breast, prostate. In developing countries, up to 25 percent of the tumors are associated with chronic infections, e.g. hepatitis B virus (liver cancer), human papillomaviruses (cervical cancer), and *Helicobacter pylori* (stomach cancer).

When incidence of cancer is compared by region wise (broad geographical areas), marked differences are appeared in terms of the sites of most common tumors in a region; equally important some similarities are evident. The validity of contrasting cancer incidence in more or less develop countries is supported, at least in part, by the similar patterns of cancer incidence recorded for North America, Northern Europe, Western Europe and Oceania. In all these regions

Table 24.3: Estimated cancer incidence and mortality figures for India by sex, 2008[9]								
Site	Men				Women			
	Incidence		Mortality		Incidence		Mortality	
	No	ASR	No	ASR	No	ASR	No	ASR
Lip and oral cavity	45445	9.8	31102	6.8	24375	5.2	16551	3.6
Nasopharynx	2460	0.5	1761	0.4	873	0.2	651	0.1
Other pharynx	36371	8.3	32446	7.2	8540	1.8	6990	1.5
Esophagus	28809	6.5	26568	6.0	19290	4.2	16783	3.6
Stomach	21077	4.7	20678	4.6	13982	2.9	12886	2.7
Large bowel	20159	4.3	14134	3.2	16317	3.5	11556	2.5
Liver	14516	3.2	12877	3.0	5628	1.2	5166	1.1
Gallbladder	5928	1.3	3666	0.8	11334	2.4	6613	1.4
Pancreas	5081	1.1	4501	1.0	3879	0.8	3265	0.7
Larynx	20320	4.6	13010	3.0	2788	0.6	1784	0.4
Lung	47010	10.9	41865	9.8	11557	2.5	10404	2.3
Melanoma of skin	500	0.1	253	0.1	445	0.1	230	0.0
Breast	-	-	-	-	115251	22.9	53592	11.9
Cervix uteri	-	-	-	-	134420	27.0	72825	15.2
Corpus uteri	-	-	-	-	8772	1.9	4851	1.1
Ovary	-	-	-	-	28080	5.7	19558	4.1
Prostate	14630	3.7	10422	2.5	-	-	-	-
Testis	3864	0.6	1665	0.3	-	-	-	-
Kidney	5453	1.1	3543	0.8	3447	0.7	2190	0.4
Bladder	11807	1.1	3543	0.8	3005	0.6	157	0.3
Brain	13085	2.5	11035	2.1	8750	1.7	6906	1.4
Thyroid	3719	0.7	840	0.2	9180	1.8	2189	0.5
Hodgkins lymphoma	5245	0.9	2528	0.5	2126	0.4	1059	0.2
NHL	14708	3.0	10074	2.1	9010	1.8	6169	1.3
Multiple myeloma	3775	0.9	3115	0.7	3014	0.7	2826	0.6
Leukemia	19491	3.5	15394	2.9	13816	2.6	10888	2.1
All sites	430096	92.9	321384	71.2	518762	105.5	312071	65.5

the predominant cancers are those of colorectal, lung, breast and prostate, the only deviation from these patterns being the immergence of melanoma as a major cancer in Australia and New Zealand. Both Central and Southern Europe differ marginally from this pattern as a result of relatively high incidence of stomach cancer. Bladder cancer occupies fifth or sixth position in all these regions.

East Asia which includes Japan and regions of China comprises nations and communities divided between the "more developed" and "less developed" categories. Accordingly, the distribution of cancer is evocative of that in more developed regions with regards to lung, colorectal and breast cancers, but different in so far as cancers of the stomach, esophagus, and liver, are major concern. In the less developed world there is no single grouping of cancers constituting a clear pattern; rather particular patterns are specific to broad regions.

Breast cancer is of importance to communities in both more and less developed countries. In contrast, cervical cancer is a particularly serious problem for much of the developing world including South Central Asia, Sub-Saharan Africa and South America. Otherwise, there are cancers that are of singular significance to certain regions. Thus, cancer of the oral cavity ranks high in South Central Asia, liver cancer is of particular relevance to Sub-Saharan Africa and parts of Asia, while bladder cancer is major problem for Northern Africa and Western Asia.

Differences in the regional distribution of cancer and its outcome as documented by worldwide network of population based cancer registries, help to identify causative factors and those influencing survival. In some western countries, cancer mortality rates have started to decline, due to a reduction in smoking prevalence, improved early detection and advances in cancer therapy.

REFERENCES

1. Curado MP, Edwards B, Shin HR, Storm H, Ferlay J, Heanue M, Boyle P. Cancer Incidence in Five Continents Vol. IX, IARC Scientific Publications No. 160, Lyon, France, 2007.
2. Three Year Report of the Population Based Cancer Registries, 2006-08, National Cancer Registry Programme, Indian Council of Medical Research, Bangalore, India, 2009.
3. Kurkure AP, Yeole BB, Koyande SS. Cancer Incidence and Patterns of Urban Maharashtra –2001, Indian Cancer Society, Mumbai, India, 2006.
4. Consolidated Report of Population Based Cancer Registries 2001-2004 Indian Council of Medical Research, Bangalore, India, 2006.
5. Population Based Cancer Registries under North Eastern Regional Cancer Registry, First Report: 2003-2004. National Cancer Registry Programmes, Indian Council of Medical Research, Bangalore, India, 2006.
6. Cancer Morbidity and Mortality in Karunagappally 2002-2003, Regional Cancer Center, Trivandrum, India, 2005.
7. Population Based Cancer Registry, Thiruvananthapuram (Urban & Rural) Kerala, India. 2001-02, Regional Cancer Center, Trivandrum, India, 2005.
8. Parkin DM, Hakulinen T. Analysis of Survival. In: Jensen OM, Parkin DM, Maclennan R, Muir C, Skeet RG (Eds). Cancer Reigstration, Principles and Methods, IARC Scientific Publications, No. 95, 159-176, Lyon, France, 1991.
9. GLOBOCAN, Cancer Fact Sheet, IARC, Lyon, France, 2010.

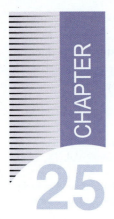

CHAPTER

25

Teasers and Tips

Arpita Vyas, Sanjay Porwal, Naveen Vyas,
Tarun Kumar, K Kant, Dinesh Vyas

Stress on Trauma, Emergency Surgery, Lymphoma, Basic Science, Breast, Endocrine Surgery, Transplant, Hepatobiliary Surgery, Esophageal, Lung cancer and Colorectal Surgery

These are quick review pages in the textbook, designed especially to address clinically most important areas to stress, depending on needs, disease prevalence and utility of surgical knowledge. Although colorectal cancer is not very common in India, but with international travel and more patients from Western world visiting India, we have incorporated it as the is second most common disease in the Western population. Breast cancer is slowly becoming more prevalent than cervical cancer as the most common cancer in females.

There is a large population with lymphoma and oral malignancy and we have tried to touch those aspects very briefly.

Cancer is second largest non-communicable disease after trauma in India

There is 25-30 percent increase expected in the registered number of cancer cases in India

TRAUMA

Trauma is one of the most common causes of death in 1-45 year age group.

Shock: Hypoperfusion of cells.

End point of shock management: Heart rate (not useful in patients on b-blocker), BP (does not drop till you lose 1-1.5 lit of blood)

End point of shock management: Physical exam, urine output, serial lactate (useful in normal renal and liver function patients)

Normalization of lactate in 24 hours has close to 100 percent survival.

Trauma patients not managed operatively needs serial exam.

Trauma care management has 3 level of management directions:
- *Option:* It means physician choice, not proven with scientific data
- *Guidelines:* Means data proven with some data, but still can be challenged
- *Standard of care:* Means very rigorously scientifically tested treatment.

Three peaks in mortality in blunt trauma:
1. Site of trauma: Rupture aorta, massive brain injury, cervical spine injury—paralyzing diaphragm, and changes in driving rules/seat belt reduces it.
2. Golden hour: Due to hemorrhage and brain injury within first hour—these can be reduced with structured trauma system and ambulance and trained paramedics,

instant OR availability, trained trauma surgeon and Emergency physicians

3. Couple of weeks with multiple system organ failure.

Damage control surgery: Prioritizing surgery and minimal surgery to manage shock and resuscitation.

Avoid dextrose for resuscitation in brain injury patient.

Trauma: Blunt and penetrating injuries have different approach.

Penetrating trauma abdomen: Liver most common, followed by small bowel, then diaphragm, and then colon.

Immediate indication for laparotomy: Hypotension, peritonitis and evisceration.

Penetrating trauma: Triple contrast CT.

Laparoscopy to determine peritoneal violation and then perform laparotomy.

Gunshot wound: Most common organ small bowel followed by colon, followed by liver.

- The damage with gunshot is dependent on size, velocity (cavitations effect, high velocity bullets have effect 5-10 times cavity diameter of the size of bullet)
- In extremity with vascular and bone injury, perform vascular shunt, followed by bone repair and finally definitive vascular repair
- Amputation of extremity is done, if atleast 3 components are damaged: Vessel, nerve, bone, muscle, and skin and is also determined by severity of damage.

In hypotensive blunt trauma patient: Always take CXR for tension pneumothorax, the benefits of cervical and pelvis X-ray is debated, as they are replaced with CT scans for better visualization and more details.

- Spine injury present in 10% of patients with head injury
- X-ray cervical spine has very low sensitivity
- Pelvis X-ray given some information, but still does it gives information of simultaneous hip joint fracture (undisplaced), bladder rupture
- Hypotensive patients need FAST or DPL (if ultrasound not available) and if criteria met are taken for abdominal exploration
- Chances of survival are minimal after 40-50 percent volume blood loss
- Vascular injury bleed very rapidly, and needs to be taken to Or immediately as high mortality in 30 minutes
- Major liver and spleen injury also needs immediate surgery/embolization and mortality within 1-2 hour

- CT scan has low sensitivity for hollow viscus/bowel injury
- Organ injured in blunt injury in order of frequency: Spleen followed by liver
- All penetrating wound needs to be taken to OR if fascia is violated
- CT scans with blush in solid organs like spleen, liver, kidney needs angiographic embolization
- Delayed CT images at 5 min differentiate active bleed (persistent blush) from pseudo aneurysm (contrast seen in initial image washed out): Both need embolization
- If there is no angioembolization service, watch if patient is stable and can be transferred to the facility with the service, any hemodynamic instability, take patient for operative procedure
- Kidney is the most common solid organ injured in blunt trauma in pediatric population.

Suspicion of Renal Injury

- Blood in urine (amount of hematuria has no relation to severity of injury, e.g. transected ureter, has no blood in urine)
- CT scan is very sensitive
- **X-ray:** Low sensitivity
- Psoas shadow loss
- Lower rib fracture: Always be suspicious of renal injury
- L1-3 transverse process fracture
- Pelvis fracture
- Extraperitoneal bladder rupture: Insert foley and wait
- Intraperitoneal bladder rupture: Surgery
- Kidney, spleen and liver injuries are mostly treated non-operatively
- Focused abdominal sonogram for trauma (FAST): Need 200 cc fluid for detection
- Focused abdominal sonogram for trauma (FAST): 4 views
- Intra-operative IVP in patients before doing nephrectomy in Or, if CT scan not done in ER, to ensure presence of contralateral kidney
- Complications of nonoperative management of renal injury: Hypertension due to renal artery stenosis, delayed occlusion and activation of rennin-angiotensin mechanism
- Endotracheal tube size in pediatric patients: (age/4) + 4.

GCS E4M6V5

- GCS is simple and reproducible evaluation of neurological status

- Mild injury (13-15), moderate (9-12) and severe (<8)
- 75 percent injuries mild to moderate
- Pupil asymmetry 1 mm or more: Intracranial mass
- CT treat should be repeated in 4-12 hr, if there is small bleed
- Helps in managing patient with neurological injury and neurological examination
- GCS 12 and less needs intubation.

Pediatric Trauma Accident

- Most common cause of death in child: Motor vehicle
- Second common: Drowning
- LD 50: Height from which child fall to cause mortality in 50 percent: 5 and ½ stories
- Children get more multiple organ injury
- Child burn is different from adult as head is big
- Rib fracture in children mean severe internal injury
- Always check any emergency surgical patient and trauma patient with ABCDE
- Narrowest part of airway in kids: Cricoids cartilage
- Intubation in kids is difficult
- Airway is anterior as compared to adults
- Nasotracheal intubation is not done in child
- Cricothyroidotomy: Successful in oxygenation in child for 20 minute
- Tachycardia most common and first parameter used in child for blood loss/shock
- Hypoxia precedes cardiac arrest in child
- Hypotension is seen in child with 45 percent blood loss
- Total blood volume in child 80 cc/kg and in adult 70 cc/kg
- Fluid bolus for resuscitation 20 cc/kg, and after 2 bolus give blood.

Neurotrauma

- Brain injury and hypotension: Give 3 percent or 7.5 percent saline. Check serum Na regularly
- Brain occupies 80 percent of volume of skull
- Unconscious if blood supply stops for 10-15 second
- Linear fracture if crosses over major vessels are concerning
- Depressed skull fractures are concerning
- Base skull is thin can be fractured even with minimal force
- Penetrating injury is concerning
- Head injury: Elevate head of bed 30 degree

- Head injury: Hyperventilation is controversial
- Head injury: Mannitol is helpful, but don't give if patient is hypotensive
- Subdural hematoma has bad outcome than epidural hematoma. Intraventricular is the worst
- Epidural hematoma has **lucid interval**, meaning episode of unconsciousness followed by normal mentation and then unconsciousness. Present in 20 percent cases
- Subdural hematoma are generally from superior sagittal sinus and has underlying brain injury as well
- Most common cause of subarachnoid hemorrhage is trauma
- Most common cause of nontrauma subarachnoid hemorrhage is aneurysm
- Epidural is like lens shaped, as duramater is stuck to bone and blood has to work to dissect it and hence get accumulated in small space
- Subdural is cresent shaped and is spread out
- Diffuse injuries are common: e.g. concussion (good outcome), diffuse axonal injury (worse outcome)
- Contrecoup injury is common in adult population as the brain get smaller and bits sharper edges inside the skull
- Epidural hematoma commonly from middle meningeal artery, **mortality has to be less than 5 percent**
- Arteriogram/MR angiogram/CT angiogram is used to identify aneurysm
- Intraventricular hemorrhage is worse than subdural
- Alcohol and drug use causes 40-50 percent of severe head trauma
- Traumatic brain injury causes immediate death in 25 percent
- Incidence of epidural—1 percent of all head injury admissions
- Penetrating intracranial injuries have the worse outcome

Intracranial pressure: Management divided into:
- Less than 20 mm Hg
- 20-40 mm Hg
- Herniation patient.

Head Injury

- Unequal puplis in ER: Temporary management till get CT
- Elevated head of bed 30 degrees
- Mannitol 0.5 gm/1gm IV, we used to give phenobarbitone, but phenobarbitone causes hypotension, hence avoided
- Hyperventilate between pCO_2 30 and 35

- 20 percent have intracranial bleed on contra lateral side, which is why needing CT scan. In past used to do burr hole on same side as dilated pupils but clinicians were wrong 20 percent times.

Neurotrauma Patient Management

- Perform hourly or 2 hourly neurovascular checks and GCS in ICU, with mean arterial pressure greater than 90 mm Hg
- Neurosurgery consult: GCS < 12.

Neurosurgical Interventions

- Midline shift from 5-10 mm
- Cerebellar lesion with mass effect
- Frontal/temporal lesion with intractable ICP greater than 25 mm Hg.

Indications for ICP—Continuous Monitoring

- GCS less than 12 with traumatic brain injury, and patient needs intubation and start phenytoin (antiseizure prophylaxis for 1 week only). Phenbarb in kids
- Goal of ICP monitoring: Keep ICP less than 15 mm Hg with external drain ventriculostomy
- Ventriculostomy kept for less than 1 week
- Remove ventriculostomy when pressure under control for 1 day
- Start high dose barbiturates (depress cardiac output) and Mannitol (contraindicated if patient is hypotensive)
- Mannitol: Follow serum osmolality and serum sodium
- If ventriculostomy fail go for paralytics and sedation
- If this fails then perform major decompressive craniectomy and bone graft implanted in abdominal wall with one side frontal lobe removal
- Neurotrauma patient needs 140 percent of calorie need as soon as possible. Early feeling encourage
- Antiepileptic >8 day. Does not help future seizures.

Evaluation of Spine Injury

- Mechanism of injury
- Presence of head injury
- Altered mental status.
  Large number of patients with vertebral injury do not have spinal cord injury
- Common spine injury: C5-7 and C1-2, hence highly advice to use cervical immobilization in trauma patient
- Central cord syndrome: More loss of power in upper extremities versus lower

- Brown-Sequard: Ipsilateral motor and proprioceptive loss and contralateral sensory loss
- Spinal cord injury below C5 has spontaneous breathing
- Spinal cord injury above C3 definitely needs ventilator and need nasotracheal intubation
- Tetanus prone injury: More than 6 hour old injury
- Fully immunized but last dose more than 10 yrs ago with tetanus prone wound: Tetanus toxoid
- If there is unknown history in tetanus prone wound: Immunoglobulin and toxoid.

ER Intubation: Rapid Sequence: LOAVES

- Lidocaine 1 mg/kg, helps easy intubation, decreases laryngeal spasticity and dysrhythmia
- Pre-Oxygenation
- Vacuronium 0.1 mg, 10 percent of paralytic dose, as it defasciculate, and prevent muscle pain from succinylcholine
- Etomidate 0.3 mg/kg or 20 mg for adult. Cannot give more than twice, causes adrenal insufficiency does not raise ICP or drop BP
- Succinylcholine, dose 1-2 mg/kg c/i: Burns, Crush injury, renal failure/hyperkalemia, old neurological damage
  In cases where succinylcholine is contraindicated give racuranium: 0.9 mg/kg.

Drugs not to give:
- Ketamine: Increases intracranial HT
- Midazolam and fentanyl causes drop in BP.

Children—LOAVES

- Add atropine, 50 percent Kids with succinylcholine get bradycardic 0.1 mg/kg
- Narrowest portion of airway in child: Cricoid cartilage
- End tidal CO_2: Gold standard for good intubation
- Difference in child chest injury than adult: Does not have external injury even with major intrathoracic injury, but in adult there is lot of bruising and other findings
- Intraosseous: 1 finger breadth below tibial tuberosity and medially
- Femoral line contraindicated in child: 20 percent of patient walk with limp later in the life, there is difference in growth—reason for intraosseous
- IV fluid in Trauma: LR is better than saline, as saline causes hypercholemic metabolic acidosis. Don't give D5 as it won't stay intravascular
- 20 cc/kg IVF bolus for child, gives another bolus, if no response. After 2-3 bolus give blood: 10 cc/kg

- In adult after 2 lit: Give blood
- 80 cc/kg blood volume in child
- Priority in correction of lytes: Calcium, potassium and magnesium first, as they are cardiac lytes, then sodium and chloride
- 60 percent weight is water in male
- 50 percent in female
- Renal failure
  - FeNa: Pre-renal less 1
  - Postrenal greater than 1
  - FENa invalidated by diuretics
- Predominant collagen in skin: Type I (80%)
- Predominant collagen in healing wound and fetus: Type III
- Stages of healing: Hemostasis and epithelialization; followed by neutrophil and macrophages; and followed by proliferation
- Wound strength: 6 month: 70 percent
- Vitamin A accelerates wound healing impaired by steroid

Classification of Shock

Class 1: 15 percent blood loss—tachycardia

Class 2: 15-30 percent blood loss—prolong capillary refill, narrow pulse pressure, orthostatic hypotension

Class 3: 30 percent blood loss—hypotension

Class 4: 40 percent blood loss—confusion

Swan-Ganz Catheter: Useful in selective patient, as the complications are more concerning then benefits from other test available as echocardiography

$$SVR = 80 \times (MAP-CVP)/CO$$

- Normal SVR is 900-1300 (dyne*sec)/cm^5
- Low SVR: Sepsis and neurogenic shock.

GENERAL TRAUMA

- Emergency help for lower extremity
  - Leg internally rotated and knee flexed: Posterior dislocated hip—reduce ASAP to prevent avascular necrosis of head of femur
  - Leg externally rotated and shortened: Fracture
- Drop of blood at urethral meatus:
  - Perform retrograde urethrogram
  - Most common injured part: Membranous urethra
  - Treatment suprapubic cystostomy or catheterize under vision with cystoscopy
- Contrast in CT in trauma is given in chest and carotids, as there is aortic dissection and carotid artery thrombosis

- Treatment of carotid thrombosis: Heparin
- Mechanism of Heparin: Stimulates antithrombin III
- Mechanism of LMWH: Inhibits factor Xa
- DDAVP for coagulation effect: 0.3 unit/kg—uremia, renal failure, von Willebrand Disease, prolonged cardiac pump time
- Stop bleeding medically in renal failure: DDAVP, Primarin(conjugated estrogen)
- Head bleed in trauma patient on Coumadin: Factor VII concentrate works in 7 minutes: But no survival advantage
- Desaturation with any local anesthetic: Methemoglobinemia
- Treatment: 1 ampoule of methylene blue
- Indication for preoperative TPN: More than 10 percent weight loss
- Protein in cirrhotic in TPN: Aliphatic, branched chain amino acid
- Protein in TPN with uremia: Nephramine contains essential amino acid
- If patient losses 20 percent weight: If you start feed—always start slow or risk refeeding syndrome
- Patients in concentration camp after World War II: High mortality in patients from refeeding syndrome
- Refeeding syndrome: Mitochondria are revved up: Marked Hypophosphatemia, leading to arrhythmia, seizures
  - RQ fat: 0.7
  - RQ Carb: 1
- General anesthesia with nuchal rigidity with masseter rigidity with end tidal CO_2 - 50: Malignant hyperthermia
- Earliest sign of malignant hyperthermia: Elevated end tidal CO_2
- Most common agent: Succynylcholine
- Next step: Dantrolene bolus
- Dantrolene dose: 2.5 mg/kg total 4 doses
- Next step: Stop surgery, cool pt with cold IV fluid, lavage stomach with NG
- Most important history: Family history
- Any kind of contracture/squint: Prone for malignant hyperthermia
- Work up: Biopsy of gastrocnemius muscle—Caffeine stimulus test—done in 3 labs in the US
- Under microscope characteristic sarcoplasmic reticulum
- Lingual thyroid: 80 percent patients don't have neck thyroid
- Treat with synthroid till they are young, then take off synthroid and they mostly do good

- Most common finding of myasthenia gravis in child: Unilateral ptosis
- Tensilon test: Ptosis resolves
- Treat patient with neostigmine
- 11 percent of patient has thymoma
- Thymectomy in case patient has rapid progression
- Plasmapharesis is done perioperatively for thymectomy in myasthenia gravis
- Indication for plasmapharesis: TTP
- Findings of TTP: FAT RN
  - Fever
  - Microangiopathic hemolytic anemia
  - Thrombocytopenia
  - Renal failure
  - Neurological sequlea
- Clinical findings of compartment syndrome: Take for surgery
- Test check for hemoglobin in urine with minimal RBC
- Brownish urine
- Treatment: Fluid, diuretic and bicarb (alkalinize urine)
- Bilateral leg motor weakness after thoracoabdominal aneurysm repair: Thrombosis of anterior spinal artery
- Traumatic aortic rupture: Most common cause of thrombosis of anterior spinal artery
- 60-yr-old male with 3 cm lesser curvature perforation: Bilroth II and truncal vagotomy
- Gastrinoma: Second part duodenum most common site
- Spontaneous bacterial peritonitis: *E. coli* most common organism
- Spontaneous bacterial peritonitis: WBC more than 500/cc
- Spontaneous bacterial peritonitis with culture showing candida is an indication for surgery
- Spontaneous bacterial peritonitis with culture with *E. coli* is not an indication of surgery
- PET scan not useful in detecting mets in brain, as brain is very bright to start
- PET scan not useful in detecting mets from renal cell carcinoma
- Barrets high grade: resection
- Barrets low grade: No treatment if symptoms controlled, nissen if there is heart burn
- Post gastrectomy: Iron deficiency anemia, as there is impaired iron absorption
- Absolute contra indication of radiation in breast cancer: Previous radiation, pregnancy, scleroderma and connective tissue disease, patient preference.

Burn

- Formula help calculate IVF resuscitation
- Parkland Formula 4 × percent burn area (only full thickness burn) × Wt in first 24 hours (50% in 8 hours)
- Curreri formula: Daily calories = 25 kcal/kg + 40 kcal/percent BSA burn
- Increased protein needs (2-3 gm/kg/day)
- Best estimate of good resuscitation: Urine output
- Best describe wound management: Early wound excision and coverage
- Early nutrition support (start within 24-48 hr) improve mortality: Burn, and severe head injury
- Lypolysis is predominant fuel in trauma
- Arginine: Increased wound healing and T-cell response in humans
- Glutamine: Enterocyte fuel, its absent in TPN
- Zinc deficiency—dermatitis around ala, lips, decreased wound healing
- Copper deficiency—neutropenia, megaloblastic anemia
- Chromium deficiency—diabetic state, neuropathy
- Essential fatty acid deficiency manifests as dermatitis and alopecia, impaired wound healing, dry, flaky rash, platelet dysfunction, anemia, respiratory distress. Occurs within two weeks

Most Common Cause of Mortality in Burn

- First peak respiratory complication: First 24 hours
- Second peak: 2-3 weeks: Infection respiratory
- CO poisoning: Cause of 70 percent of death (shift oxygen dissociation curve to left), inhibit cytochrome enzyme
- Close space burn: High COHb, carbonaceous sputum, Hydrogen cyanide
- Intubate patient with findings of close space airway injury for atleast 2 days.

Admission Criteria of Burn Patient

- Full thickness burn greater than 2 percent, as patient will develop contracture
- Perineum, face, hand
- Partial 15 percent in adult, 10 percent in children
- Inhalation, electrical burn
- Escharotomy needed for circumferential extremity and chest
- Sulfamylon: Not sulphur drug, penetrates eschar, and inhibits carbonic anhydrase
- Silver drug: Neutropenia

Changes in Starvation

- Decreased insulin
- GH increased then decreases after 10 days
- Increase free plasma cortisol
- Decrease in complement proteins (except C4).

Colon and GI Cancer

- Western culture patients have higher incidence of colon cancer. Not seen frequently in India and Southeast Asia, but is extremely important
- National polyp study: 7-10 years for polyp to turn into cancer
- 1 percent polyp turn malignant
- 4 types polyps: Hyperplastic (nonmalignant), tubular, tubulo-villous, villous adenoma (greater than 2 cm has 50 percent chance of malignancy)
  - Stage 1: Early local disease, node neg
  - Stage 2: Local advance with local nodes neg
  - Stage 3: Any T, local node
  - Stage 4: Mets, N3 (portal node)
- Difference in staging between colon and rectal ca: Stage 3
- Stage IIIa T1/T2 with N1 and IIIb T3/T4 with any N in rectal has difference in survival outcome
- Screening colonoscopy: 50 years
- 70-75 percent colon cancer distal to splenic flexure
- FAP: APC gene, autosomal dominant, 100 percent will have cancer by 40 yrs, less than 1 percent colon ca, most common cause of death now is desmoids tumor, as most patients already have total colectomy by 20 yrs of age, interestingly have **thyroid cancer**
- Proctocolectomy is treatment at 20 yr with ileal pouch with anal anastomosis. Still need annual pouch scope.
- Attenuated FAP: Less invasive, late presentation
- HNPCC: Mismatch repair gene abnormality, 80 percent with colon cancer by 60 yrs, autosomal dominant, 5 percent of colon cancer, right side colon cancer common, better prognosis than other cancer, 80-90 percent have known genetic defect identified
- Lynch syndrome 1: Only colon ca
- Lynch syndrome 2: Colon, endometrial (life time risk 60%), ovarian, urinary tract transitional cell, stomach.

Amsterdam criteria for lynch syndrome: 3,2,1
- 3 family members, two first degree relative
- 2 generation
- 1 member less than 50 years.

Screening: Colonoscopy every 1 to 3 years starting at 20-25.

Pelvic examination annualy at age 18 and annual endometrial biopsy at age 25-35 and urinalysis for hematuria.

Pedunculated polyp malignancy classification:
1. Invades head of polyp
2. Junction head and neck
3. Neck
4. Muscularis mucosa invasion.
   4 will need resection, to examine lymph node.
   1-3 need 2 mm margin of polyp. Poor differentiation and lymphovascular invasion need resection.
- Adenomiatory polyp:
  Seen in 33 percent population: Age 50
  Seen in 50 percent population: Age 70
- <5 percent tubular adenoma: Malignant
- 20-25 percent tubulovillous: Malignant
- 35% villous: Malignant
- Rectal polyp: 30 percent of all colorectal cancer in rectum
- Transanal excision: Lesion within 8-10 cm tru the anal verge and less than 4 cm in size. Mobile nonulcerate well differentiate negative nodes (<5% meet the criteria)
- Chemotherapy in node positive patient:
  - FolFox: 5FU, leucovorin and oxaloplatin is main treatment
  - FolFiri: Irinotecan instead of oxaloplatin second line treatment
- Avastin (bevacizumab, VEGF receptor antagonist) is added to FolFox for better results in metastatic disease
- Avastin is also used for another malignancy like metastatic lung cancer, kidney and brain
- Surgery should be delayed for 6 weeks in patients on Avastin as they bleed intraoperative.
- 60-70 percent patient have CEA elevation on recurrence.
- Patient with CEA greater than 10 is an indication for investigation.

Rectal Cancer: Different with Colon in Certain Ways

- Always need staging with CT for metastasis in liver and lung, as there is option of giving minimal transanal surgery, if disease is localized
- T1/2 and node negative-surgery
- Advance local disease (T3/4) or positive LN on transanal ultrasound/MRI needs neoadjuvant and then extensive surgery
- Local excision criteria: All T1 well- or moderate

- Anal margin and anal canal cancer are treated differently: Anal canal is treated with nigro protocol. Dentate line is middle of anal canal. Anal canal—lower end buttocks. Upper end of anal canal is levators.
- Anal margin cancer is 5 cm outside anal canal and is treated with wide excision like regular squamous cell cancer.
- Avoid using O'clock system for anatomical description, as it is confusing, so recommend using anterior, posterior, right, left.

CONGENITAL ANOMALIES

Most common tracheoesophageal fistula TEF-EA— Tracheoesophageal fistula and esophageal atresia (85%)
- TEF: 50-75 percent have associated anomalies
- TEF: VACTERL anomaly 25 percent
- TEF: Also associated with trisomy 18
- TEF: Can have both oligo and polyhydroamnios. Oligohydroamnios is worse than polyhydroamnios. Potter syndrome is with oligohydroamnios
- H-type fistula: Recurrent right upper lobe pneumonia, present as choking with meals, may present in older children
- Gastroschisis: Right of umbilical, umbilicus anomaly, 10 percent intestinal atresia due to vascular compromise, not associated with major anomaly
- Gastroschisis: Staged treatment
- Omphalocele: Herniation in umbilical cord, there are multiple anomalies, cardiac problems
- Omphalocele: Silo treatment
- Congenital diaphragmatic hernia: Pulmonary and cardiac anomaly
- Congenital diaphragmatic hernia: Infant has pulmonary hypoplasia, due to pressure on lung from abdominal content
- Congenital diaphragmatic hernia: Mortality from pulmonary reason
- Congenital cystadenomatoid malformation (CCAM): Proliferation of bronchus without alveoli, most of them resolve *in utero*, but can have malignancy in future
- Umbilical cord has 2 artery and one vein (remember it is better to have more blood coming in)
- Jejunoileal atresia is the most common bowel atresia in infants followed by duodenal atresia
- Duodenal atresia: 33 percent have trisomy 21, needs cardiac echo, most common reconstruction is duodenoduodenostomy, as minimal follow-up complication

- Jejunoileal atresia: **Multiple atresias may be present**, distal ileum most common, rule out cystic fibrosis, rule out meconium ileus with barium enema
- One bubble: Pyloric obstruction/atresia
- Double bubble: Duodenal atresia
- Multiple bubble: Distal atresia
- Cystic fibrosis: Study genetic mutation in newborn, and by one month, perform the gold standard test, sweat chloride test
- Cystic fibrosis: 95 percent meconium ileus child, treat with water soluble enema, plug the terminal ileum, mucomyst also used
- Meconium peritonitis: Calcification on KUB
- Meconium cyst: Leaking bowel, resect bowel and give stoma
- Hirschsprungs disease: Aganglionosis, it can be of any length, but generally terminal (85% rectosigmoid). Dilated segment is healthy bowel and normal diameter bowel is diseased bowel
- Hirschsprungs disease: Rectosigmoid ratio on barium enema of less than 1 is also helpful.
- Hirschsprungs disease: Suction rectal biopsy with histological examination. Absent Auerbach plexus (muscular), with hypertrophic nerve trunk, also can perform acetylcholine esterase stain.
- Hirschsprungs disease: Swenson, Soave, and Duhamel procedures
- Choledochal cyst: Type 1, dilatation of cyst, most common (85-90%)
- Choledochal cyst: 10 percent chance malignancy, type 3/choledochocele does not develop cancer
- Choledochal cyst: No histological finding to differentiate cyst from normal duct. More of clinical finding with dilatation greater than 1 cm
- Biliary atresia: Liver biopsy finding—histology finding of proliferation of biliary duct in portal triad
- Biliary atresia: Kasai procedure—perform before 8 weeks, after 12 weeks need liver transplant
- Biliary atresia: Kasai procedure—33 percent benefited long-term, 33 percent short-term benefit and then need liver transplant and last 33 percent fail postoperative and need transplant
- Biliary atresia: Complication of cholangitis post-Kasai procedure—needs transplant
- Imperforated anus: Infant needs colostomy, if there is no meconium stain in perineum
- Imperforated anus: In males especially perform delayed surgery, as there are male reproductive problems

- Imperforated anus: Females have cloacal (rectum and uretera together) anomaly. Need colostomy
- Imperforated anus: Female with posterior foucette (vaginal) fistula—initial dilatation and interval (delayed) posterior saggital anoplasty, hence prevent colostomy
- Imperforated anus: Always perform end colostomy with mucous fistula; avoid loop colostomy, to prevent recollection in distal segment
- Imperforated anus: Three stage surgery once baby is grown—colostomy, posterior sagittal anoplasty (extraperitoneal mobilization) with urethral repair, and colostomy closure
- Meckels diverticulum: Rule of 2, usually asymptomatic
- Claudication is not indication for bypass surgery
- Rest pain is an indication for bypass as that limb may need amputation
- Air bubble in arterial line: Dampens the waves, but no change in mean pressure
- Right atrium is the most common chamber involved in blunt trauma
- Cullen sign is periumbilical (peritoneal) sign and is late sign
- Grey-Turner is flank (retroperitoneal) discoloration
- Brain death: Two physicians needed. Angiography with no blood flow in brain—definite
- In the US: Living and deceased kidney donation is equal
- In India: Living nonrelated donor kidney transplant is common
- Best way to diagnose small bowel perforation: Serial abdominal examination by same surgeon
- End tidal CO_2: In death goes down
- End tidal CO_2: Increases in malignant hyperthermia
- End tidal CO_2: Decreases in pulmonary embolism
- Lidocaine dose 3-5 mg/kg without epinephrine
- Lidocaine dose 7 mg/kg with epinephrine
- Rectal, breast and thyroid glands are routinely examined with ultrasound by surgeons in their office.

Transplant

- Unrelated match living kidney graft survival 18.5 years
- Identical match kidney transplant survival 30 years plus
- Deceased kidney transplant 10 years
- Brain death: Important to know cause of death.

Conditions Mask Brain Death

- Barbiturate or other drug use
- Hypothermia
- Wait 6 hrs in adult before declaring death
- Wait 24 hrs in child before declaring death

Contraindication of Kidney Transplant

- Cancer (active) except skin and 2-5 years after curative cancer surgery
- Active infection
- Advance cardiac (post-CABG can perform) or liver disease or stroke
- Psychotic
- HIV patients can be transplanted if on protocol
- ABO incompatilibility is absolute contraindication of transplant (there are cases done postplasmaphresis)
- HLA matching (identical/nonidentical): Identical have 10 percent more graft survival
- HLA: Mixed lymphocyte reaction—put lymphocytes of both recipient and donor—watch for 5 days—done in living donation
- HLA-A, B, DR on chromosome 6 are use for matching serum v/s cell
- No mismatch: Kidney graft half life 16 years
- All others except total mismatch: Half life 10 years
- Identical donors: 25 percent of sibling
- Child kidney increase in size in 4-6 weeks when transplanted in adult
- No compensation/payment is allowed for donation
- Spouse donation is increasing in renal transplant
- Right kidney is difficult for transplant surgery as the vein is short
- Most critical area in liver transplant: Biliary leak or stricture
- Early complication in liver transplant: Hepatic artery thrombosis
- Liver does not have hyperacute rejection hence, can be transplanted in incompatible blood group and zero cross match
- Hyperacute rejection has no treatment, preformed antibody
- Kidney removal after hyperacute rejection
- Acute rejection: Most common, and is after 4 days, due to T cell, secondary to IL-2
- Chronic rejection: Newly formed antibody
- Kidney chronic rejection: Glomerular and arteriolar sclerosis
- Liver chronic rejection: Vanishing bile duct syndrome
- Lung chronic rejection: Obliterative bronchiolitis
- Heart chronic rejection: Concentric coronary artery stenosis
- Steroid decreases IL-1
- Cyclosporine suppress bone marrow, mycophenolate suppress lymphocyte in peripheral circulation
- IL-2 Causes proliferation of active T cells

- Mycophenolate: GI side effect (dose related)
- Sirolimus: Wound healing impaired (fibroblast proliferation), given 1 month after transplant
- Sirolimus: Hypertriglyceridemia and needs treatment
- Side effect—cyclosporine and tacrolimus—nephrotoxic and hypertension
- Side effect: Cyclosporine—hirsutism and gingival hyperplasia
- Side effect: Tacrolimus—tremor, alopecia and headache
- Last resort in rejection: OKT3 and thymoglobulin
- OKT3 causes cytokine storm and needs steroid priming before injection
- CMV was the most common infection, but is becoming rare as there is prophylaxis treatment with ganciclovir
- EBV is common infection in child: 4 percent in transplant
- EBV: Causes PTLD and Burkitts lymphoma
- PTLD: Treated with Rituxin, anti B cell antibody
- *Pneumocystis carinii* is reducing with decreasing use of steroid and use of prophylaxis with Bactrim
- Malignancy: B-cell lymphoma, cervical cancer (pap smear 6 months), skin cancer (100% patient 20 years after transplant).

Endocrine Surgery

There are 2 arteries (superior from external carotid and inferior from thyrocervical trunk) and 3 veins for thyroid.
- Left recurrent laryngeal nerve is constant in place for identification—trachea-esophageal groove
- Right recurrent laryngeal nerve is variable in location
- Superior laryngeal nerve supplies cricothyroid muscle
- Toxic multinodular goiter is the most common cause of hyperthyroidism in the world
- Common in female older than 50
- Most common treatment is near-total thyroidectomy
- Using radio-iodine does not decrease size of the gland
- Plummer's nodule/solitary toxic nodule: Young females and greater than 3 cm nodule
- Nodules have autodestruction with central necrosis and may become euthyroid
- Radio-iodine followed by lobectomy if surgery needed
- Grave's disease in the US is the most common cause of hyperthyroidism
- Treatment of Grave's disease: First treatment—anti thyroid medication, followed by radio-iodine and last treatment is near-total thyroidectomy to bring patient to euthyroid state
- Eye changes do not regress but arrest after treatment

- Trauma/emergency surgery/treatment with Grave's patient: Start β blocker and then take for surgery
- Solitary thyroid nodule: 4 percent population has nodule and half are diagnosed by physical exam
- Findings suggestive of malignancy: LN enlargement, involved muscles, voice change, irregular borders
- 1 cm is cut-off for workup of nodule
- Malignant nodules are generally cold nodule
- Best diagnostic tool is ultrasound guided FNA.

Work-up: Perform TSH, microsomal antibody and then ultrasound guided FNA.

If FNA is benign, offer TSH suppression and 50 percent of the nodule recedes:
- Regressing tumors are less likely malignant
- Hashimoto disease: Antimicrosomial and antithyroglobulin antibody for diagnosis
- Lack of iodine organification
- Episode of hyper followed by hypo and neck mass (not always)
- Low incidence of malignancy
- Treatment is hormone replacement
- Surgeon should diagnose and not offer surgery
- Subacute thyroiditis: Young women with respiratory infection followed by acute thyroid pain with minimal enlargement
- Treated with anti-inflammatory NSAIDs
- Surgery not needed until very resistant case
- Thyroid carcinoma: Incidence is increasing, may be due to better diagnostic test
- Papillary cancer: Most common 60 percent of all thyroid cancers, and 30 percent of all papillary cancers have lymph nodes positive and 10 percent have distant mets especially lung metastasis
- In papillary worry about neck nodes
- Papillary cancer less than 1 cm in size—lobectomy with isthmectomy
- Papillary cancer—intrathyroid papillary cancer: 1-4 cm in size—total thyroidectomy and perform central lymphadenectomy if palpable LN extend to lateral neck dissection
- Papillary cancer-extrathyroid-thru capsule-total thyroidectomy
- Papillary cancer: All patients are given thyroid replacement regimen postsurgery
- Papillary cancer: Lung mets are treated with radio-iodine
- Radio-iodine: Malignant nodule greater than 2 cm
- Radio-iodine: Regional mets

- Radio-iodine: Trans-capsular spread
- Radio-iodine: Distant mets
- Radio-iodine: Age older than 45 years (variable among medical centers)
- Radio-iodine: Given once TSH greater than 30
- Thyroid scan is technetium scan and radio-iodine is beta emitting from I-131
- Radio-iodine: Side effect—leukemia and bone marrow suppression, and pregnancy avoided for 1 year
- Follicular carcinomas are second common with 20 percent of all thyroid cancers, and lung mets (hematogenous) most common and in work-up get CXR always
- Follicular carcinomas: Not diagnosed by FNA (lymphovascular and capsular invasion)
- Workup for FNA for follicular cells: Lobectomy and 15 percent will have malignancy and need completion thyroidectomy
- Follicular carcinomas–microinvasive–less than 1 cm–lobectomy
- Follicular carcinomas–macroinvasive–total thyroidectomy
- Medullary cancer are 5-10 percent of all thyroid cancers and 10 percent of them familial syndrome
- Serum marker calcitonin is present in 100 percent and histopath characteristic of amyloid
- Medullary cancer: Can have both lymph and blood metastasis
- **All patients with MEN2 have medullary cancer**
- 90 percent patients with MEN1 have medullary cancer
- Medullary cancer surgery is performed after pheochromocytoma surgery in MEN2
- Markers medullary cancer: CEA and calcitonin
- Medullary cancer: More aggressive than papillary and follicular, as mets more common
- Medullary cancer: No role of radio-iodine
- Medullary cancer: Treatment greater than 1 cm—total thyroidectomy with ipsilateral neck dissection
- Medullary cancer **in MEN**: Perform b/l neck dissection
- Medullary cancer **in MEN: If greater than stage 4a— external beam radiation**
- Medullary cancer: **RET proto-oncogene**
- Medullary cancer: **c cell hyperplasia**
- Anaplastic are 1-2 percent with very bad prognosis (**life expectancy few weeks**) and affect very old population with underlying thyroid disease like multinodular goiter
- Follicular cancer may be precursor of anaplastic
- Patients get tracheotomy for respiratory help

- Hurthle cell cancer is subtype of follicular cancer and does not take iodine
- Hurthle cell cancer: No role of radio-iodine
- Hurthle cell cancer: Treatment—total thyroidectomy - surgery with TSH suppression
- Renal cell carcinoma is the most common mets in thyroid
- Staging thyroid cancer: Multiple systems—TNM, AMES, AGES, and others
- TNM: All patients less than 45 yrs **without distant mets** are stage 1, as they have same prognosis (0% mortality at 20 years)
- AMES classification: Endocrinologist use it.

Risk Factors for Thyroid Cancer

- Radiation in intermediate dose (thymus, acne): 15 year lag period—papillary cancer
  Minimal surgery for patient with radiation neck: Always perform total thyroidectomy—as multifocal disease
- Iodine deficiency
- Papillary
- Extremes of age less than 20 yrs (40% chance of malignancy in nodule) and greater than 60 years
- Recurrent cyst after aspiration
- Thyroglobulin is a marker for differentiated thyroid cancer but is not very sensitive (check pre-op, post-op and has to be zero, and then of some significance)
- Near total thyroidectomy: 90 percent thyroid removal. **Survival is equal to total thyroidectomy**, although increase chances of local recurrence.
- Near total thyroidectomy: Prevents major complications of hypoparathyroidism and recurrent laryngeal nerve injury
- Intraoperative: Ligate and divide inferior thyroid artery close to the thyroid gland to prevent nerve injury
- Most patients die from locoregional disease
- Bilateral RLN injury during thyroid surgery may need temporary trachestomy
- RLN paresis 20 percent and permanent paralysis 1-1.5 percent
- Respiratory distress postoperative is due to edema of glottis and hematoma compression
- Respiratory distress postoperative: Patient needs awake fiber optic intubation
- Hypoparathyroid postoperative is treated only if symptomatic, as hypocalcemia is stimulus for parathyroid hormone production

- Parathyroid gland—superior (fourth pouch) and inferior with thymus (third pouch)
- PTH half-life 3-5 minute
- PTH excreted by kidney
- Primary hyperparathyroidism HPTH (adenoma and hyperplasia): High PTH and high calcium
- Most patients with primary hyperparathyroidism: 75 percent with no or mild symptoms
- Peak age 50-60 years
- Rarely patients have **pentad of HPTH:** Renal stones, painful bones, psychogenic moanes, abdominal groans, fatigue, overtones
- 1 percent primary hyperparathyroidism has malignancy of parathyroid
- Symptomatic primary hyperparathyroidism needs surgery
- Asymptomatic primary hyperparathyroidism: The new studies show there is quality of life symptoms, and there bone diseases decrease, and prevent future bone fractures
- Genetic testing for MEN 1: Menin
- Genetic testing for MEN 2: RET protooncogene
- Secondary hyperparathyroidism: chronic renal failure
- Tertiary hyperparathyroidism: Persistent hyperparathyroidism due to **autonomous parathyroid**, after correction of cause of secondary hyperparathyroidism, i.e. postrenal transplant
- Hypercalcemia of malignancy: Low PTH
- Benign familial hypocalciuric hypercalcemia: Urine calcium for 24 hr less than 100, but PTH can be slightly elevated. They have family members with parathyroid excision, with no benefits
- Primary hyperparathyroidism: Increased calcium and parathyroid hormone, commoner than diagnosed
- Intraoperative: Both parathyroids are located within 1 cm radius of crossing of RLN and inferior thyroid artery
- Superior parathyroid is posterior to RLN
- Inferior parathyroid is anterior to RLN
- Missing upper gland is above upper pole and can be in posterior mediastinum
- Missing inferior gland can be in thymus, anterior mediastinum
- 5 percent patients have fifth parathyroid
- 4 gland hyperplasia: Take 3 and half gland and leave half of normal looking gland or autotransplant/implant in forearm muscle (brachioradialis) of nondominant hand
- Familial/MEN/secondary HPTH has hyperplasia
- Most common form of primary hyperparathyroidism: Adenoma 80-90 percent

- Hyperplasia associated with MEN syndrome
- Parathyroid carcinoma less than 1 percent, its diagnosed intraoperative and need lobectomy (thyroid)
- Familial hypocalciuric hypercalcemia: Low 24 hour urine calcium—**Do not offer surgery.** Rarely have renal stone
- Thiazide and lithium also cause hypercalcemia
- Hypercalcemic crisis: Calcium greater than 14—emergency surgery
- Calciphylaxis: 50 percent mortality—emergency parathyroid excision
- Hypercalcemic crisis: Hydrate and use loop diuretic like lasix
- Parathyroid adenoma removed by focused exploration using sestamibi scan or USG
- Sestamibi scan is serendipity, need to localize intrathoracic localization of parathyroid
- Intraoperative PTH monitoring: 50 percent drop in 5-10 min (postoperative) from baseline
- All parathyroid get blood supply from inferior thyroid artery
- Adrenals are 5 gm in weight with 3 arteries and 1 vein (right to IVC and left to left renal vein)
- Blood supply in adrenals goes to medulla from cortex
- Mets in adrenals are common due to rich blood supply
- Most mets are in medulla
- Adrenal incidentaloma: 2 important questions—are they functional and malignant
- Adrenal incidentaloma: 1 percent of CT scans
- Adrenal incidentaloma: 7 percent are pheochromocytoma
- Adrenal incidentaloma: 7 percent are aldosteronoma
- Adrenal incidentaloma: Greater than 4-5 cm needs surgery
- 25 percent malignancy size greater than 6 cm
- 2 percent malignancy size less than 4 cm
- Adrenal incidentaloma: Always do workup for functional tumor before surgery
- Adrenal has 3 layers (outer to inner GFR—glomerulosa-mineralocort, fasciculate-glucocorticoids and reticularis) of cortex and central medulla
- Hyperaldosterone: Can be from adenoma and hyperplasia
- Adrenal hyperplasia is treated with medicine not surgery: Spironolactone
- Adrenal adenoma: Surgery
- Adrenal malignancy: Bimodal age distribution
- Adrenal malignancy: Presents at late stage

- Aldosteronoma: Plasma aldosterone concentration/plasma renin activity greater than 25
- Aldosteronoma: Mostly benign tumor
- Aldosteronoma: Hypokalemia is very helpful, but found less often
- Screening for Cushings disease: Low dose dexamethasone suppression test
- Feminizing tumors are almost always malignant tumors
- Virilizing tumors are malignant in 33 percent patient
- Hypercortisolism: 24 hr urine cortisol sensitive test, other test plasma cortisol
- Nelson syndrome: Patient with pituitary mass with excessive ACTH production treated with bilateral adrenalectomy
- Conn syndrome: Hyperaldosteronism—hypokalemia
- Pheochromocytoma: 10 percent rule
- Pheochromocytoma: Serum metanephrine for diagnosis
- Pheochromocytoma: 10 percent bilateral in sporadic form, but in MEN 75 percent are bilateral
- Pheochromocytoma: **Never perform** needle biopsy on adrenal tumor, always do serum test
- Patient with mets in adrenal after complete removal of primary—perform adrenalectomy
- Pheochromocytoma: Presentation
  - 25 percent silent hypertension
  - 25 percent paroxysm hypertension
  - 25 percent sustained with paroxysm hypertension
  - 25 percent sustained hypertension
- Pheochromocytoma: Management—alpha blocker for 10 days followed by beta-blocker and hydration
- Pheochromocytoma: Intraoperative, if BP does not drop, look for other places of pheochromocytoma
- MEN 1: HPTH (100%), pancreatic tumor (60%) (gastrinoma—most common), pituitary adenoma (prolactinoma—most common) and other tumors like adrenal, thyroid, thymic carcinoids
- Gastrinoma: Serum gastrin greater than 1000
- PPI cause elevation of serum gastrin
- Secretin test causes elevation of gastrin greater than 200
- Octreotide scan is most helpful in localizing the gastrinoma
- MEN1 patient with HPTH and gastrinoma: Operate HPTH first as this control calcium level
- MEN 1 has multiple gastrinomas
- Gastrinoma most commonly in duodenal wall
- Insulinoma: 90 percent benign and are in pancreas
- Insulinoma treated with enucleation
- Glucagonoma: 50 percent patient dies from PE and DVT
- Somatostatinoma get gall stones and need prophylactic cholecystectomy
- MEN 2A: Medullary thyroid cancer (100%), HPTH (33%) four gland hyperplasia, pheochromocyoma
- MEN 2A: 2-5 percent Hirshsprung disease
- MEN 2A: Most patient die of MTC
- MEN 2B: MTC (100%), mucosal neuroma (100%), pheochromocytoma (50%), marfanoid habitus, skeletal abnormalities, megacolon
- MEN 2B: Aggressive MTC tumor as compared to MEN 2A
- MEN 2B: Prophylactic thyroid surgery before 6 months of age.

Liver and Portal Hypertension

- 3.9 men per 100,000 with primary liver (HCC/hepatoma) cancer in India
- 44.5 men per 100,000 with primary liver (HCC/hepatoma) cancer in Japan
- Resection can not be done in HCC with both lobes (T4) involved
- HCC is one of the most prevalent diseases in the world
- 70 percent patient with HCC has elevated AFP, but is not a good marker
- Normal AFP is of no value
- Elevated AFP in 5000 in HCC needs diagnostic laparoscopy before resection, as they have metastatic disease
- HCC can be diagnosed with imaging
- TACE (trans-arterial chemo-embolization) used for HCC locoregional measure
- AFP greater than 400 and 2 imaging suggestive of HCC: diagnosis is 95 percent
- If AFP less than 400, and 2 imaging suggestive of HCC- perform biopsy to diagnosis
- 5 year survival with HCC 30 percent (noncirrhotic) and 5 percent (cirrhotic)
- Sorefinib (tyrosine kinase inhibitor) is new drug in liver cancer HCC
- It is not useful preoperative
- Other application for Sorafinib is kidney cancer
- HCC incidence is rising in western culture, as cirrhotics are living longer and developing HCC
- HCC treated with resection or transplant
- HCC needs preoperative workup like EGD for varicose veins or get portal pressure, and evaluate severity of cirrhosis.

- 5 years survival of liver transplant better than resection in HCC
- MELD score online tool for liver allocation, for transplant in the US
- Young patient with cirrhosis and HCC needs transplant
- Old patient with HCC and early cirrhosis: Perform resection
- Contraindication of liver transplant: Sepsis, recent cancer (patient with old cancer that is cured, can have transplant)
- HCC is only malignancy indication for liver transplant
- Experimental study for cholangiocarcinoma as an indication for liver transplant
- HCC: T1 or T2/single tumor less than 5 cm or 3 tumors each less than 3 cm are indication for transplant
- Cholangiocarcinoma has neurovascular invasion and hence, they are spread before becoming identified or become symptomatic
- Locoregional therapy is not curative
- 80 percent of colorectal cancer metastasizes to liver
- 25 percent of these patients present at the same time as colorectal cancer (synchronous)
- The liver met resection has been evolving every year—with resection acceptable for multiple lesions, large size, in both lobes, and with cirrhosis.
- Resection is acceptable as long as enough liver is left behind after resection: For example, close to 40 percent liver left after resection in non-cirrhotic liver and close to 60 percent in cirrhotics (class A and B)
- Alcohol is the most common cause of HCC in the USA
- Hepatitis B is the most common cause of HCC in India
- Cholangiocarcinoma are 10-20 percent of liver cancer
- MRI can differentiate benign from malignant tumor
- PET scan is very good for colon cancer
- PET scan also useful in—head and neck, lung, melanoma, breast, lymphoma, ovary and musculoskeletal
- Best modality for liver cancer: Intra-operative ultrasound
- Intraoperative ultrasound: Changes operative plan in 40 percent liver resection
- Median survival colorectal cancer metastasizes to liver is 6-8 month without any chemotherapy
- Median survival colorectal cancer metastasizes to liver is 16 months with FoLFOx (best chemotherapy combination at this point)
- Anti-VEGF antibody, Bevacizumab, add 4 months to survival when added to FoLFOx
- Another anti-VEGF antibody, Erbitux/Cetuximab can be given if there is wild type K-Ras mutation in colon cancer

- Current trends in management is neoadjuvant to down stage cancer, current therapy is very effective, followed by surgery
- Lobectomy gives same results as wedge resection, if margins are free
- Repeat hepatic resection is as good as primary tumor
- Age is no contraindication for surgery, as long as patient has good health
- Preoperative survival predictor of worse outcome: Size greater than 5 cm, synchronous mets, CEA greater than 200
- Operative mortality of liver mets less than 5 percent
- Preoperative chemotherapy/Neoadjuvant therapy with FoLFOx and another anti-VEGF antibody can convert nonoperative liver mets to resectable in 30 percent cases
- There are techniques to shrink lobe of liver by selective embolization
- Variation in liver arterial supply: Right hepatic artery arise from SMA in 15-20 percent of patients
- Variation in liver arterial supply: Left hepatic artery arise from left gastric in 15 percent of patients
- Secondaries in liver from other primaries are also resectable
- *E-coli* is the most common cause of pyogenic abscess worldwide, treated with surgery
- In India, a large number patient have amebic liver abscess from *Entamoeba histolytica*, treated with metronidazole, choloroquine
- Fungal liver abscess: Patients with cholangitis treated with multiple stents and workup for HIV or malignancy done
- Left lobe cyst is more symptomatic than right side
- Polycystic liver disease: Symptomatic patient need liver transplant
- Echinococcal liver cyst disease: Serology test and then albendazole followed by excision
- Hemangioma is the most common benign tumor of liver
- Hemangioma liver: They have characteristic imaging character, they rarely grow and do not need intervention until major symptoms
- Hemangioma liver: Can sometimes cause gastric outlet symptoms/mass effect, need few serial scans to ensure no hemangiocarcinoma
- Hepatic adenoma is seen in young female on oral contraceptive, and can cause surgical emergency if they rupture and bleed
- Hepatic adenoma: Resection needed, inoperable patient needs embolization
- Hepatic adenoma: Can rupture and bleed

- Hepatic adenoma: Patient on birth control pill and 30-40 percent adenoma involute. If no involution then needs surgery
- Hepatic adenoma: If they become pregnant, they need ultrasound in first and third trimester and needs embolization in third trimester, if greater than 3 cm
- Intra-abdominal bleeding during pregnancy: Most common rupture ectopic, followed by rupture splenic artery aneurysm followed by hepatic adenoma
- Hepatic adenoma: Can develop malignancy (2-3%)
- Hepatic adenoma: Only hepatocytes in biopsy no biliary element
- Hepatic adenoma: Does not respond to radiation
- Focal nodular hyperplasia FNH: Characteristic finding of central scar (it is not scar actually but vascular supply and feeds mass inside out) on imaging with CT and MRI
- Focal nodular hyperplasia FNH: Normal liver tissue abnormally distributed
- Focal nodular hyperplasia FNH: Does not need surgery unless large
- Treatment of fulminant liver failure: Liver transplant
- Hepatic trauma with massive hepatic vein injury has minimal chance of survival: Perform atria-caval shunt
- Penetrating portal vein injury: Try to repair, if fail ligate the vein
- Patient with cirrhosis from hepatitis B undergoing major surgery can have better surgical outcome, if pre-operative viral load is brought to minimal.

Lymphoma and Hematological Issues for Surgeons

- Screening preoperative for bleeding: Previous history of profuse bleeding, bruising and family history
- Arterial bleed needs surgery
- aPTT is used for heparin therapy
- aPTT have false elevations commoner than other tests
- Alcoholics, liver disease are also one of cause of coagulation problem
- Platelet transfusion in thrombocytopenic is avoided unless patient is symptomatic
- Patients postheart valve replacement needing lifelong warfarin, if needing reversal for surgery give oral/IV vitamin K, as IM/SC vitamin K injections make postoperative management of warfarin challenging
- vWD is the most common disease
- Factor XI deficiency is the most common cause of litigations in the US

- Lupus anticoagulants are prone to clotting not bleeding
- Hypothermia causes platelet dysfunction and coagulation cascade disorder
- Hemophilia A: Factor VIII deficiency, treat with factor 40 units/kg preoperative, postoperative give half dose in 12 hours
- Hemophilia B: Factor IX deficiency; treat with 80 units/kg
- Fibrinogen levels are checked in liver disease patients as synthesis is impaired
- Dilution coagulopathy: Lose 4 liters of blood in 6-12 hours
- 30 percent of clotting factors are good for surgical intervention
- 4-6 units FFP give 30-40 percent of clotting product
- Cryoprecipitate: Concentrated FFP, increase fibrinogen level, 10 units increase to clotting products to 100 percent
- Postheart lung bypass machine: Platelet dysfunction issue
- Recombinant VIIa: Hemophila, head injury/intracranial bleed on warfarin for quick reversal
- More than 1 dose of recombinant VIIa causes thrombotic problems
- Heparin does not dissolve clot already formed
- Heparin should be given per protocol and the levels must be achieved within 24-48 hours
- Heparin single dose can casue HIT (heparin induced thrombocytopenia)
- Reversal of heparin with protamine
- LMWH: High bioavailability, do not bind to prothrombin and hence aPTT not useful, can check Xa level
- LMWH: Low incidence of HIT and osteopenia
- LMWH: Renal excretion and long half-life, renal failure patients not suitable for it
- HIT: Drop in platelet to 50 percent and generally takes place 5 days, but can happen early
- HIT: Prothrombotic condition
- HIT: Tested with antibody against PF4 (platelet factor)
- HIT treated with Argatroban (direct thrombin inhibitor)
- Warfarin causes hypercoagulable (inhibition of protein C and S) in first 24 hours
- Factor V leiden D deficiency has prothrombotic problem
- Homocystinemia is a prothrombotic disease.

Thoracic Surgery, Head and Neck, Esophageal Cancer and Lung Cancer

- Tracheal obstruction: Perform awake fiberoptic bronchoscopy

- Most common cause of massive hemoptysis: Pneumonia and bronchitis with erosion of bronchial artery, in India can be from tuberculosis
- Empyema: Chest tube first step, if no improvement—VATS with pleurodesis. No chest tube/drainage in tuberculosis effusion
- Amount of blood to drown: 350 cc blood
- Protect airway with disease side of lung down
- Tracheostomy can cause trachea-innominate fistula
- Trachea-innominate fistula is a rare disease in tracheostomy
- Hemoptysis in Swan catheter due to rupture of small arteries
- Treat with removal of Swan with ballon down and disease side down
- Spontaneous pneumothorax: Chest pain most common presentation
- Tension pneumothorax: Hypotension, tachycardia, shock
- Spontaneous pneumothorax: Due to bleb rupture
- 30 percent of primary pneumothorax recurs
- Spontaneous pneumothorax: First time managed with chest tube
- Nonthoracic cause of malignant pleural effusion: Breast and ovarian cancer
- Traumatic hemothorax: Indication for exploration—unstable patients, bleeding 200 cc/hr for 3 hrs. 1500 cc on initial placement of chest tube
- Pericardiac temponade: Becks triad—narrow pulse pressure, increase JVD, distant heart sound
- Traumatic diaphragm hernia: 2-3 percent of chest and abdominal hernia (may present many years after trauma)
- Thymoma: 80 percent are benign
- 20 percent of thymoma patients have myasthenia
- 20 percent of myasthenia patients have thymoma
- 85 percent myasthenia patients respond to thymectomy
- Substernal thyroid: Greater than 50 percent of thyroid intrathoracic
- Substernal thyroid: Patient can have trachoemalacia
- Posterior mediastinal tumor: Should be evaluated with MRI to ensure no spinal cord extension
- Esophageal perforation: Early diagnosis is crucial and intervention
- Benign lung tumor: Granuloma from tuberculosis
- Malignant lung tumor: Carcinoid and typical lung cancer
- Malignant lung nodule in lobe other than lung cancer is M1 disease
- CT and PET are standard preoperative workup
- Postresection volume 800 cc is ok for surgery
- Patient with stage 1 lung cancer: Operation give 70 percent 5 years survival and nonoperative management gives 10 percent survival
- Achalasia: Degeneration of myenteric plexus
- Achalasia: Lack of peristalsis (please see they may contract, but the contraction is not coordinated, meaning the whole esophagus contract at the same time) of esophagus and nonrelaxation of LES
- Achalasia: Treatment—Heller myotomy (open/laparoscopic)
- Achalasia: Liquid to solid dysphagia, in contrast to malignancy where solid dysphagia followed by liquid
- Achalasia: Increased chances of malignancy in mid esophagus
- Achalasia: Barium study (bird-beak appearance), manometry (best test) and endoscopy needed for workup
- DES/nutcracker esophagus: High amplitude contraction
- Esophageal perforation serious complication from dilatation of achalasia
- Perforation diagnosed with gastrograffin swallow
- Surgery is performed through left thoracotomy
- The larynx is divided into three anatomical regions and they are supraglottic, glottis and subglottis and is an important and most common malignancy in India with very strong association between smoking, excess alcohol ingestion, and the development of squamous cell cancers
- Malignancy presents as sore throat, painful swallowing, referred ear pain, change in voice, enlarged neck nodes
- The increased risk of malignancy persists for several years after cessation of smoking
- Other risk factors: HPV and EBV infection, Plummer-Vinson syndrome, metabolic polymorphisms, malnutrition, and occupational exposure
- Most important prognostic factor: Increasing T and N stage
- Early stage laryngeal malignancy has cure rate of 70-90 percent (very important that its recognized early)
- Lip and oral cavity malignancy also has a good cure rate for stage 1 and 2
- It responds like most squamous malignancy to radiation therapy or surgery; radiation therapy—preferable to preserve the voice
- Supraglottic larynx: The epiglottis, false vocal cords, ventricles, aryepiglottic folds, and arytenoids and rich in lymphatic drainage and more than 50 percent patients present with LN mets
- Glottis: True vocal cords (have no lymphatics) and the anterior and posterior commissures.

- Subglottic region: about 1 cm below the true vocal cords to the lower border of the cricoid cartilage/the first tracheal ring, quite rare to have malignancy
- Oropharynx: Between the soft palate and the hyoid bone and includes (Base of the tongue, tonsillar region, soft palate, pharyngeal walls)
- Most common location for a primary tumor of the oropharynx: Anterior tonsillar pillar and tonsil
- Precancerous lesions: Leukoplakia (most common, and diagnosed by exclusion of lichen, candida and other conditions), erythroplakia, and mixed erythro-leukoplakia
- The recent data suggests oropharyngeal malignancy associated with HPV has better outcome than those from alcohol and tobacco
- Recurrences after 5 years represent new primary malignancies
- A tumor detected within 6 months is a synchronous second primary lesion
- A second primary lesion more than 6 months after is a metachronous tumor
- Patients have high likelihood of second primary of orodigestive system and hence daily treatment with moderate doses of isotretinoin (13-cis-retinoic acid) for 1 year helps reduce it. Although there is no survival advantage as patient dies from the primary tumor.

Transplantation

- Three types of graft rejection occur: Hyperacute, acute and chronic
- Hyperacute rejection occurs within minutes to days after transplantation
- It is mediated by preformed IgG antibodies which causes thrombotic occlusion of the transplanted allograft
- Hyperacute rejection: Prevented by screening the recipient serum for preformed antibodies
- Hyperacute rejection is irreversible
- Acute rejection: T lymphocytes mediated and generally within 1 and 3 weeks, if no rejection medication given, but most common before 3 to 6 months after transplantation
- Chronic rejection takes months to years and is mediated by both T- and B cell responses.
- Chronic rejection: Fibrosis and scarring seen in organ
- Findings are: Accelerated atherosclerosis (heart); bronchiolitis obliterans (lung); vanishing bile duct syndrome (liver); and fibrosis and glomerulopathy (kidney).

- Risk factors of chronic rejection: Previous acute rejection episodes, inadequate immunosuppression, initial delayed graft function, donor age, reperfusion injury, diabetes, and infections.
- 1 year patient survival after kidney transplant is 95 percent
- Survival has improved significantly in diabetic patient with renal failure
- Diabetic patient with renal failure has 20 percent 5 year survival without renal transplant
- 10 year survival after kidney transplant is 40-50 percent
- Test for donor specific antibody is called crossmatch
- Positive crossmatch is an absolute contraindication for deceased/cadaveric transplant, but not for living transplant, as new technique of plasmapheresis have shown 75 percent–5 year survival
- Crossmatch is performed to prevent hyperacute rejection
- Presence of donor specific antibody is determined by PRA test
- Higher PRA result means higher chances of acute rejection
- ABO incompatibility is no longer a contraindication for transplant (Done in few centers)
- Patient becomes anuric immediately after renal transplant: Thrombosis of vessel or ureter flow obstruction
- Delayed graft function: Low urine output after transplant
- Most common cause of DGF: ATN
- Pancreas transplant: FNA or urinary amylase detect early rejection
- Pancreas transplant: Elevated blood sugar is a late finding of rejection
- Pancreas transplant: Can be done with kidney or solitary
- Pancreas transplant: Two types of drainage procedure used—enteric and bladder (infection complications same)
- Pancreas transplant: Enteric drainage more common
- Pancreas transplant: Prevent secondary complications and arrest already existing complications of diabetes
- Pancreas transplant: Bladder drainage can be done is solitary transplant
- Liver transplant: Hepatitis C causes cirrhosis and HCC in 20-30 years
- Liver transplant: All patients with transplant get re-infected
- Liver transplant: Cirrhosis develops early in transplanted liver (30% in 5 years)
- Hepatitis C is most common indication of liver transplant, followed by alcoholic cirrhosis and sclerosing cholangitis

- In pediatric population: Biliary atresia is a common indication
- Hepatocellular carcinoma without metastasis are treated with liver transplant
- Hyperacute rejection is very rare in liver
- Usual postoperative infection is common is first month
- Opportunistic infection like pneumocystis and aspergillosis are common 2-6 months postoperative period
- Infection is uncommon 6 months posttransplant

- Skin tumors are most common with squamous cell carcinoma most common followed by BCC
- Post-transplant lymphoproliferative disorder (PTLD) is common and is precursor of lymphoma
- PTLD: Discontinue cyclosporine
- PTLD: Treat with ganciclovir for EBV
- Postrenal transplant mortality: First year—infection followed by CVS
- Postrenal transplant mortality: After 1 year—CVS, followed by malignancy followed by infection
- Breast.

INDEX

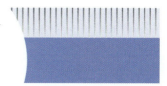

Page numbers followed by *f* refer to figure and *t* refer to table

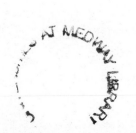